Recent Advances in Pancreatic Neoplasms

Recent Advances in Pancreatic Neoplasms

Editor

Cosimo Sperti

MDPI • Basel • Beijing • Wuhan • Barcelona • Belgrade • Manchester • Tokyo • Cluj • Tianjin

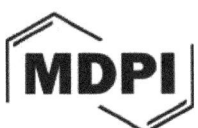

Editor
Cosimo Sperti
University of Padua
Italy

Editorial Office
MDPI
St. Alban-Anlage 66
4052 Basel, Switzerland

This is a reprint of articles from the Special Issue published online in the open access journal *Journal of Clinical Medicine* (ISSN 2077-0383) (available at: https://www.mdpi.com/journal/jcm/special_issues/Pancreatic_Neoplasms).

For citation purposes, cite each article independently as indicated on the article page online and as indicated below:

LastName, A.A.; LastName, B.B.; LastName, C.C. Article Title. *Journal Name* **Year**, *Volume Number*, Page Range.

ISBN 978-3-0365-3499-2 (Hbk)
ISBN 978-3-0365-3500-5 (PDF)

© 2022 by the authors. Articles in this book are Open Access and distributed under the Creative Commons Attribution (CC BY) license, which allows users to download, copy and build upon published articles, as long as the author and publisher are properly credited, which ensures maximum dissemination and a wider impact of our publications.

The book as a whole is distributed by MDPI under the terms and conditions of the Creative Commons license CC BY-NC-ND.

Contents

About the Editor . . . . **vii**

Cosimo Sperti, Simone Serafini and Lucia Moletta
Recent Advances in Pancreatic Neoplasms
Reprinted from: *J. Clin. Med.* **2021**, *10*, 4724, doi:10.3390/jcm10204724 . . . . **1**

Munseok Choi, Na Won Kim, Ho Kyoung Hwang, Woo Jung Lee and Chang Moo Kang
Repeated Pancreatectomy for Isolated Local Recurrence in the Remnant Pancreas Following Radical Pancreatectomy for Pancreatic Ductal Adenocarcinoma: A Pooled Analysis
Reprinted from: *J. Clin. Med.* **2020**, *9*, 3945, doi:10.3390/jcm9123945 . . . . **5**

Elisa Sefora Pierobon, Lucia Moletta, Sandra Zampieri, Roberta Sartori, Alessandra Rosalba Brazzale, Gianpietro Zanchettin, Simone Serafini, Giovanni Capovilla, Michele Valmasoni, Stefano Merigliano and Cosimo Sperti
The Prognostic Value of Low Muscle Mass in Pancreatic Cancer Patients: A Systematic Review and Meta-Analysis
Reprinted from: *J. Clin. Med.* **2021**, *10*, 3033, doi:10.3390/jcm10143033 . . . . **17**

Weiyao Li, Javier Martinez-Useros, Nuria Garcia-Carbonero, Maria J. Fernandez-Aceñero, Alberto Orta, Luis Ortega-Medina, Sandra Garcia-Botella, Elia Perez-Aguirre, Luis Diez-Valladares, Angel Celdran and Jesús García-Foncillas
The Clinical Significance of PIWIL3 and PIWIL4 Expression in Pancreatic Cancer
Reprinted from: *J. Clin. Med.* **2020**, *9*, 1252, doi:10.3390/jcm9051252 . . . . **35**

Anna Caterina Milanetto, Matteo Fassan, Alina David and Claudio Pasquali
Serotonin-Secreting Neuroendocrine Tumours of the Pancreas
Reprinted from: *J. Clin. Med.* **2020**, *9*, 1363, doi:10.3390/jcm9051363 . . . . **57**

Woohyung Lee, Yejong Park, Jae Woo Kwon, Eunsung Jun, Ki Byung Song, Jae Hoon Lee, Dae Wook Hwang, Changhoon Yoo, Kyu-pyo Kim, Jae Ho Jeong, Heung-Moon Chang, Baek-Yeol Ryoo, Seo Young Park and Song Cheol Kim
Reduced and Normalized Carbohydrate Antigen 19-9 Concentrations after Neoadjuvant Chemotherapy Have Comparable Prognostic Performance in Patients with Borderline Resectable and Locally Advanced Pancreatic Cancer
Reprinted from: *J. Clin. Med.* **2020**, *9*, 1477, doi:10.3390/jcm9051477 . . . . **67**

Cosimo Sperti, Alberto Friziero, Simone Serafini, Sergio Bissoli, Alberto Ponzoni, Andrea Grego, Emanuele Grego and Lucia Moletta
Prognostic Implications of 18-FDG Positron Emission Tomography/Computed Tomography in Resectable Pancreatic Cancer
Reprinted from: *J. Clin. Med.* **2020**, *9*, 2169, doi:10.3390/jcm9072169 . . . . **77**

Natalia Gablo, Karolina Trachtova, Vladimir Prochazka, Jan Hlavsa, Tomas Grolich, Igor Kiss, Josef Srovnal, Alona Rehulkova, Martin Lovecek, Pavel Skalicky, Ioana Berindan-Neagoe, Zdenek Kala and Ondrej Slaby
Identification and Validation of Circulating Micrornas as Prognostic Biomarkers in Pancreatic Ductal Adenocarcinoma Patients Undergoing Surgical Resection
Reprinted from: *J. Clin. Med.* **2020**, *9*, 2440, doi:10.3390/jcm9082440 . . . . **89**

Yejong Park, Jae Hyung Ko, Dae Ryong Kang, Jun Hyeok Lee, Dae Wook Hwang, Jae Hoon Lee, Woohyung Lee, Jaewoo Kwon, Si-Nae Park, Ki-Byung Song and Song Cheol Kim
Effect of Flowable Thrombin-Containing Collagen-Based Hemostatic Matrix for Preventing Pancreatic Fistula after Pancreatectomy: A Randomized Clinical Trial
Reprinted from: *J. Clin. Med.* **2020**, *9*, 3085, doi:10.3390/jcm9103085 . . . . **101**

Anna Caterina Milanetto, Luca Morelli, Gregorio Di Franco, Alina David, Donata Campra, Paolo De Paolis and Claudio Pasquali
A Plea for Surgery in Pancreatic Metastases from Renal Cell Carcinoma: Indications and Outcome from a Multicenter Surgical Experience
Reprinted from: *J. Clin. Med.* **2020**, *9*, 3278, doi:10.3390/jcm9103278 . . . . **113**

Jessica Allen, Colin Cernik, Suhaib Bajwa, Raed Al-Rajabi, Anwaar Saeed, Joaquina Baranda, Stephen Williamson, Weijing Sun and Anup Kasi
Association of Neutrophil, Platelet, and Lymphocyte Ratios with the Prognosis in Unresectable and Metastatic Pancreatic Cancer
Reprinted from: *J. Clin. Med.* **2020**, *9*, 3283, doi:10.3390/jcm9103283 . . . . **125**

Martina Catalano, Giuseppe Aprile, Monica Ramello, Raffaele Conca, Roberto Petrioli and Giandomenico Roviello
Association between Low-Grade Chemotherapy-Induced Peripheral Neuropathy (CINP) and Survival in Patients with Metastatic Adenocarcinoma of the Pancreas
Reprinted from: *J. Clin. Med.* **2021**, *10*, 1846, doi:10.3390/jcm10091846 . . . . **131**

Simone Serafini, Alberto Friziero, Cosimo Sperti, Lorenzo Vallese, Andrea Grego, Alfredo Piangerelli, Amanda Belluzzi and Lucia Moletta
The Ratio of C-Reactive Protein to Albumin Is an Independent Predictor of Malignant Intraductal Papillary Mucinous Neoplasms of the Pancreas
Reprinted from: *J. Clin. Med.* **2021**, *10*, 2058, doi:10.3390/jcm10102058 . . . . **143**

Marco V. Marino, Adrian Kah Heng Chiow, Antonello Mirabella, Gianpaolo Vaccarella and Andrzej L. Komorowski
Rate of Post-Operative Pancreatic Fistula after Robotic-Assisted Pancreaticoduodenectomy with Pancreato-Jejunostomy versus Pancreato-Gastrostomy: A Retrospective Case Matched Comparative Study
Reprinted from: *J. Clin. Med.* **2021**, *10*, 2181, doi:10.3390/jcm10102181 . . . . **155**

About the Editor

Cosimo Sperti is a member of the pancreatic surgical team at the 1st General Surgery Institute, Department of Surgery, Oncology and Gastroenterology, University of Padua, Padua, Italy. After receiving his medical degree from the University of Padua in 1979, he received a post-graduate degree in general Surgery (1984) and Oncology (1987) at the University of Padua. He was appointed the Associate Professor of Surgery (2014-present) at the University of Padua. Prof. Sperti has a strong research and clinical interest in pancreatic cancer and hepatobiliary malignancies. He is involved in the testing of innovative technology for diagnosing and staging pancreatic tumors and pancreatic cystic neoplasms, and in evaluating the results of surgical treatment and follow-up for patients with pancreatic cancer.

Publications and presentations: 155 full, peer-reviewed publications (listed in PUBMED), 25 book chapters, 600 presentations at international or national meetings.

He is a member of the Editorial Board of *World Journal of Gastroenterology, World Journal of Surgery, Cancers, Journal of Clinical Medicine, Surgery Res Practice*. He is a reviewer for 40 academic journals, mainly in the surgical, oncological and gastroenterological sciences.

He is member of the Italian Association for the Study of the Pancreas (A.I.S.P.); Italian Society of Surgical Oncology (SICO), European Society of Surgical Oncology (ESSO), Italian Society of Surgery (SIC); European Pancreatic Club (EPC); International Association of Pancreatology (IAP); International Society of Surgery (ISS).

Editorial

Recent Advances in Pancreatic Neoplasms

Cosimo Sperti *, Simone Serafini and Lucia Moletta

Department of Surgery, Oncology and Gastroenterology, 3rd Surgery Clinic, University of Padua, Via Giustiniani 2, 35128 Padua, Italy; simone.serafini@ymail.com (S.S.); lucia.moletta@unipd.it (L.M.)
* Correspondence: csperti@libero.it; Tel.: +39-049-821-8823

Pancreatic neoplasms, both primary and secondary, include different pathological entities with variable biological behavior and, consequently, different treatment modalities. Pancreatic adenocarcinoma is the fourth cause of cancer-related death in Western countries, and, in the coming years, it is estimated to become the second cause of gastrointestinal cancer death [1]. Surgery and adjuvant therapy are the cornerstones of the therapeutic approach; however, even after radical resection, the majority of patients experience disease recurrence. A multimodal therapeutic approach based on the combination of neoadjuvant therapy, chemotherapy, radiotherapy, immunotherapy, and surgery, appears fundamental in order to improve the outcomes, but the prognosis of pancreatic cancer remains dismal [2]. This Special Issue of the *Journal of Clinical Medicine*, entitled "Recent Advances in Pancreatic Neoplasms", focuses on new possible strategies to treat pancreatic neoplasms, especially pancreatic adenocarcinoma (PDCA). This Special Issue contains 13 articles, 11 studies and 2 review articles, focusing on the pancreatic ductal adenocarcinoma ($n = 10$), intraductal papillary mucinous neoplasm (IPMN) ($n = 1$), neuroendocrine tumors ($n = 1$) and secondary tumor to the pancreas ($n = 1$) [3–15]. Seven papers [4–6,9–11,14] explored new prognostic factors potentially able to stratify patients with pancreatic cancer and different survival rates in order to select the adequate treatment. Allen et al. [6] examined the relationship between the daily rate of change in CA 19-9 over the first 90 days of chemotherapy for unresectable and metastatic pancreatic cancer and the pretreatment levels of neutrophils, lymphocytes and platelets with an overall progression-free survival. They found that the ratio of absolute neutrophils count to the absolute platelet count (NLR) was associated with a shorter overall survival (OS) and progression-free survival (PFS). As in other tumors, NLR could be considered a prognostic marker.

Gablo et al. [9] from the Czech Republic, studied miRNAs as prognostic biomarkers in the preoperative blood plasma specimen of patients with PDCA. A population of patients with a poor prognosis (OS < 16 months) and patients with a good prognosis (>20 months) were considered in the study. Two miRNAs were confirmed to have lower levels and one miRNA was confirmed to have higher levels in the plasma sample of poor prognosis cases. By combining these three miRNA levels, poor prognosis cases were identified with a sensitivity of 85% and a specificity of 80%.

In a multicentric retrospective study, Catalano et al. [5] evaluated the correlation between the occurrence of treatment-related peripheral neuropathy and the efficacy of the nab-P/Gem combination in patients with metastatic pancreatic adenocarcinoma. Peripheral neuropathy was the most frequent treatment-related adverse event and, in this study, patients developing peripheral neuropathy seemed to experience more favorable outcomes compared to patients without neuropathy.

Li et al. [13] from Madrid, Spain, evaluated the expression of several proteins (PIWIL1, PIWIL2, PIWIL3, PIWIL4) in pancreatic cancer-derived cell lines and in healthy control in one non-tumor cell line. These proteins played a role in regulating gene expression through the complementary recognition and guidance of short RNAs against their target genes. They also played a role in recognizing and binding a specific type of non-coding small RNAs: the piRNAs (PIWI-interacting RNAs), constituting the piRNA-induced silencing complex (piRISC). PIWI proteins are fundamental for epigenetic regulation, silencing transposable elements, protecting genome integrity, gametogenesis and piRNA biogenesis. The authors investigated the PIWI protein functions and their controversial role in tumorigenesis. According to this paper, PIWIL3 and PIWIL4 seemed to have a crucial role in the regulation of cell motility, stem cell maintenance and drug resistance both in tumorous and healthy pancreatic cells. Furthermore, a low PIWIL4 expression predicted a shorter survival time for patients with a pancreatic carcinoma.

The tumor marker CA 19-9 was proven to be useful in the clinical management of patients with PDAC, especially in monitoring the effects of treatment. Lee et al. [11] evaluated the association of CA 19-9 concentrations after neoadjuvant therapy (NACT) and the prognosis in a large number of patients with border-line resectable or locally advanced PDCA who underwent subsequent surgery. The authors considered the CA 19-9 concentrations before and after NACT, and after surgery, and calculated the relative difference (RDC) as follows: [(CA19-9 after NACT) − (CA 19-9 before NACT)]/(CA 19-9 before NACT). By constructing prognostic models for the overall survival and recurrence of free survival, the authors found RDC to be independently associated with a better prognosis in patients with border-line resectable or locally advanced PDCA.

Sperti et al. [10] from the University of Padua (Italy) retrospectively evaluated the prognostic implication of 18-FDG PET in resectable pancreatic cancer. One hundred and forty-four patients with PDCA who underwent pancreatic resection were enrolled in this study: the maximum standardized uptake value (SUVmax) was able to identify two populations with a different prognosis. The patients with a lower SUVmax ($\leq$3.65) had a significantly better survival rate than those with a higher SUVmax ($p < 0.001$). The SUVmax was an independent predictor of survival on multivariate analysis; therefore, it had the potential use in patients' therapeutic management (i.e., the selection of patients for neoadjuvant therapy before surgery).

Another emerging and important factor impacting the outcome of oncologic patients is the cancer cachexia. In recent years, there has been a growing interest in the possible role of sarcopenia in influencing the morbidity and mortality of patients undergoing pancreatectomy for pancreatic adenocarcinoma [16,17]. In fact, among solid tumors, pancreatic cancer carries the highest prevalence of cancer cachexia and involuntary weight loss [18]. Pierobon et al. [14] from the University of Padua reviewed the literature and performed a meta-analysis comparing the outcomes of patients, with or without low muscle mass, undergoing pancreatic surgery for PDCA. These authors found that patients with a low muscle mass experienced a reduced OS ($p < 0.001$). However, the meta-analysis did not demonstrate the influence of low muscle mass on postoperative outcomes.

Most pancreatic cancer recurs after a tumor resection. Despite the fact that surgery for recurrent cancer is not recommended and rarely feasible, a series of patients with recurrent pancreatic cancer who underwent re-resection were increasingly reported in the English literature. Choi et al. [15] from Korea, reviewed the literature to assess the role of repeated pancreatectomy for patients with recurrent pancreatic cancer in the remnant pancreas. The median overall survival was 60 months after repeated pancreatectomy for isolated local recurrence. Although surgery cannot replace adjuvant chemotherapy, repeated pancreatectomy has a potential role in selected local recurrent PDAC.

Two studies [3,8] focused on the pancreatic fistula rate after pancreatic resection. Park et al. [8] evaluated the use of a flowable hemostatic matrix in preventing postoperative pancreatic fistula (POPF). Fifty-three patients were enrolled in a randomized trial, and the use of the flowable hemostatic matrix was found to be an independent negative risk factor for POPF at multivariate logistic regression analysis, particularly after distal pancreatectomy. In the study of Marino et al. [3], the incidence of POPF was evaluated in a minimally invasive pancreatectomy performed with robotic approach, an emerging surgical technique which has gained increased interest worldwide. After pancreatic resection, the pancreatic stump was anastomosed to the jejunum ($n = 40$) (PJ) or to the stomach ($n = 20$) (PG). The rate of clinically relevant POPF (12.5% vs. 10%, $p = 0.82$) did not differ between the two groups. Patients with PJ experienced more frequently intra-abdominal collections (7.5% vs. 0%, $p = 0.002$), but in this group there was a lower rate of post-pancreatectomy hemorrhage (2.5% vs. 10%, $p = 0.003$). On the contrary, patients with PG experienced a lower rate of POPF (33.3% vs. 50%, $p = 0.003$) in the high-risk group of patients.

Over the years, a growing number of patients were diagnosed with IPMNs, most likely as a consequence of a more extensive use of cross-sectional imaging. However, the management of this clinical entity remains controversial. Different clinical and radiological variables have been proposed in order to stratify the risk of the malignant degeneration of pancreatic IPMNs, and thus to guide their management. International consensus guidelines (ICG) recommend pancreatic resection for IPMNs with one or more "high-risk stigmata" (HRS), while patients with "worrisome features" (WF) should undergo a further assessment with endoscopic ultrasonography [19]. However, there is still a lack of accuracy in detecting the early invasive carcinoma in IPMNs. Serafini et al. [4] from the University of Padua (Italy) investigated the role of some systemic, inflammatory biomarkers in the diagnosis and prognosis of malignant, intraductal, papillary, mucinous neoplasms (IPMNs) of the pancreas. In 83 patients with histologically proven IPMN, the ratio of the C-reactive protein to the albumin ratio (CAR) was an independent predictor of high- grade dysplasia or invasive carcinoma in a multivariate analysis, and therefore, it could be useful to stratify the patients' prognosis.

Two studies from the same institution focused on non-ductal neoplasms. Milanetto et al. [12] reported a series of seven patients with rare neuroendocrine tumors of the pancreas: the serotonin-secreting tumors. Six out of seven patients presented high urinary 5-HIAA and two patients presented with a carcinoid syndrome. In all cases, liver metastases were present at diagnosis and none of the patients underwent resection, but after a multimodality treatment (chemotherapy, somatostatin analogues and/or loco-regional liver ablation) a 5-year survival rate of 42.9% was achieved.

The same author [7] conducted an Italian, retrospective, multicentric study concerning the treatment of the pancreatic metastases of renal cell cancer (RCC-PMs), the most frequent secondary tumors of the pancreas. The authors considered the clinical-pathological characteristics, the therapeutic management and the DFS/OS, and they discussed the potential indications of pancreatic resection. They concluded that surgery could be considered for radically resectable RCC-PMs; both single and multiple PMs. There were no differences in disease recurrence when comparing limited pancreatic resections to standard pancreatectomies. A splenectomy and lymph node surgery could be avoided, since lymph node metastases were uncommon. In experienced hands, surgical resection was safe and effective, with more than one third of cases showing no disease recurrence after a median follow-up longer than 12 years. New studies are needed in order to establish how to combine the newly available target therapies with the surgical resection.

In conclusion, this Special Issue brings new insights on the outcomes and potential problems connected to multimodality therapy for pancreatic adenocarcinoma, potential prognostic factors influencing both surgery and chemotherapy, and novel strategies for the individualized treatment of patients with pancreatic neoplasms.

Funding: This research received no external funding.

Institutional Review Board Statement: Not applicable.

Informed Consent Statement: Not applicable.

Data Availability Statement: Not applicable.

Conflicts of Interest: The authors declare no conflict of interest.

References

1. Sung, H.; Ferlay, J.; Siegel, R.L.; Laversanne, M.; Soerjomataram, I.; Jemal, A.; Bray, F. Global Cancer Statistics 2020: GLOBOCAN estimates of incidence and mortality worldwide for 36 cancers in 185 countries. *CA Cancer J. Clin.* **2021**, *71*, 209–249. [CrossRef] [PubMed]
2. Neoptolemos, J.P.; Kleeff, J.; Michl, P.; Costello, E.; Greenhalf, W.; Palmer, D.H. Therapeutic developments in pancreatic cancer: Current and future perspectives. *Nat. Rev. Gastroenterol. Hepatol.* **2018**, *15*, 333–348. [CrossRef] [PubMed]
3. Marino, M.V.; Heng Chiow, A.K.; Mirabella, A.; Vaccarella, G.; Komorowski, A.L. Rate of post-operative pancreatic fistula after robotic-assisted pancreaticoduodenectomy with pancreato-jejunostomy versus pancreato-gastrostomy: A retrospective case matched comparative study. *J. Clin. Med.* **2021**, *10*, 2181. [CrossRef] [PubMed]
4. Serafini, S.; Friziero, A.; Sperti, C.; Vallese, L.; Grego, A.; Piangerelli, A.; Belluzzi, A.; Moletta, L. The ratio of C-reactive protein to albumin is an independent predictor of malignant intraductal papillary mucinous neoplasms of the pancreas. *J. Clin. Med.* **2021**, *10*, 2058. [CrossRef] [PubMed]
5. Catalano, M.; Aprile, G.; Ramello, M.; Conca, R.; Petrioli, R.; Roviello, G. Association between low-grade Chemotherapy-Induced Peripheral Neuropathy (CINP) and survival in patients with metastatic adenocarcinoma of the pancreas. *J. Clin. Med.* **2021**, *10*, 1846. [CrossRef] [PubMed]
6. Allen, J.; Cernik, C.; Bajwa, S.; Al-Rajabi, R.; Saeed, A.; Baranda, J.; Williamson, S.; Sun, W.; Kasi, A. Association of Neutrophil, Platelet, and Lymphocyte Ratios with the Prognosis in unresectable and metastatic pancreatic cancer. *J. Clin. Med.* **2020**, *9*, 3283. [CrossRef] [PubMed]
7. Milanetto, A.C.; Morelli, L.; Di Franco, G.; David, A.; Campra, D.; De Paolis, P.; Pasquali, C. A Plea for surgery in pancreatic metastases from renal cell carcinoma: Indications and outcome from a multicenter surgical experience. *J. Clin. Med.* **2020**, *9*, 3278. [CrossRef] [PubMed]
8. Park, Y.; Ko, J.H.; Kang, D.R.; Lee, J.H.; Hwang, D.W.; Lee, J.H.; Lee, W.; Kwon, J.; Park, S.N.; Song, K.B.; et al. Effect of flowable thrombin-containing collagen-based hemostatic matrix for preventing pancreatic fistula after pancreatectomy: A randomized clinical trial. *J. Clin. Med.* **2020**, *9*, 3085. [CrossRef] [PubMed]
9. Gablo, N.; Trachtova, K.; Prochazka, V.; Hlavsa, J.; Grolich, T.; Kiss, I.; Srovnal, J.; Rehulkova, A.; Lovecek, M.; Skalicky, P.; et al. Identification and validation of circulating micrornas as prognostic biomarkers in pancreatic ductal adenocarcinoma patients undergoing surgical resection. *J. Clin. Med.* **2020**, *9*, 2440. [CrossRef] [PubMed]
10. Sperti, C.; Friziero, A.; Serafini, S.; Bissoli, S.; Ponzoni, A.; Grego, A.; Grego, E.; Moletta, L. Prognostic implications of 18-FDG positron emission tomography/computed tomography in resectable pancreatic cancer. *J. Clin. Med.* **2020**, *9*, 2169. [CrossRef] [PubMed]
11. Lee, W.; Park, Y.; Kwon, J.W.; Jun, E.; Song, K.B.; Lee, J.H.; Hwang, D.W.; Yoo, C.; Kim, K.-p.; Jeong, J.H.; et al. Reduced and normalized carbohydrate antigen 19-9 Concentrations after neoadjuvant chemotherapy have comparable prognostic performance in patients with borderline resectable and locally advanced pancreatic cancer. *J. Clin. Med.* **2020**, *9*, 1477. [CrossRef] [PubMed]
12. Milanetto, A.C.; Fassan, M.; David, A.; Pasquali, C. Serotonin-secreting neuroendocrine tumours of the pancreas. *J. Clin. Med.* **2020**, *9*, 1363. [CrossRef] [PubMed]
13. Li, W.; Martinez-Useros, J.; Garcia-Carbonero, N.; Fernandez-Aceñero, M.J.; Orta, A.; Ortega-Medina, L.; Garcia-Botella, S.; Perez-Aguirre, E.; Diez-Valladares, L.; Celdran, A.; et al. The clinical significance of PIWIL3 and PIWIL4 expression in Pancreatic cancer. *J. Clin. Med.* **2020**, *9*, 1252. [CrossRef] [PubMed]
14. Pierobon, E.S.; Moletta, L.; Zampieri, S.; Sartori, R.; Brazzale, A.R.; Zanchettin, G.; Serafini, S.; Capovilla, G.; Valmasoni, M.; Merigliano, S.; et al. The prognostic value of low muscle mass in pancreatic cancer patients: A systematic review and meta-analysis. *J. Clin. Med.* **2021**, *10*, 3033. [CrossRef] [PubMed]
15. Choi, M.; Kim, N.W.; Hwang, H.K.; Lee, W.J.; Kang, C.M. Repeated Pancreatectomy for isolated local recurrence in the remnant pancreas following radical pancreatectomy for pancreatic ductal adenocarcinoma: A pooled analysis. *J. Clin. Med.* **2020**, *9*, 3945. [CrossRef] [PubMed]
16. Levolger, S.; Van Vugt, J.L.A.; De Bruin, R.W.F.; Ijzermans, J.N.M. Systematic review of sarcopenia in patients operated on for gastrointestinal and hepatopancreatobiliary malignancies. *Br. J. Surg.* **2015**, *102*, 1448–1458. [CrossRef] [PubMed]
17. Joglekar, S.; Nau, P.N.; Mezhir, J.J. The impact of sarcopenia on survival and complications in surgical oncology: A review of the current literature. *J. Surg. Oncol.* **2018**, *112*, 503–509. [CrossRef] [PubMed]
18. Siegel, R.L.; Miller, K.D.; Jemal, A. Cancer statistics, 2020. *CA Cancer J. Clin.* **2020**, *70*, 7–30. [CrossRef] [PubMed]
19. Tanaka, M.; Fernández-del Castillo, C.; Kamisawa, T.; Jang, J.Y.; Levy, P.; Ohtsuka, T.; Salvia, R.; Shimizu, Y.; Tada, M.; Wolfgang, C.L. Revisions of international consensus Fukuoka guidelines for the management of IPMN of the pancreas. *Pancreatology* **2017**, *17*, 738–753. [CrossRef] [PubMed]

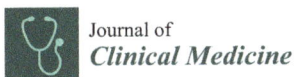

Review

Repeated Pancreatectomy for Isolated Local Recurrence in the Remnant Pancreas Following Radical Pancreatectomy for Pancreatic Ductal Adenocarcinoma: A Pooled Analysis

Munseok Choi [1], Na Won Kim [2], Ho Kyoung Hwang [1], Woo Jung Lee [1] and Chang Moo Kang [1,*]

[1] Division of Hepatobiliary and Pancreatic Surgery, Department of Surgery, Yonsei University College of Medicine, Seoul 03722, Korea; cms2598@yuhs.ac (M.C.); DRHHK@yuhs.ac (H.K.H.); wjlee@yuhs.ac (W.J.L.)
[2] Yonsei University of Medical Library, Seoul 03722, Korea; NWKIM@yuhs.ac
* Correspondence: CMKANG@yuhs.ac; Tel.: +82-2-2228-2135

Received: 20 October 2020; Accepted: 1 December 2020; Published: 5 December 2020

Abstract: The mainstream treatment for recurrent pancreatic cancer is potent chemotherapy or chemoradiotherapy. However, recent clinical investigations have suggested a potential oncologic role of local resection of recurrent pancreatic cancer. This systemic review with a pooled analysis aimed to assess the potential role of local repeated pancreatectomy with respect to the survival outcomes for patients with recurrent pancreatic ductal adenocarcinoma (PDAC) in the remnant pancreas. The PubMed database was searched, and 15 articles reporting on repeated pancreatectomy for local recurrence of PDAC in the remnant pancreas were identified. The pooled individual data were examined for the clinical outcomes of repeated pancreatectomy for recurrent PDAC. The survival analysis was performed using the Kaplan–Meier method. In the pooled analysis, the mean time interval from initial pancreatectomy to repeated pancreatectomy was 41.3 months (standard deviation (SD), 29.09 months). Completion total pancreatectomy was most commonly performed as repeated pancreatectomy (46 patients, 92.0%), and partial pancreatic resection was performed for only 4 (10.3%) patients. Twenty (40.9%) patients received postoperative chemotherapy following repeated pancreatectomy. The median overall survival was 60 months (95% confidential interval (CI): 45.99–74.01) after repeated pancreatectomy for isolated local recurrence in the remnant pancreas. Overall survival was markedly longer considering the timing of the initial pancreatectomy for pancreatic cancer (median, 107 months (95% CI: 80.37–133.62). The time interval between the initial and subsequent repeated pancreatectomy for pancreatic cancer was not associated with long-term oncologic outcomes ($p = 0.254$). Repeated pancreatectomy cannot completely replace adjuvant chemotherapy but should be considered for patients with isolated local recurrent PDAC in the remnant pancreas.

Keywords: completion total pancreatectomy; pancreatic ductal adenocarcinoma; pooled analysis; recurrent pancreatic cancer; repeated pancreatectomy; survival

---

1. Introduction

Despite low resection rates at the initial diagnostic stage, margin-negative resection is the only strategy to ensure long-term survival when treating patients with pancreatic cancer. However, recurrence is high in patients with resected pancreatic cancer. Up to 80% of patients who undergo curative pancreatectomy will experience systemic or local recurrence within 2 years [1]. According to the available literature, isolated local recurrence without systemic metastasis is reported in up to 30% of patients [2,3].

International consensus concerning the role of surgical management for patients with isolated local recurrence of pancreatic ductal adenocarcinoma (PDAC) in the remnant pancreas has not been achieved. Importantly, an adequate number of cases of treatment for isolated local recurrence of PDAC in the remnant pancreas have not been documented; therefore, the treatment required for recurrent PDAC has not been discussed in detail. The mainstream treatment for isolated local recurrence of PDAC in the remnant pancreas was potent chemotherapy or chemoradiotherapy. However, recent clinical investigations have suggested a potential oncologic role of local resection of recurrent pancreatic cancer [4–6]. This study aimed to evaluate the potential role of repeated pancreatectomy for isolated local recurrence of PDAC in the remnant pancreas using a pooled analysis, and to scrutinize the oncologic significance of the reported studies on repeated pancreatectomy so far.

2. Materials and Methods

2.1. Search Strategy and Data Sources

An extensive literature review was conducted according to the 2009 Preferred Reporting Items for Systematic Reviews and Meta-Analyses (PRISMA) guidelines [7]. The PubMed (MEDLINE) database was searched for articles published between January 2000 and April 2020 using the following terms: remnant pancreatic cancer, pancreatic cancer, pancreatectomy, pancreatic resection, local neoplasm recurrence, completion pancreatectomy, remnant pancreas, pancreatic ductal adenocarcinoma, recurrent pancreatic cancer, and second pancreatectomy. The variables of interest included sex, age, surgical procedures, disease-free interval between the initial pancreatectomy and appearance of remnant PDAC, R status (Resection margin status), adjuvant chemotherapy, 30-day mortality, and overall survival (OS). Isolated local recurrence of PDAC was defined as first recurrence limited to the remnant pancreas.

2.2. Inclusion and Exclusion Criteria

The inclusion criteria were (1) repeated pancreatectomy for isolated locally recurrent pancreatic cancer limited to the remaining pancreas after pancreatic resection, (2) evaluation of at least one of the clinicopathological or survival characteristics, (3) published original articles or case reports that contained original data, and (4) cases with pathologically confirmed ductal adenocarcinoma and with data available on both individualized long-term survival and time interval. All studies that did not meet the inclusion criteria were excluded. In addition, the following exclusion criteria were applied: (1) absence of data for individual patients, (2) other types of pancreatic cancer except pancreatic ductal adenocarcinoma, and (3) written in languages other than English. Two independent reviewers (MSC and CMK) reviewed all the retrieved studies that met the inclusion and exclusion criteria by manually screening the articles. Discrepancies between the two reviewers were resolved by discussion and achieving a team consensus.

2.3. Statistical Analysis

All statistical analyses were performed using SPSS Statistical software (version 25.0; SPSS Inc., Chicago, IL, USA). The continuous variables were expressed as means ± standard deviations or ranges, and the categorical variables were expressed as frequencies or percentages. The Student's t-test was used to compare the continuous variables, and the chi-square tests and Fisher's exact tests were used to compare the categorical data. The Kaplan–Meier method was used for the analysis of the OS. To identify the potential factors predicting the OS, univariate and multivariate analyses of the clinicopathological variables were performed using Cox-proportional hazard regression models with backward elimination. A p-value < 0.05 was considered statistically significant.

3. Results

3.1. General Characteristics of the Patients

A total of 727 potential studies were identified. Overall, 692 studies were excluded on reviewing the title and abstract. Thirty-five studies were selected for full-text review [3,4,6,8–38]. Of these, 15 studies met the inclusion criteria and were included in our pooled analysis [8,11–15,17,21,23–25,29–31,39] (Figure 1). The 15 studies are summarized in Table 1.

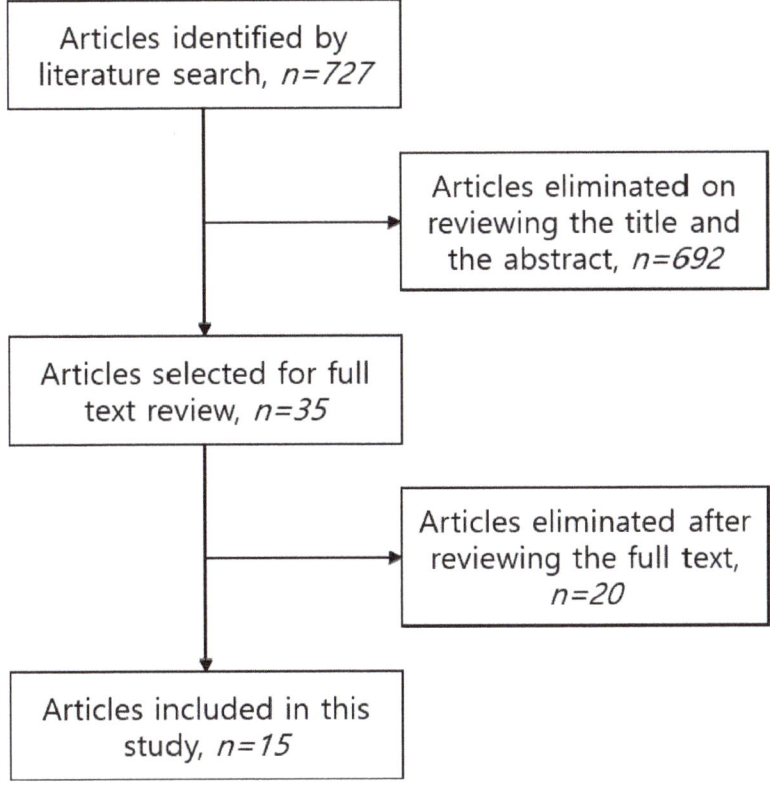

Figure 1. Flow chart for study selection.

The overall incidence of isolated local recurrence in the remnant pancreas was reported in 8 of 15 articles and showed a distribution of 0.3–5.3%. Among 50 patients, 18 male and 32 female patients with a mean age of 65.0 (range 57.15–72.85) years were identified. Pancreaticoduodenectomy was performed for 32 (64.0%) patients, distal pancreatectomy for 17 (34.0%) patients, and partial pancreatic resection for 1 (2.0%) patient as the initial pancreatectomy for pancreatic cancer. The mean time interval from initial pancreatectomy to repeated pancreatectomy was 41.3 (range 12.21–70.39) months. Completion total pancreatectomy was most commonly performed as repeated pancreatectomy (46 patients, 92.0%), and partial pancreatic resection was performed for only 4 (10.3%) patients. Twenty (40.9%; missing data, 17 patients, 34.0%) patients received postoperative chemotherapy following repeated pancreatectomy (Table 2).

Table 1. Characteristics of the selected studies.

Author, Year	Study Design	Incidence [†], %	n	1st Operation PD/DP/PP	Time Interval (Months, Mean)	2nd Operation CTP/PP	OS (Months, Median)
Eriguchi, 2000 [8]	Case report	NA	1	0/1/0	88.0	1/0	8.0
Takamatsu, 2005 [11]	Case report	NA	1	1/0/0	47.0	1/0	10.0
Dalla Valle, 2006 [12]	Case report	NA	1	1/0/0	15.0	1/0	24.0
Miura, 2007 [13]	Case series, single center	2.3	1	1/0/0	20.0	1/0	44.0
Tajima, 2008 [14]	Case report	NA	1	1/0/0	37.0	1/0	38.0
Koizumi, 2010 [15]	Case report	NA	2	1/1/0	59.5	2/0	9.0
Lavu, 2011 [17]	Case series, single center	1.3	3	2/1/0	68.0	3/0	8.0
Shimoike, 2013 [21]	Case report	NA	2	1/1/0	18.0	2/0	24.0
Boone, 2013 [23]	Case series, single center	NA	6	6/0/0	29.9	4/2	31.0
Hashimoto, 2014 [24]	Case series, single center	2.6	6	3/3	29.7	6/0	15.5
Miyazaki, 2014 [25]	Case series, single center	5.3	9	6/3/0	32.7	8/1	28.0
Shima, 2015 [39]	Case series, single center	3.2	6	4/2/0	28.8	5/1	27.5
Ishida, 2016 [29]	Case series, single center	0.8	1	0/1/0	53.0	1/0	21.0
Sahakyan, 2016 [30]	Case report	0.3	1	1/0/0	36.0	1/0	4.0
Suzuki, 2016 [31]	Case series, single center	1.1	9	4/4/1	64.7	9/0	15.0

PD, pancreaticoduodenectomy; DP, distal pancreatectomy with or without splenectomy; CTP, completion total pancreatectomy; PP, partial pancreatectomy. [†] Incidence, isolated local recurrence in the remnant pancreas/total resected pancreatic cancer.

Table 2. Characteristics of the patients undergoing repeated pancreatectomy for recurrent pancreatic ductal adenocarcinoma included in the pooled analysis.

	$n = 50$
Age	65.0 ± 7.85
Sex, male	18 (40.9)
Type of 1st OP	
PD	32 (64.0)
DP	17 (34.0)
TP	0 (0.0)
PP	1 (2.0)
Combined resection	11 (22.0)
R status, 1st OP	
R0	43 (91.5)
R1 or R2	4 (8.5)
Adjuvant CTx., 1st OP	25 (58.1)
Time interval	41.3 ± 29.09
Type of 2nd OP	
CTP	46 (92.0)
PP	4 (10.3)
R status, 2nd OP	
R0	32 (84.2)
R1 or R2	6 (15.8)
30-day mortality	0 (0.0)
90-day mortality	1 (2.0)
Adjuvant CTx., 2nd OP	20 (40.9)

OP, operation; PD, pancreaticoduodenectomy; DP, distal pancreatectomy with or without splenectomy; TP, total pancreatectomy; PP, partial pancreatectomy; CTx, chemotherapy; CTP, completion total pancreatectomy.

3.2. Long-Term Oncologic Outcomes

The median OS was 60 (95% confidential interval (CI): 45.9–74.0) months after repeated pancreatectomy for isolated local recurrence in the remnant pancreas (Figure 2A). The median OS was markedly longer if the follow-up duration was calculated from the time of the initial pancreatectomy (107 months, 95% CI: 80.3–133.0, Figure 2B). The time interval between the initial and repeated pancreatectomy was not associated with the long-term oncologic outcome of repeated pancreatectomy ($p = 0.254$; Figure 2C). In univariate analysis, the time interval between the initial and repeated pancreatectomy, R1 resection, and adjuvant chemotherapy were not associated with the OS after repeated pancreatectomy (Table 3).

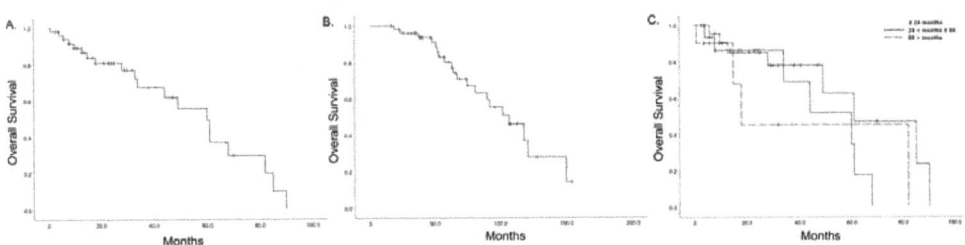

Figure 2. (**A**) Overall survival after repeated pancreatectomy. (**B**) Overall survival calculated from the time of the initial pancreatectomy. (**C**) Overall survival according to the time interval from the initial radical pancreatectomy.

Table 3. Univariate analysis of the predictors of overall survival after repeated pancreatectomy.

Variables	HR	95% CI	p-Value
Time interval			0.280
≤24 months			
24 < months ≤ 60	0.460	0.152–1.390	0.169
>60 months	1.096	0.308–3.907	0.887
R1 resection, repeated pancreatectomy	2.785	0.287–27.007	0.377
Adjuvant CTx after repeated pancreatectomy	3.704	0.788–17.418	0.097

CTx, chemotherapy; CI, confidence interval.

3.3. Short-Term Operative Outcomes

Of those 50 patients, none experienced 30-day mortality, and only one patient died within 90 days after repeated pancreatectomy. Postoperative complications mentioned explicitly in the literature were delayed gastric emptying ($n = 2$), intra-abdominal abscess ($n = 4$), sepsis ($n = 1$), focal hepatic infarction ($n = 1$), and subcutaneous abscess ($n = 1$). Among all 50 cases, 11 did not mention postoperative complications.

4. Discussion

In this study, we aimed to evaluate the potential role of local repeated pancreatectomy for recurrent PDAC in the remnant pancreas, and we found that repeated pancreatectomy improved the survival outcomes for patients with isolated local recurrent PDAC in the remnant pancreas. Pancreatic cancer is considered one of the dismal malignant diseases in the gastrointestinal system. Only margin-negative resection is essential for long-term survival; however, the resection rate at diagnostic stage is low, and recurrence is commonly noted within 2 years, even after radical pancreatectomy [40]. Finally, disease progression leading to cancer-related mortality during chemotherapy is inevitable in patients with recurrence. However, this clinical scenario may not always hold true owing to the recent changes in clinical oncology, such as the development of advanced surgical techniques, perioperative management strategies, and improved potent chemotherapeutic agents.

Unlike systemic recurrence, isolated local recurrence of pancreatic cancer is considered a topic of interest for pancreatic surgeons because recurrence can be controlled by local treatment, such as repeated pancreatectomy, in selected patients. Especially, considering the potential role of neoadjuvant chemotherapy in treating pancreatic cancer, chemotherapy for local recurrence in the remnant pancreas followed by repeated pancreatectomy may potentially be an option for treating isolated local recurrent pancreatic cancer [41]. Neoadjuvant chemotherapy is used for treating isolated recurrence of pancreatic cancer in the remnant pancreas with the aim of treating possible microscopic systemic metastasis that cannot be detected, and assessing tumor biology for selecting the appropriate patients.

With respect to the long-term oncologic outcomes of repeated pancreatectomy for isolated local recurrence of pancreatic cancer, Yamada, et al. reported 114 patients with remnant pancreatic cancer after initial pancreatectomy [6]. Ninety patients underwent repeated pancreatectomy; the median survival was 26 months, which was superior to that noted for patients who did not undergo resection (hazard ratio (HR): 0.56, $p = 0.012$). Hashimoto et al. reviewed 12 published studies reporting on recurrent pancreatic cancer in the remnant pancreas following initial pancreatectomy, and they showed that the OS after repeated pancreatectomy for remnant pancreatic cancer was 14–35.5 months, which was markedly longer than that noted for patients with unresectable pancreatic cancer in recent studies [24]. Groot et al. performed a systemic review of the treatment of isolated local recurrence of pancreatic cancer. Based on eight published studies including 100 patients who underwent re-resection of recurrent pancreatic cancer, they concluded that local re-resection of recurrent pancreatic cancer may be feasible, safe, and effective in the selected patients [33]. They demonstrated that the postoperative morbidity and mortality rates were 29% and 1%, respectively. In addition, the median survival was markedly higher (32 months) compared to that for other treatment modalities, such as chemotherapy

(19 months) and radiotherapy (16 months). Zhou et al. reported that repeated pancreatectomy can be safely performed in recurrent PDAC and showed good long-term results by conducting a literature review from 2000 to 2016 with pooled analysis, which is the same analysis method as the present study [32]. The present study was conducted for a literature review by adding case reports or case series for the extended period.

The reason why patients with isolated local recurrence of pancreatic cancer have better prognosis than those with other sites of distant dissemination of the disease is a matter of debate. What is the reasonable basis for better survival in isolated local recurrence of pancreatic cancer? At first, taking into account the biological background of isolated local recurrence patients, obtaining a survival benefit through surgical treatment could be a well-founded treatment strategy. Research has shown that pancreatic cancer is likely to be exposed to distant metastasis prior to surgical resection [42]. In an autopsy series, Haeno et al. revealed that a small subset of patients died with only locally advanced disease, suggesting that some tumors may lack metastasis-promoting factors (or have metastasis-suppressing factors) or may have metastases that are especially sensitive to systemic chemotherapy [43]. This is thought to be directly related to the high median OS highlighted in the present study. Furthermore, the role of adjuvant therapy is also significant. In the ESPAC-4 trial, the patient group using the combination of gemcitabine with capecitabine showed a better DFS and OS than the group of patients using gemcitabine alone [44]. This result should be considered for one factor that improves survival. Although further study is necessary, the first surgery dissects the soft tissue (nerve, lymphatics) and blocks the route to propagate the tumor to the surrounding area. Besides, most patients recur in a highly attenuated state of potential residual cancer cells by adjuvant chemotherapy after the first surgery. Therefore, there is a possibility that it remains purely isolated recurrence, and there is room for improvement in oncologic outcome through repeated pancreatectomy.

Operating on a recurrent PDAC in the remnant pancreas is challenging as the procedure may be associated with high morbidity or mortality due to adhesion of the tumor with the surrounding tissue and anatomical deformation after the surgery. However, according to recent reports, repeated pancreatectomy is safe [4]. According to our limited experiences, completion total pancreatectomy for isolated recurrence in the remnant pancreas after initial pancreaticoduodenectomy is technically demanding as a safe surgical procedure, especially when the previous pancreatic division line is above the Superior mesenteric vein-splenic vein-portal vein confluence. Pancreaticojejunostomy associated postoperative pancreatic fistula (POPF) may result in severe adhesion around these venous vascular systems and the celiac axis where the remnant distal pancreas and these major vascular structures should be dissected safely; thus, difficulties are encountered in performing repeated pancreatectomy. Therefore, as Fortner suggested, the pancreatic division may be performed distal to the splenic artery origin during the initial pancreaticoduodenectomy for resectable pancreatic cancer, considering the possibility of subsequent repeated pancreatectomy for isolated recurrent pancreatic cancer in the remnant pancreas [45].

Although long-term follow-up is required to address the potential role of repeated pancreatectomy for recurrent pancreatic cancer, recent studies and the present pooled analysis strongly suggest the oncologic benefits of this approach [36,37]. In the present study, the median OS was estimated to be 60 months from the time of repeated pancreatectomy and 107 months from the time of initial radical pancreatectomy. Although the R1 resection rate after repeated pancreatectomy was higher than that noted after the first pancreatectomy (8.5% vs. 15.5%, Table 2), the R1 resection rate was not associated with the OS after pancreatectomy in univariate analysis (Table 3). Therefore, repeated pancreatectomy is a challenging procedure, but preparing for R1 resection and attempting surgical treatment may benefit the patient with respect to the OS.

In addition, it is quite difficult to differentiate between local recurrence and de novo carcinogenesis, especially when the duration from the initial pancreatectomy is quite long. However, regardless of the duration, the present pooled analysis showed that there was no difference with respect to survival after repeated pancreatectomy was successfully performed. Therefore, medical oncologists and pancreatic surgeons should consider that the patients with isolated local recurrence in the remnant pancreas following initial radical pancreatectomy may not show poor prognosis but may be able to survive long-term if repeated pancreatectomy can be safely performed.

When reviewing the literature, it was found that isolated local recurrence is rare compared to systemic recurrence following radical pancreatectomy for pancreatic cancer. Therefore, it is thought that very selected cases were collected and analyzed, resulting in difficulty for generalization. However, despite a rare recurrent pattern of resected pancreatic cancer, these patients are potentially encountered in clinical practice. In addition, with the advance of laparoscopic technique, even laparoscopic repeated pancreatectomy seems to be feasible in recurred pancreatic cancer [46]. What shall we do for them? The present analysis may not be generalized but can at least provide potential treatment options for the patients. Further experiences and investigations are mandatory to reveal the potential oncologic role of local resection in isolated local recurrence of resected pancreatic cancer.

A limitation of the present study is that potential clinically important factors, such as tumor differentiation, lymph node metastasis, and perineural invasion, were not considered in this analysis. A more reliable analysis would have been possible if the original data of the cohort study, including a relatively larger number of cases specifying clinic-pathological variables, could be obtained. In the near future, a risk model for predicting isolated local recurrence following initial pancreatectomy for pancreatic cancer should be developed based on data from a well-designed multicenter collaborative study.

In conclusion, we revealed that repeated pancreatectomy for isolated local recurrence in the remnant pancreas could improve survival outcomes based on the pooled analysis of data from published studies. Hence, a case-specific surgical approach for repeated pancreatectomy for recurrent pancreatic cancer, such as indications, the extent of surgery, and prognostic factors, should be established based on consensus and more reliable, convincing data.

5. Conclusions

Repeated pancreatectomy cannot completely replace the role of adjuvant chemotherapy but should be considered for patients with isolated local recurrent PDAC in the remnant pancreas.

Author Contributions: Conceptualization, C.M.K. and M.C.; methodology, C.M.K.; software, N.W.K.; validation, M.C.; formal analysis, M.C.; data curation, N.W.K., M.C., C.M.K.; writing—original draft preparation, M.C.; writing—review and editing, H.K.H., W.J.L., C.M.K.; visualization, M.C.; supervision, C.M.K. All authors have read and agreed to the published version of the manuscript.

Funding: This research received no external funding.

Conflicts of Interest: The authors declare no conflict of interest.

References

1. Garcea, G.; Dennison, A.R.; Pattenden, C.J.; Neal, C.P.; Sutton, C.D.; Berry, D.P. Survival following curative resection for pancreatic ductal adenocarcinoma. A systematic review of the literature. *Jop* **2008**, *9*, 99–132.
2. Van den Broeck, A.; Sergeant, G.; Ectors, N.; Van Steenbergen, W.; Aerts, R.; Topal, B. Patterns of recurrence after curative resection of pancreatic ductal adenocarcinoma. *Eur. J. Surg. Oncol.* **2009**, *35*, 600–604. [CrossRef]
3. Hishinuma, S.; Ogata, Y.; Tomikawa, M.; Ozawa, I.; Hirabayashi, K.; Igarashi, S. Patterns of recurrence after curative resection of pancreatic cancer, based on autopsy findings. *J. Gastrointest. Surg.* **2006**, *10*, 511–518. [CrossRef]
4. Hashimoto, D.; Arima, K.; Nakagawa, S.; Negoro, Y.; Hirata, T.; Hirota, M.; Inomata, M.; Fukuzawa, K.; Ohga, T.; Saeki, H.; et al. Pancreatic cancer arising from the remnant pancreas after pancreatectomy: A multicenter retrospective study by the kyushu study group of clinical cancer. *J. Gastroenterol.* **2019**, *54*, 437–448. [CrossRef]
5. Groot, V.P.; Rezaee, N.; Wu, W.; Cameron, J.L.; Fishman, E.K.; Hruban, R.H.; Weiss, M.J.; Zheng, L.; Wolfgang, C.L.; He, J. Patterns, timing, and predictors of recurrence following pancreatectomy for pancreatic ductal adenocarcinoma. *Ann. Surg.* **2018**, *267*, 936–945. [CrossRef]

6. Yamada, S.; Kobayashi, A.; Nakamori, S.; Baba, H.; Yamamoto, M.; Yamaue, H.; Fujii, T. Resection for recurrent pancreatic cancer in the remnant pancreas after pancreatectomy is clinically promising: Results of a project study for pancreatic surgery by the japanese society of hepato-biliary-pancreatic surgery. *Surgery* **2018**, *164*, 1049–1056. [CrossRef]
7. Moher, D.; Liberati, A.; Tetzlaff, J.; Altman, D.G. Preferred reporting items for systematic reviews and meta-analyses: The prisma statement. *PLoS Med.* **2009**, *6*, e1000097. [CrossRef]
8. Eriguchi, N.; Aoyagi, S.; Imayama, H.; Okuda, K.; Hara, M.; Fukuda, S.; Tamaie, T.; Kanazawa, N.; Noritomi, T.; Hiraki, M.; et al. Resectable carcinoma of the pancreatic head developing 7 years and 4 months after distal pancreatectomy for carcinoma of the pancreatic tail. *J. Hepato-Biliary-Pancreat. Surg.* **2000**, *7*, 316–320. [CrossRef] [PubMed]
9. Wada, K.; Takada, T.; Yasuda, H.; Amano, H.; Yoshida, M. A repeated pancreatectomy in the remnant pancreas 22 months after pylorus-preserving pancreatoduodenectomy for pancreatic adenocarcinoma. *J. Hepato-Biliary-Pancreat. Surg.* **2001**, *8*, 174–178. [CrossRef] [PubMed]
10. Doi, R.; Ikeda, H.; Kobayashi, H.; Kogire, M.; Imamura, M. Carcinoma in the remnant pancreas after distal pancreatectomy for carcinoma. *Eur. J. Surg. Suppl.* **2003**, *588*, 62–65.
11. Takamatsu, S.; Ban, D.; Irie, T.; Noguchi, N.; Kudoh, A.; Nakamura, N.; Kawamura, T.; Igari, T.; Teramoto, K.; Arii, S. Resection of a cancer developing in the remnant pancreas after a pancreaticoduodenectomy for pancreas head cancer. *J. Gastrointest. Surg.* **2005**, *9*, 263–269. [CrossRef] [PubMed]
12. Dalla Valle, R.; Mancini, C.; Crafa, P.; Passalacqua, R. Pancreatic carcinoma recurrence in the remnant pancreas after a pancreaticoduodenectomy. *J. Pancreas* **2006**, *7*, 473–477.
13. Miura, F.; Takada, T.; Amano, H.; Yoshida, M.; Isaka, T.; Toyota, N.; Wada, K.; Takagi, K.; Kato, K. Repeated pancreatectomy after pancreatoduodenectomy. *J. Gastrointest. Surg.* **2007**, *11*, 179–186. [CrossRef] [PubMed]
14. Tajima, Y.; Kuroki, T.; Ohno, T.; Furui, J.; Tsuneoka, N.; Adachi, T.; Mishima, T.; Kosaka, T.; Haraguchi, M.; Kanematsu, T. Resectable carcinoma developing in the remnant pancreas 3 years after pylorus-preserving pancreaticoduodenectomy for invasive ductal carcinoma of the pancreas. *Pancreas* **2008**, *36*, 324–327. [CrossRef] [PubMed]
15. Koizumi, M.; Sata, N.; Kasahara, N.; Morishima, K.; Sasanuma, H.; Sakuma, Y.; Shimizu, A.; Hyodo, M.; Yasuda, Y. Remnant pancreatectomy for recurrent or metachronous pancreatic carcinoma detected by fdg-pet: Two case reports. *J. Pancreas* **2010**, *11*, 36–40.
16. Kinoshita, H.; Yamade, N.; Nakai, H.; Sasaya, T.; Matsumura, S.; Kimura, A.; Shima, K. Successful resection of pancreatic carcinoma recurrence in the remnant pancreas after a pancreaticoduodenectomy. *Hepatogastroenterology* **2011**, *58*, 1406–1408. [CrossRef]
17. Lavu, H.; Nowcid, L.J.; Klinge, M.J.; Mahendraraj, K.; Grenda, D.R.; Sauter, P.K.; Rosato, E.L.; Kennedy, E.P.; Yeo, C.J. Reoperative completion pancreatectomy for suspected malignant disease of the pancreas. *J. Surg. Res.* **2011**, *170*, 89–95. [CrossRef]
18. Katz, M.H.; Wang, H.; Balachandran, A.; Bhosale, P.; Crane, C.H.; Wang, X.; Pisters, P.W.; Lee, J.E.; Vauthey, J.N.; Abdalla, E.K.; et al. Effect of neoadjuvant chemoradiation and surgical technique on recurrence of localized pancreatic cancer. *J. Gastrointest. Surg.* **2012**, *16*, 68–78. [CrossRef]
19. Kobayashi, T.; Sato, Y.; Hirukawa, H.; Soeno, M.; Shimoda, T.; Matsuoka, H.; Kobayashi, Y.; Tada, T.; Hatakeyama, K. Total pancreatectomy combined with partial pancreas autotransplantation for recurrent pancreatic cancer: A case report. *Transplant. Proc.* **2012**, *44*, 1176–1179. [CrossRef]
20. Thomas, R.M.; Truty, M.J.; Nogueras-Gonzalez, G.M.; Fleming, J.B.; Vauthey, J.N.; Pisters, P.W.; Lee, J.E.; Rice, D.C.; Hofstetter, W.L.; Wolff, R.A.; et al. Selective reoperation for locally recurrent or metastatic pancreatic ductal adenocarcinoma following primary pancreatic resection. *J. Gastrointest. Surg.* **2012**, *16*, 1696–1704. [CrossRef]
21. Shimoike, N.; Fujikawa, T.; Maekawa, H.; Tanaka, A. Aggressive secondary surgery for local recurrence of pancreatic cancer. *BMJ Case Rep* **2013**, *2013*, bcr2013009914. [CrossRef] [PubMed]
22. Akabori, H.; Shiomi, H.; Naka, S.; Murakami, K.; Murata, S.; Ishida, M.; Kurumi, Y.; Tani, T. Resectable carcinoma developing in the remnant pancreas 7 years and 10 months after distal pancreatectomy for invasive ductal carcinoma of the pancreas: Report of a case. *World J. Surg. Oncol.* **2014**, *12*, 224. [CrossRef] [PubMed]
23. Boone, B.A.; Zeh, H.J.; Mock, B.K.; Johnson, P.J.; Dvorchik, I.; Lee, K.; Moser, A.J.; Bartlett, D.L.; Marsh, J.W. Resection of isolated local and metastatic recurrence in periampullary adenocarcinoma. *HPB* **2014**, *16*, 197–203. [CrossRef] [PubMed]

24. Hashimoto, D.; Chikamoto, A.; Ohmuraya, M.; Sakata, K.; Miyake, K.; Kuroki, H.; Watanabe, M.; Beppu, T.; Hirota, M.; Baba, H. Pancreatic cancer in the remnant pancreas following primary pancreatic resection. *Surg. Today* **2014**, *44*, 1313–1320. [CrossRef] [PubMed]
25. Miyazaki, M.; Yoshitomi, H.; Shimizu, H.; Ohtsuka, M.; Yoshidome, H.; Furukawa, K.; Takayasiki, T.; Kuboki, S.; Okamura, D.; Suzuki, D.; et al. Repeat pancreatectomy for pancreatic ductal cancer recurrence in the remnant pancreas after initial pancreatectomy: Is it worthwhile? *Surgery* **2014**, *155*, 58–66. [CrossRef] [PubMed]
26. Sunagawa, H.; Mayama, Y.; Orokawa, T.; Oshiro, N. Laparoscopic total remnant pancreatectomy after laparoscopic pancreaticoduodenectomy. *Asian J. Endosc. Surg.* **2014**, *7*, 71–74. [CrossRef]
27. Balaj, C.; Ayav, A.; Oliver, A.; Jausset, F.; Sellal, C.; Claudon, M.; Laurent, V. Ct imaging of early local recurrence of pancreatic adenocarcinoma following pancreaticoduodenectomy. *Abdom. Radiol.* **2016**, *41*, 273–282. [CrossRef]
28. Hardacre, J.M. Completion pancreaticoduodenectomy for a second primary pancreatic cancer: A case report. *Case Rep. Pancreat. Cancer* **2016**, *2*, 50–52. [CrossRef]
29. Ishida, J.; Toyama, H.; Matsumoto, I.; Asari, S.; Goto, T.; Terai, S.; Nanno, Y.; Yamashita, A.; Mizumoto, T.; Ueda, Y.; et al. Second primary pancreatic ductal carcinoma in the remnant pancreas after pancreatectomy for pancreatic ductal carcinoma: High cumulative incidence rates at 5 years after pancreatectomy. *Pancreatology* **2016**, *16*, 615–620. [CrossRef]
30. Sahakyan, M.A.; Yaqub, S.; Kazaryan, A.M.; Villanger, O.; Berstad, A.E.; Labori, K.J.; Edwin, B.; Røsok, B.I. Laparoscopic completion pancreatectomy for local recurrence in the pancreatic remnant after pancreaticoduodenectomy: Case reports and review of the literature. *J. Gastrointest. Cancer* **2016**, *47*, 509–513. [CrossRef]
31. Suzuki, S.; Furukawa, T.; Oshima, N.; Izumo, W.; Shimizu, K.; Yamamoto, M. Original scientific reports: Clinicopathological findings of remnant pancreatic cancers in survivors following curative resections of pancreatic cancers. *World J. Surg.* **2016**, *40*, 974–981. [CrossRef] [PubMed]
32. Zhou, Y.; Song, A.; Wu, L.; Si, X.; Li, Y. Second pancreatectomy for recurrent pancreatic ductal adenocarcinoma in the remnant pancreas: A pooled analysis. *Pancreatology* **2016**, *16*, 1124–1128. [CrossRef] [PubMed]
33. Groot, V.P.; van Santvoort, H.C.; Rombouts, S.J.; Hagendoorn, J.; Borel Rinkes, I.H.; van Vulpen, M.; Herman, J.M.; Wolfgang, C.L.; Besselink, M.G.; Molenaar, I.Q. Systematic review on the treatment of isolated local recurrence of pancreatic cancer after surgery; re-resection, chemoradiotherapy and sbrt. *HPB* **2017**, *19*, 83–92. [CrossRef] [PubMed]
34. Kim, N.H.; Kim, H.J. Preoperative risk factors for early recurrence in patients with resectable pancreatic ductal adenocarcinoma after curative intent surgical resection. *Hepatobiliary Pancreat. Dis. Int.* **2018**, *17*, 450–455. [CrossRef]
35. Nakayama, Y.; Sugimoto, M.; Gotohda, N.; Konishi, M.; Takahashi, S. Efficacy of completion pancreatectomy for recurrence of adenocarcinoma in the remnant pancreas. *J. Surg. Res.* **2018**, *221*, 15–23. [CrossRef]
36. Kim, Y.I.; Song, K.B.; Lee, Y.J.; Park, K.M.; Hwang, D.W.; Lee, J.H.; Shin, S.H.; Kwon, J.W.; Ro, J.S.; Kim, S.C. Management of isolated recurrence after surgery for pancreatic adenocarcinoma. *Br. J. Surg.* **2019**, *106*, 898–909. [CrossRef]
37. Moletta, L.; Serafini, S.; Valmasoni, M.; Pierobon, E.S.; Ponzoni, A.; Sperti, C. Surgery for recurrent pancreatic cancer: Is it effective? *Cancers* **2019**, *11*, 991. [CrossRef]
38. Suzuki, S.; Shimoda, M.; Shimazaki, J.; Maruyama, T.; Nishida, K. Clinical outcome of resected remnant pancreatic cancer after resection of the primary pancreatic cancer. *J. Investig. Surg.* **2019**, *32*, 670–678. [CrossRef]
39. Shima, Y.; Okabayashi, T.; Kozuki, A.; Sumiyoshi, T.; Tokumaru, T.; Saisaka, Y.; Date, K.; Iwata, J. Completion pancreatectomy for recurrent pancreatic cancer in the remnant pancreas: Report of six cases and a review of the literature. *Langenbeck Arch. Surg.* **2015**, *400*, 973–978. [CrossRef]
40. Rahib, L.; Smith, B.D.; Aizenberg, R.; Rosenzweig, A.B.; Fleshman, J.M.; Matrisian, L.M. Projecting cancer incidence and deaths to 2030: The unexpected burden of thyroid, liver, and pancreas cancers in the united states. *Cancer Res.* **2014**, *74*, 2913–2921. [CrossRef]
41. Katz, M.H.; Pisters, P.W.; Evans, D.B.; Sun, C.C.; Lee, J.E.; Fleming, J.B.; Vauthey, J.N.; Abdalla, E.K.; Crane, C.H.; Wolff, R.A.; et al. Borderline resectable pancreatic cancer: The importance of this emerging stage of disease. *J. Am. Coll. Surg.* **2008**, *206*, 833–846, discussion 846–838. [CrossRef] [PubMed]

42. Tuveson, D.A.; Neoptolemos, J.P. Understanding metastasis in pancreatic cancer: A call for new clinical approaches. *Cell* **2012**, *148*, 21–23. [CrossRef] [PubMed]
43. Haeno, H.; Gonen, M.; Davis, M.B.; Herman, J.M.; Iacobuzio-Donahue, C.A.; Michor, F. Computational modeling of pancreatic cancer reveals kinetics of metastasis suggesting optimum treatment strategies. *Cell* **2012**, *148*, 362–375. [CrossRef] [PubMed]
44. Jones, R.P.; Psarelli, E.E.; Jackson, R.; Ghaneh, P.; Halloran, C.M.; Palmer, D.H.; Campbell, F.; Valle, J.W.; Faluyi, O.; O'Reilly, D.A.; et al. Patterns of recurrence after resection of pancreatic ductal adenocarcinoma: A secondary analysis of the espac-4 randomized adjuvant chemotherapy trial. *JAMA Surg.* **2019**, *154*, 1038–1048. [CrossRef]
45. Fortner, J.G. Surgical principles for pancreatic cancer: Regional total and subtotal pancreatectomy. *Cancer* **1981**, *47*, 1712–1718. [CrossRef]
46. Choi, M.; Lee, S.J.; Shin, D.M.; Hwang, H.K.; Lee, W.J.; Kang, C.M. Laparoscopic repeated pancreatectomy for isolated local recurrence in remnant pancreas following laparoscopic radical pancreatectomy for pancreatic ductal adenocarcinoma: Two cases report. *Ann. Hepatobiliary Pancreat. Surg.* **2020**, *24*, 542–546. [CrossRef]

Publisher's Note: MDPI stays neutral with regard to jurisdictional claims in published maps and institutional affiliations.

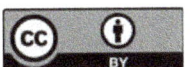

© 2020 by the authors. Licensee MDPI, Basel, Switzerland. This article is an open access article distributed under the terms and conditions of the Creative Commons Attribution (CC BY) license (http://creativecommons.org/licenses/by/4.0/).

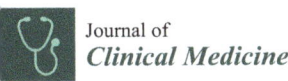

Review

The Prognostic Value of Low Muscle Mass in Pancreatic Cancer Patients: A Systematic Review and Meta-Analysis

Elisa Sefora Pierobon [1,†], Lucia Moletta [1,†], Sandra Zampieri [1,2], Roberta Sartori [2,3,*], Alessandra Rosalba Brazzale [4], Gianpietro Zanchettin [1], Simone Serafini [1], Giovanni Capovilla [1], Michele Valmasoni [1], Stefano Merigliano [1] and Cosimo Sperti [1]

1. Department of Surgery, Oncology and Gastroenterology, 3rd Surgical Clinic, University of Padua, Via Giustiniani 2, 35128 Padua, Italy; elisaseforapierobon@gmail.com (E.S.P.); lucia.moletta@unipd.it (L.M.); sanzamp@unipd.it (S.Z.); gianpietro.zanchettin@gmail.com (G.Z.); simone.serafini@ymail.com (S.S.); giovannicapovilla88@gmail.com (G.C.); michele.valmasoni@unipd.it (M.V.); stefano.merigliano@unipd.it (S.M.); cosimo.sperti@unipd.it (C.S.)
2. Department of Biomedical Sciences, University of Padua, Via U. Bassi 58/B, 35121 Padua, Italy
3. Veneto Institute of Molecular Medicine (VIMM), Via Orus 2, 35129 Padua, Italy
4. Department of Statistical Sciences, University of Padua, Via C. Battisti 241, 35121 Padua, Italy; brazzale@stat.unipd.it
* Correspondence: roberta.sartori@unipd.it; Tel.: +39-(0)-4-9792-3268
† These Authors contributed equally to this work.

Abstract: Low muscle mass is associated with reduced survival in patients with different cancer types. The interest in preoperative sarcopenia and pancreatic cancer has risen in the last decade as muscle mass loss seems to be associated with poorer survival, higher postoperative morbidity, and mortality. The aim of the present study was to review the literature to compare the impact of low muscle mass on the outcomes of patients undergoing surgery for pancreatic adenocarcinoma. An extensive literature review was conducted according to the 2009 Preferred Reporting Items for Systematic Reviews and Meta-Analyses (PRISMA) guidelines and 10 articles were analyzed in detail and included in the meta-analysis. Data were retrieved on 2811 patients undergoing surgery for pancreatic cancer. Meta-analysis identified that patients with low muscle mass demonstrated a significantly reduced OS when compared to patients without alterations of the muscle mass (ROM 0.86; 95% CI: 0.81–0.91, $p < 0.001$), resulting in a 14% loss for the former. Meta-analysis failed to identify an increase in the postoperative complications and length of stay of patients with low muscle mass. Our analysis confirms the role of low muscle mass in influencing oncologic outcomes in pancreatic cancer. Its role on surgical outcomes remains to be established.

Keywords: low muscle mass; sarcopenia; pancreatic adenocarcinoma; pancreatic cancer; pancreatic surgery; body composition

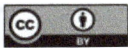

1. Introduction

Skeletal muscle accounts for 40–50% of the total mass in healthy-weight individuals [1] and serves as a body protein reservoir [2]. It is a plastic and highly adaptive organ that can increase or decrease its size, functional capacity, and metabolism in response to different pathophysiological stimuli. Since the muscle is an endocrine and exocrine organ, its adaptations have an impact on the entire organism's well-being and the muscle metabolic state has been proposed as a disease modifier [2–4].

Pathological conditions such as cancer compromise the mechanisms that regulate muscle homeostasis, resulting in severe muscle wasting, functional impairment, and altered metabolism, impacting profoundly on the health of the host and leading to cancer cachexia syndrome.

Low muscle mass ('secondary' or disease-related sarcopenia) [5] is part of the diagnostic criteria to define cancer cachexia in association with body weight loss and body mass index (BMI) [6], and is associated with increased treatment toxicity and reduced survival in patients with different cancer types. In addition to low muscle mass, low muscle quality characterized by fatty infiltration (myosteatosis) is a predictor of poor outcomes after resection of various malignancies including pancreatic cancer [7–15].

The prognosis for pancreatic cancer is generally poor, with five-year survival rates in the range of 6% to 10% [16,17]. Radical surgical resection represents the only potential cure. Over the years, advances in surgical technique and perioperative care have led to progressive improvements of outcomes after pancreatectomy for cancer. However, postoperative morbidity rates remain high; up to 40% of patients will experience complications after surgical resection [18]. Several studies have focused on investigating preoperative factors that are able to influence postoperative course and secondary sarcopenia has been proposed as a patient-related condition with potential impacts on short and long-term surgical outcomes [19]. In fact, the interest in preoperative sarcopenia and pancreatic cancer has risen in the last decade as muscle mass and adipose tissue loss seems to be associated with higher postoperative morbidity and increased mortality [8,20,21]. Moreover, among solid tumors, pancreatic cancer carries the highest prevalence of cancer cachexia and involuntary weight loss [22]. Patients with cancer are prone to metabolic modifications, such as the Warburg effect, leading to a dramatically altered nutrient utilization [19]. Furthermore, in the case of pancreatic cancer patients, malnutrition is worsened by the exocrine insufficiency that might ensue [10].

There are multiple radiological methods that have been approved to perform body composition analysis, evaluate muscle mass, and define sarcopenia such as computed tomography (CT), magnetic resonance imaging (MRI), and dual energy X-ray absorptiometry (DXA). DXA is not usually available in cancer settings, though, and it cannot discriminate visceral adipose tissue, decipher changes between tumor mass and lean muscle mass, and it has decreased precision in obese patients [23]. Computed tomography (CT) scans have been used and proposed as the gold standard to evaluate cancer-associated changes in body composition and its association with the prognosis [11,24]. Indeed, the imaging resolution of adipose, skeletal muscles, and the precision of measures of a tissue cross-sectional area of a CT scan is excellent. Moreover, it is a practical choice as CT images are routinely acquired in the standard care of cancer patients and can provide information on body composition over time without incremental cost or radiation exposure [24]. CT scan analyses quantify skeletal muscle mass and other tissues, such as adipose or connective tissue, allowing the detection of low mass and decreased muscle radiodensity due to myosteatosis. CT image analyses reveal low levels of muscle also in individuals who are overweight or obese (sarcopenic obesity) [24–27].

The aim of the present study was to review the published literature to compare the impact of low muscle mass (evaluated by CT scan) on the short and long-term outcomes in patients with pancreatic ductal adenocarcinoma (PDAC) undergoing surgery.

2. Materials and Methods

2.1. Literature Search Strategy

Eligibility criteria were established a priori. A systematic search of literature published in English from January 2010 to September 2020 was performed to identify all original articles on patients undergoing surgical resection of PDAC in which a preoperative abdominal CT scan was used to assess skeletal muscle mass. The Preferred Reporting Items for Systematic Reviews and Meta-Analyses (PRISMA) guidelines were followed [28]. The following terms were used to search through the literature (PubMed and Web of Science databases): 'sarcopenia', 'analytic morphomics', 'body composition', 'muscle depletion', 'muscle mass', 'psoas area', 'myopenia', 'core muscle', 'lean body mass', or 'muscular atrophy', and 'pancreatic cancer', 'surgery', 'pancreatic resection', or 'pancreatectomy'. The "related articles" function and all citations were used to broaden the search. Three independent researchers (ESP, LM, and GZ) reviewed the relevant titles. After excluding duplicates, abstracts were reviewed and included for initial analysis if the inclusion criteria were met. Records without abstracts, case reports, review articles, opinion articles, and experimental studies were excluded. In case of disagreement, a fourth author (MV) participated in the discussion. A manual search of the reference lists in precedent reviews and eligible articles was also performed.

2.2. Inclusion and Exclusion Criteria

Inclusion criteria were: (1) studies reporting the assessment of body composition by CT scan in human subjects with PDAC receiving surgical treatment; (2) body composition defined as total muscle area or total psoas area/volume at the lumbar level; (3) studies reporting on the prevalence of muscle alterations and at least one of the following outcomes: postoperative mortality, postoperative complications, length of hospital stay (LOS), disease-free survival (DFS), and overall survival (OS); and (4) studies published in English.

Exclusion criteria were: (1) review articles or case series (<5 patients); (2) publications comprising of patients with either a benign or malignant disease in which the surgical and oncological outcome were not presented separately; and (3) body composition analyzed using methods other than those described in the inclusion criteria (e.g., MRI, DEXA, etc.).

2.3. Measured Outcomes and Data Extraction

Data were registered in digital sheets. Data regarding authors, year of publication, country of publication, study type, characteristics of populations and of their present disease, muscle mass evaluated, cut-offs' selection, muscle loss prevalence, incidence of major complications (graded ≥ 2 according to Clavien–Dindo classification [29]), DFS, and OS were retrieved. When reported by the authors, data regarding sarcopenic obesity, myosteatosis prevalence, and impact on outcomes were collected.

2.4. Terminology and Definitions

Regarding low muscle mass, the CT scan-determined muscle parameters, cut-off values used, muscles, and vertebral level analyzed to define low muscle mass (secondary sarcopenia) in the papers considered are reported in Table 1 and discussed in the results section. Sarcopenic obesity is defined as sarcopenia accompanied by obesity (an increase in the adipose tissue) [30]. The definitions of sarcopenic obesity used in the papers considered are reported in Table 1. Myosteatosis is the skeletal muscle fat infiltration diagnosed by CT scan-determined low muscle radiodensity (radiation attenuation in Hounsfield units). The cut-off values used to define myosteatosis in the papers considered are reported in Table 1.

Table 1. Terminology and definitions of sarcopenia in the included studies.

Author	Measurements of Skeletal Muscle	Criteria to Define Sarcopenia	Cut-Off Values Males	Cut-Off Values Females	Definition of Sarcopenic Obesity	Definition of Myosteatosis
Peng P et al. [31]	TPA (L3)	Quartiles	Lowest quartile: 492 mm^2/m^2	Lowest quartile: 362 mm^2/m^2	Sarcopenia + BMI $\geq$ 30 kg/m^2	-
Amini et al. [32]	TPA (L3) and TPV (L3)	Quartiles	Lowest quartile TPA: 564.2 mm^2/m^2; TPV: 17.2 cm^3/m^3	Lowest quartile TPA: 414.5 mm^2/m^2; TPV: 12.0 cm^3/m^3	Sarcopenia + BMI $\geq$ 30 kg/m^2	-
Clark et al. [33]	CSAPM/CSAL5	Linear regression analysis with survival				
Delitto et al. [34]	CSAPM/CSAL3	Linear regression analysis and Median	CSAPM/CSAL3 < 0.58	CSAPM/CSAL3 < 0.58		
Okumura et al. [35]	SMI	Self-determined cut-offs (in relation to 3-year mortality)	47.1 cm^2/m^2	36.6 cm^2/m^2	Low SMI + VFA $\geq$ 100 cm^2	<35.1 HU (Male) <30.7 HU (Female)
Ninomiya et al. [36]	SMI	Prado 2008 [26] (only for females)	43.75 cm^2/m^2	38.5 cm^2/m^2	Sarcopenia + BMI $\geq$ 22 kg/m^2	-
Sugimoto et al. [37]	SMI	Quartiles	Lowest quartile	Lowest quartile		
Choi et al. [38]	SMI	Tertiles	Lowest tertile 45.3 cm^2/m^2	Lowest tertile 39.3 cm^2/m^2		<40.8 HU (Male) <33.9 HU (Female)
Gruber et al. [39]	SMI	Prado 2008 [26]	52.4 cm^2/m^2	38.5 cm^2/m^2	Sarcopenia + BMI $\geq$ 25 kg/m^2	-
Peng YC et al. [40]	SMI	Choi 2015 [41]	42.2 cm^2/m^2	33.9 cm^2/m^2	Sarcopenia +VAT/TAMA $\geq$ 2	<41 HU with BMI <25 kg/m^2 <33 HU with BMI $\geq$ 25 kg/m^2

TPA (L3): total psoas area measured at the level of L3 normalized for the square of the height; TPV (L3): total psoas volume measured at the level of L3 normalized for the square of the height. A total of 55 cm of the total psoas length was assessed in Amini et. al.; CSAPM/CSAL5: cross-sectional area of the psoas muscle at the L5 vertebral level standardized to the L5 cross-sectional area of the body (CSAL5); CSAPM/CSAL3: cross-sectional area of the psoas muscle at the L3 vertebral level standardized to the L3 cross-sectional area of the body (CSAL3); SMI (skeletal muscle index): cross-sectional area of the muscle at the L3 level normalized for the square of the height; VFA: visceral fat area; VAT/TAMA: visceral adipose tissue area/total abdominal muscle area at the L3 vertebral level.

2.5. Statistical Analysis

Three meta-analyses were conducted in line with the Cochrane Collaboration guidelines on the meta-analysis of observational studies in epidemiology [42,43]. The first analysis focused on OS in months, the second on the prevalence of major complications according to the Clavien–Dindo classification ($\geq$2), and the third on the length of hospital stay after pancreatic surgery in patients with or without muscle loss.

A fixed-effect meta-analytical model was used for OS and major complications, whereas a random-effects meta-analytical model was used for LOS. OS was retrieved from the published studies as median values and ranges and converted into means and standard deviations (SD) using appropriate statistical algorithms according to Hozo et al [44]. The analysis requires the specification of maximal and minimal survival which was extrapolated from the figures for the purpose of this study when not clearly reported in the paper. LOS was already reported in means and SDs. Major complications are reported as percentages. The effect on the endpoints were meta-analyzed either as mean difference (MD) or as ratio of means (ROM) [43]. Values of MD < 0 or ROM < 1 indicate a disadvantage in the survival for patients with low muscle mass. The opposite holds true for the prevalence of major complications and mean LOS. Cochran's Q statistic and the I^2 statistic were used to test between-study heterogeneity [45]. If the Q statistic was significant at the 0.5 level, the summary effect and corresponding 95% confidence interval (CI) were obtained with the Mantel–Haenszel random effects model [46]. For I2 < 50%, between-study heterogeneity was judged to be low-moderate, while for I2 $\geq$ 50% it was considered substantial. The point estimate of MD and ROM was considered statistically significant when p was <0.05. Publication bias was assessed visually using a funnel plot and the number of missing studies was estimated using the trim-and-fill method [43].

All analyses were conducted using R version 3.5.2 [47].

3. Results

The search flowchart is presented in Figure 1. A total of 5711 article titles were reviewed by following the inclusion and exclusion criteria set beforehand and after a related article and cross-reference search, a total of ten original articles in English were included in the present review. All articles were single-center retrospective cohort studies with a total of 2811 patients with PDAC undergoing surgery with curative intent. Amini et al. [32] ran two separate analyses with two different low muscle mass definitions according to the total psoas area (TPA) or total psoas volume (TPV), hence they were included individually in the meta-analysis. Studies' characteristics are depicted in Table 2, while data used for the meta-analyses are reported in Table 3.

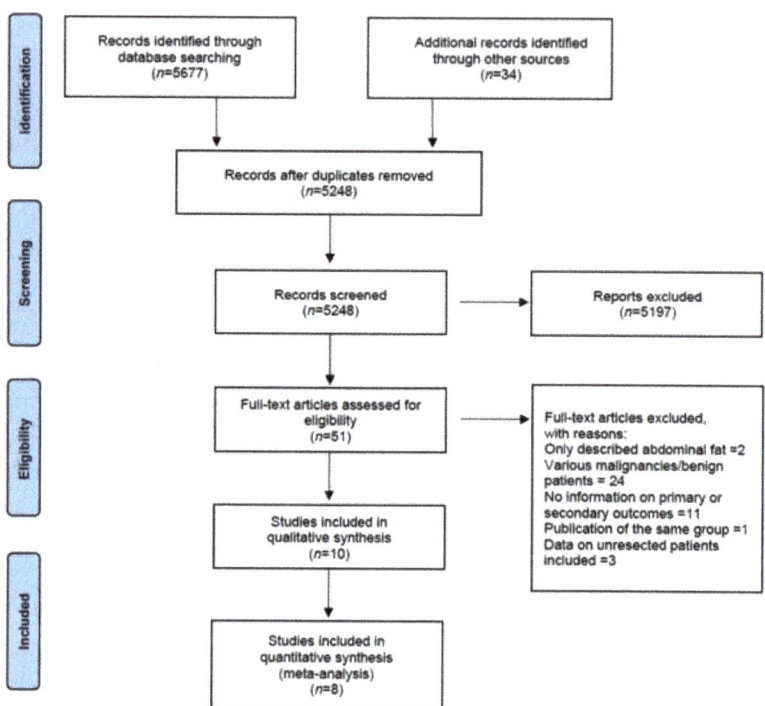

Figure 1. Studies' inclusion flowchart according to the Preferred Reporting Items for Systematic Reviews and Meta-Analyses (PRISMA) guidelines [28].

Table 2. Characteristics of the studies included in the systematic review.

Author	Year	Country	Study Accrual Period	Study Type	Patients (n)
Peng P et al. [31]	2012	Baltimore, USA	1999–2010	RCS	557
Amini et al. [32]	2015	Baltimore, USA	1996–2014	RCS	763
Clark et al. [33]	2016	Tampa, USA	2004–2012	RCS	100
Delitto et al. [34]	2016	Gainesville, FL, USA	2010–2014	RCS	73
Okumura et al. [35]	2017	Kyoto, Japan	2004–2015	RCS	301
Ninomiya et al. [36]	2017	Nagoya, Japan	2005–2014	RCS	265
Sugimoto et al. [37]	2018	Rochester, MN, USA	2000–2015	RCS	323
Choi MH et al. [38]	2018	Seoul, Korea	2008–2015	RCS	180
Gruber et al. [39]	2019	Vienna, Austria	2005–2010	RCS	133
Peng YC et al. [40]	2020	Taipei, Taiwan	2005–2018	RCS	116

RCS = retrospective cohort study.

Table 3. Studies included in the quantitative analyses and outcomes used for the three meta-analyses.

Author	Low Muscle Mass	N pts	OS Mo (Range)	p	Major Complications n (%)	p	LOS Days (Range)	p
Peng P et al. [31]	Yes	139	13.7	0.01	21 (15.1)	NS	12	0.980
	No	418	18		83 (19.9)		12	
Amini et al. (TPA) [32]	Yes	192	18.0	<0.001	38 (19.8)	0.16	9 (7–15)	0.05
	No	571	28.4		88 (15.4)		8 (7–13)	
Amini et al. (TPV) [32]	Yes	152	17.0	<0.001	34 (22.4)	0.03	10 (7–15.5)	0.002
	No	611	26.7		92 (15.1)		8 (7–13)	
Clark et al. [33]	Yes	NA	NR		NR		NR	
	No	NA	NR		NR		NR	
Delitto et al. [34]	Yes	NA	NA	0.001	NR		NR	
	No	NA	NA		NR		NR	
Okumura et al. [35]	Yes	120	NA	<0.001	12 (10)	0.493	NR	
	No	181	NA		14 (7.7)		NR	
Ninomiya et al. [36]	Yes	170	23.7	0.185	91 (53.5)	0.541	NR	
	No	95	25.8		54 (56.8)		NR	
Sugimoto et al. [37]	Yes	80	23	0.075	NR		NR	
	No	243	26		NR		NR	
Choi et al. [38]	Yes	60	13.9	0.031	5 (8.3)	0.402	15.6 ±7.9	0.303
	No	120	21.9		15 (12.5)		17.2 ±10.8	
Gruber et al. [39]	Yes	78	14 (11–17)	0.016	13 (16.7)	0.531	14	0.243
	No	55	20 (14–26)		7 (12.7)		11	
Peng YC et al. [40]	Yes	20	11.6	0.009	4 (20)	0.630	32 ±22.5	0.51
	No	96	26.6		15 (15.6)		27.6 ±27.5	

OS: overall survival; Mo: months; LOS: length of hospital stay; NA: not available; NR: not reported; and NS: non-significant p value.

3.1. Low Muscle Mass Definitions

Six articles defined muscle mass as the area occupied by all the muscles at the level of L3 normalized for height (L3-SMI) [35–40]. Four articles defined muscle mass as the total psoas area normalized for height [31,32] or normalized for the cross-sectional area of the body at the level of L3 [34] or L5 [33]. Amini et al. also evaluated the total psoas volume normalized for height at the level of L3 (see Table 1 for details) [32]. Three articles defined low muscle mass as sarcopenia using predefined cut-offs already published in the literature [36,39,40]. Six articles [31,32,34,35,37,38] used self-determined cut-offs, whereas Delitto et al. [34] and Clark et al. [33] conducted correlation analyses as depicted in Table 1.

3.2. Prevalence of Low Muscle Mass in Patients with Pancreatic Adenocarcinoma

The reported prevalence of low muscle mass varies from 17.2% to 64.2% [31,32,35–40]. Two authors did not report any percentage [33,34] and one [33] did not define a cut-off as they conducted a correlation analysis to identify the relationship between low muscle mass and long-term survival. Moreover, three authors [35,38,40] reported data also regarding the prevalence of myosteatosis, ranging from 33.3% to 47.8%. Six studies [31,32,35,36,39,40] reported the numbers of sarcopenic obese patients, whose prevalence ranges from 2.5% to 25.6%.

3.3. Preoperative Patients' Characteristics

Eight studies [31,32,34–36,38–40] investigated a relationship between age and low muscle mass but only 3 authors [34,36,40] found that patients with low muscle mass were significantly older. All studies reported data regarding the gender distribution of patients but only two authors [36,39] found a difference in the prevalence of low muscle mass between male and female patients with contrasting results. Specifically, higher rates of prevalence of sarcopenia were found in males by Gruber et al. [39] and in females by Ninomiya et al [36].

Six studies [34,35,37–40] reported data regarding the albumin levels and three studies [34,35,39] found significant lower levels of pre-operative albumin in the group with low muscle mass. The prevalence of diabetes was reported in two studies [38,40]. No significant difference was found in SMI values in patients with or without diabetes but sex-specific standardized skeletal muscle density was lower in diabetic patients [40]. BMI stratified according to muscle mass status was reported in five articles [35,36,38–40]. In four studies [35,36,38,40] BMI was significantly lower in the low muscle mass group.

Three authors [34,35,39] reported data regarding the neoadjuvant treatment. Delitto et al. reported that even if the neoadjuvant treatment was not associated with differences in the mean psoas index, a decrease in the psoas index during therapy is associated with a poor prognosis [34]. A higher rate of treated patients was found in the sarcopenic group by Gruber et al. [39] but not by Okumura et al [35].

3.4. Low Muscle Mass and Postoperative Outcomes

Data regarding postoperative outcomes were reported in nine studies [31,32,34–40]. The comparison of overall morbidity rates between patients who have low muscle mass and non-low muscle mass were reported in seven papers [31,32,35,36,38–40]. An increased postoperative morbidity rate in low muscle mass patients was found only by Amini et al. [32] and patients with a lower TPV were at a higher risk for postoperative complications (OR: 1.79, 95% CI: 1.25–2.56; p = 0.002). Moreover, in a multivariate logistic regression model, TVP-sarcopenia was confirmed to be independently associated with a higher risk for postoperative complications (OR: 1.69, 95% CI: 1.16–2.46; p = 0.006). Regarding specific postoperative complications, two papers [35,39] reported the rate of pancreatic fistula between the sarcopenic and non-sarcopenic group, although no correlation was found with low muscle mass. Data on 90-day postoperative mortality were reported in four papers [31,32,35,36] and no differences were noted in regard to muscle mass status. Complete data on major postoperative complications and on postoperative LOS were reported by seven [31,32,35,36,38–40] and four papers [31,32,38,40], respectively, and were included in the meta-analysis. Meta-analysis failed to identify a higher prevalence ratio of major complications after pancreatic surgery in the low muscle mass group (PR: 1.07; 95% CI: 0.93–1.24, $p = 0.22$) (Figure 2). There was no heterogeneity between studies ($I^2 = 0\%$, $p = 0.70$) and publication bias analysis estimated one study missing, nonetheless obtaining comparable results (PR: 1.00; 95% CI: 0.88–1.15, $p = 0.95$) (Figure 3). The difference in the prevalence of major complications in patients with vs. without low muscle mass was 0.02 (95% CI: −0.01–0.04, $p = 0.32$) (Figure 4). There was some heterogeneity between studies ($I^2 = 18.8\%$, $p = 0.28$). There was no evidence of publication bias (Figure 5).

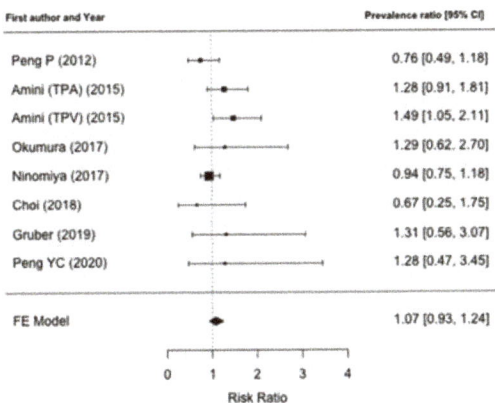

Figure 2. Forest plot for the prevalence ratio of major complications. Meta-analysis did not identify a higher prevalence ratio of major complications after pancreatic surgery in the low muscle mass group.

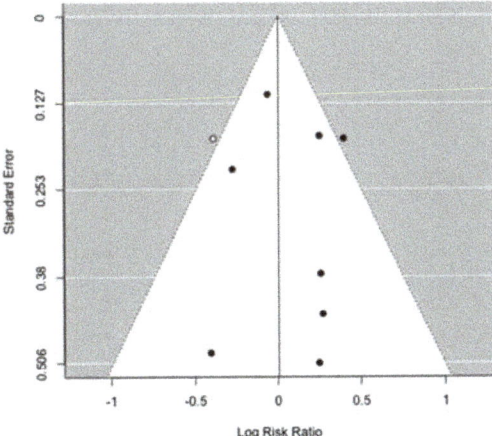

Figure 3. Funnel plot for the prevalence ratio of major complications after pancreatic resection. Black circles identified studies included in the meta-analysis. Publication bias analysis estimated one study missing (white circle).

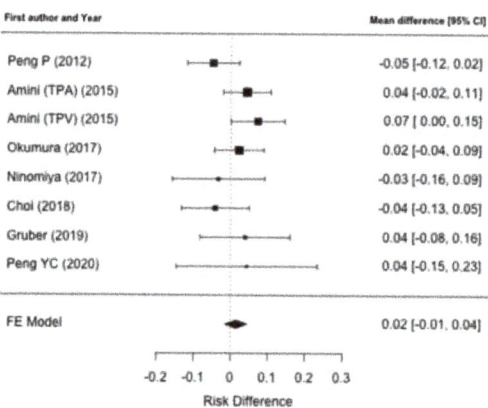

Figure 4. Forest plot for the difference in the prevalence of major complications. The difference in prevalence of major complications in patients with vs. without low muscle mass was not significant.

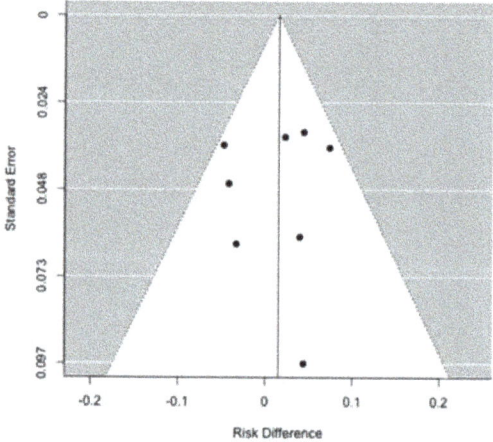

Figure 5. Funnel plot for the difference in the prevalence of major complications. No publication bias was evident.

Meta-analysis failed to identify an increase in the mean LOS of patients with or without low muscle mass (ROM: 1.08; 95% CI: 0.97–1.20, $p = 0.17$). There was heterogeneity between the studies ($I^2 = 64.3\%$, $p = 0.02$) without any publication bias. Similarly, the difference of the mean LOS was not significantly different between the two groups (low muscle mass vs. non-low muscle mass) (MD: 0.8; 95% CI: −0.3–1.9, $p = 0.14$). There was heterogeneity ($I^2 = 52.6\%$, $p = 0.076$) and no publication bias was present.

Moreover, some authors investigated the correlation between postoperative outcomes and sarcopenic obesity or muscle attenuation. Amini et al. reported that patients with sarcopenic obesity based on TPV had a more pronounced risk of complications compared with patients who did not have sarcopenia (TPV-sarcopenic obesity, 74.1% vs. non-sarcopenia 42.2%, $p = 0.003$) [32]. Peng YC et al. found no significant differences between sarcopenic patients and sarcopenic obese patients in terms of LOS and major complications [40]. Okumura compared patients with or without sarcopenic obesity and found no correlation in terms of major complications or postoperative pancreatic fistula incidence [35]. Furthermore, Okumura investigated the correlation between muscle attenuation and the postoperative outcomes, finding no correlation between myosteatosis and major complications or pancreatic fistula [35]. Apart from the study of Okumura et al. [35], Choi et al. also found no correlation between low muscle attenuation and the overall morbidity rate [38].

3.5. Low Muscle Mass and Survival

The effects of alterations of preoperative muscle mass on OS were reported in nine studies [31,32,34–40]. Seven studies were included in the meta-analysis [31,32,36–40], in which two studies' [34,35] data on survival required for meta-analysis could not be retrieved in the text. Meta-analysis identified that patients with low muscle mass who underwent pancreatic resection demonstrated a significantly reduced OS when compared to patients without alterations of the muscle mass (ROM: 0.86; 95% CI: 0.82–0.91, $p < 0.001$), resulting in a 14% loss for the former (Figure 6). There was no heterogeneity between studies ($I^2 = 0\%$, $p = 0.46$) and publication bias analysis estimated one study missing, nonetheless obtaining comparable results (ROM: 0.87; 95% CI: 0.82–0.92, $p < 0.001$) (Figure 7). The mean survival loss for patients with low muscle mass was 3.4 months (95% CI: -4.62, -2.18 $p < 0.001$) (Figure 8). There was some heterogeneity between studies ($I^2 = 14.6\%$, $p = 0.32$) with no publication bias identified (Figure 9). Nine studies performed multivariate analysis, identifying low muscle mass as a significant independent risk factor for mortality [31,32,34–40].

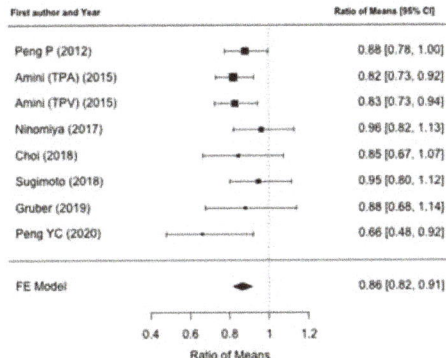

Figure 6. Forest plot for the difference ratio of overall survival. Meta-analysis identified that patients with low muscle mass who underwent pancreatic resection demonstrated a significantly reduced OS when compared to patients without alterations of the muscle mass.

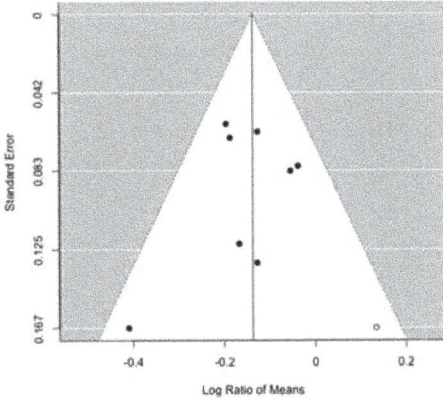

Figure 7. Funnel plot for the difference ratio of overall survival. Publication bias analysis estimated one study missing (white circle).

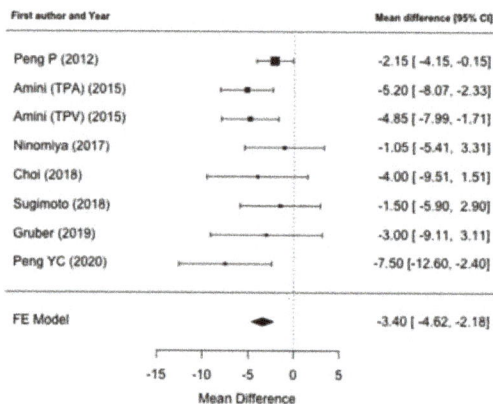

Figure 8. Forrest plot for the mean difference of overall survival. The mean survival loss for patients with low muscle mass was 3.4 months.

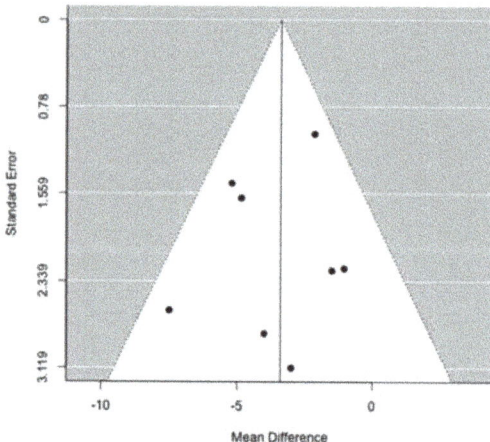

Figure 9. Funnel plot for the mean difference of overall survival. No publication bias was identified.

Moreover, five studies [35,37–40] analyzed the impact of low muscle mass on the DFS. Okumura determined that DFS rates were significantly lower in patients with low muscle mass [35] and Sugimoto et al. reported that a smaller sex-standardized SMI was independently associated with a shorter DFS [37]. On the contrary, three studies found that DFS was not significantly different between patients with or without sarcopenia [38–40]. As data were missing, meta-analysis was not possible. Regarding sarcopenic obesity, three authors [35,39,40] reported data regarding the OS and DFS. Peng YC et al. [40] found an association in the univariate analysis between sarcopenic obesity and OS (HR = 3.19, 95% CI = 0.98–10.37, p = 0.041), although data were not confirmed in the multivariate analysis (HR = 1.29, 95% CI = 0.23–7.19, p = 0.768). Okumura et al. [35] found a correlation between sarcopenic obesity and OS both in the univariate (HR = 1.91, 95% CI = 1.30–2.75, p = 0.001) and multivariate analysis (HR = 2.01, 95% CI = 1.31–3.03, p = 0.002). Gruber et al. reported an impaired OS in the obese sarcopenic patients compared to non-sarcopenic obese [39]. While Peng YC et al. [40] and Gruber at al. [39] found no association between sarcopenic obesity and DFS, Okumura et al. [35] found the association to be relevant both in the univariate (HR = 1.83, 95% CI = 1.31–2.53, p = 0.001) and multivariate analysis (HR = 1.87, 95% CI = 1.32–2.61, p = 0.001). Two authors [38,40] found no association between muscle attenuation and OS or DFS. On the contrary, Okumura et al. [35] found a significantly reduced OS and DFS in patients with preoperative reduced muscle attenuation both in the univariate (HR = 1.93, 95% CI = 1.40–2.67, $p < 0.001$ for OS; HR = 1.56, 95% CI = 1.18–2.07, $p = 0.002$ for DFS) and multivariate analysis (HR = 1.63, 95% CI = 1.13–2.36, $p = 0.01$ for OS; HR = 1.37, 95% CI = 1.02–1.84, $p = 0.037$ for DFS).

4. Discussion

Cancer cachexia is defined as a multifactorial syndrome characterized by ongoing loss of skeletal muscle mass (with or without loss of fat mass) that can be partially but not entirely reversed by conventional nutritional support [6]. This muscle loss is defined as secondary sarcopenia, also known as disease-related sarcopenia, in which a causal factor other than (or in addition to) aging is evident [5]. As opposed to primary sarcopenia, secondary sarcopenia has predominantly focused on the loss of muscle mass without an emphasis on muscle function [48]. Indeed, none of the retrospective studies considered in this review documented muscle strength or performance. Secondary sarcopenia could represent an individual characteristic to target in order to improve the outcome. In fact, patients with solid tumors frequently experience malnutrition due to reduced food intake, malabsorption, energy expenditure, and altered metabolism. Treatment options include physical training, modifications of nutritional intake (including appetite stimulants), and pharmacological treatment tested in clinical trials [49]. Among solid tumors, pancreatic cancer carries the highest prevalence of cancer cachexia and weight loss [49]. Its overall survival rate is still dismal with little improvements over the last decade [50] and postoperative complications remain an important burden after pancreatic surgery, with morbidity rates still up to 40% [18]. Surgical complications such as pancreatic fistula, hemorrhage, and delayed gastric emptying not only affect patient convalescence and quality of life but negatively impact oncological outcomes, delay adjuvant treatment, and affect survival [51]. Sarcopenia has been proposed as an indicator of frailty and therefore as a potential mean to predict the risk of postoperative morbidity [52]. In fact, low muscle mass or radiodensity can lead to impaired wound healing, depressed immunity, and inability to mobilize after surgery, thus affecting postoperative outcomes [53]. While several studies have reported the association between sarcopenia and outcomes following surgery for various oncologic diseases [54], the actual impact of sarcopenia on surgical morbidity after pancreatic surgery and on survival remains poorly defined with a high heterogeneity of results. As depicted by our meta-analysis, sarcopenia plays a significant role in the OS, while the influence on postoperative outcomes remains uncertain. The meta-analyses we conducted failed to demonstrate a certain relationship between low muscle mass and major complications or LOS. On the contrary, other authors have found a correlation between low muscle mass and postoperative outcomes [55]. The inhomogeneity among the considered populations could be a possible explanation of the different results reported. Another potential bias to be considered is the different assessment parameters used to define the presence of low muscle mass. Similarly to Amini et al. [32], previous studies reported divergent results when using different assessment parameters. In addition, Pecorelli et al. [9] reported that sarcopenia using the total abdominal muscle area (TAMA) was not a significant prognostic factor for 60-day postoperative mortality ($p = 0.224$). However, the ratio of visceral fat area (VFA) to TAMA was found to be a significant predictor for 60-day mortality when the ratio was 3.2 in the multivariate analysis [OR 6.76, 95% CI: 2.42–18.99; $p < 0.001$]. The lack of a univocal definition of sarcopenia and, even worse, too many different self-determined cut-offs, obtained by means of optimum stratification in populations with different ethnicities, BMI results, age, and cancer types, determine a void in research and clinical practice. For instance, it is worth noticing that cut-offs from previous western studies, such as in Prado et al. [26], might be inappropriate for Asian populations such as that studied by Ninomiya et al [36]. Moreover, the cut-offs described by Prado et al. were obtained in a subset of obese patients (BMI > 30) and therefore their application on non-obese patients may be inappropriate.

In fact, the study of sarcopenia in humans is complicated by the large variability among individual and multiple factors affecting muscle (comorbidities, drugs, lifestyle, nutritional aspects, and environmental influences), which can vary in different populations. This muscle loss (secondary sarcopenia) is caused or worsened by cancer treatments and the tumor itself. Moreover, different studies are focused on different muscles and presently there is no consensus in the methodology of the assessment of muscle mass in the diagnosis of sarcopenia or cancer cachexia. Despite the importance of evaluating muscle mass in cancer, the definition of "low" muscle mass is difficult to be standardized when different cut-off values are applied. As depicted in our literature review, all included studies used a different cut-off to define sarcopenia and the reported prevalence of low muscle mass varied from 17.2% to 64.2%. Hence, more collective and coordinated efforts are required to compile and compare data obtained in different populations of cancer patients.

The rising subject in the field of muscle wasting and frailty regards the quality of the muscle rather than the quantity. Akahori et al. [56] focused on the muscle density as a possible prognostic factor in pancreatic patients and found a significant association between reduced muscle attenuation after chemo-radiotherapy and overall survival. Similarly, other authors found a correlation of a progression/outcome of cancer with muscle attenuation [7,15,27,53,57]. Moreover, some recent results demonstrated that sarcopenia and myosteatosis represent two separate and distinct clinical phenotypes accompanied by different biological profiles in patients with pancreatic adenocarcinomas [53]. Yet again, there are no standardized cut-offs and thus it is difficult to compare the literature results.

Our study has some limitations to consider. The relatively small number of studies analyzed and their heterogeneity and retrospective nature could represent a significant risk of selection bias. Moreover, due to the lack of data in some studies, we could not measure outcomes such as overall postoperative morbidity rates or specific complications of pancreatic surgery. Therefore, we were unable to fully investigate the potential role of low muscle mass on postoperative short-term outcomes. New prospective and multicentric studies are necessary in order to draw more definitive results.

5. Conclusions

Although we cannot draw unequivocal conclusions, we can expect sarcopenia to have an impact on the surgical and oncological outcomes of cancer patients. Our meta-analysis on patients with PDAC undergoing surgery demonstrates a reduced survival in those with sarcopenia; however, a clear correlation with the short-term postoperative outcomes was not evident. We believe results can be compromised by the diverse definitions and cut-off values utilized. We advocate a joint effort to standardize body composition evaluation methods, assessment parameters, and cut-off values. This enables risk stratification in order to implement nutritional and pre-/re-habilitation interventions with the aim of reducing physical disability, improving the quality of life, and prolonging survival.

Author Contributions: Conceptualization, C.S., R.S., L.M., and E.S.P.; methodology, R.S., L.M., S.Z., and E.S.P.; software, A.R.B.; validation, C.S., S.M., and M.V.; formal analysis, A.R.B., L.M., and E.S.P.; investigation, E.S.P. and L.M.; resources, C.S.; data curation, G.Z, G.C., and S.S.; writing—original draft preparation, E.S.P., L.M., and R.S.; writing—review and editing, C.S., L.M., E.S.P., and R.S.; visualization, G.C., G.Z., and S.S.; supervision, C.S.; project administration, C.S.; funding acquisition, C.S. All authors have read and agreed to the published version of the manuscript. E.S.P. and L.M. equally contributed to the work.

Funding: This research received no external funding.

Institutional Review Board Statement: Not applicable.

Informed Consent Statement: Not applicable.

Data Availability Statement: The data presented in this study are available within the article.

Conflicts of Interest: The authors declare no conflict of interest.

References

1. Rolfe, D.F.S.; Brown, G.C. Cellular energy utilization and molecular origin of standard metabolic rate in mammals. *Physiol. Rev.* **1997**, *77*, 731–758. [CrossRef] [PubMed]
2. Baskin, K.K.; Winders, B.; Olson, E.N. Muscle as a "mediator" of systemic metabolism. *Cell Metab.* **2015**, *21*, 237–248. [CrossRef] [PubMed]
3. Demontis, F.; Piccirillo, R.; Goldberg, A.L.; Perrimon, N. The influence of skeletal muscle on systemic aging and lifespan. *Aging Cell* **2013**, *12*, 943–949. [CrossRef] [PubMed]
4. Karstoft, K.; Pedersen, B.K. Skeletal muscle as a gene regulatory endocrine organ. *Curr Opin Clin. Nutr. Metab. Care* **2016**, *19*, 270–275. [CrossRef] [PubMed]
5. Cruz-Jentoft, A.J.; Bahat, G.; Bauer, J.; Boirie, Y.; Bruyère, O.; Cederholm, T. Sarcopenia: Revised European consensus on definition and diagnosis. *Age Ageing* **2019**, *48*, 16–31. [CrossRef] [PubMed]
6. Fearon, K.; Strasser, F.; Anker, S.D.; Bosaeus, I.; Bruera, E.; Fainsinger, R.L. Definition and classification of cancer cachexia: An international consensus. *Lancet Oncol.* **2011**, *12*, 489–495. [CrossRef]
7. Van Dijk, D.P.J.; Bakens, M.J.A.M.; Coolsen, M.M.E.; Rensen, S.S.; van Dam, R.M.; Bours, M.J.L. Low skeletal muscle radiation attenuation and visceral adiposity are associated with overall survival and surgical site infections in patients with pancreatic cancer. *J. Cachexia Sarcopenia Muscle* **2017**, *8*, 317–326. [CrossRef]
8. Levolger, S.; Van Vugt, J.L.A.; De Bruin, R.W.F.; IJzermans, J.N.M. Systematic review of sarcopenia in patients operated on for gastrointestinal and hepatopancreatobiliary malignancies. *Br. J. Surg.* **2015**, *102*, 1448–1458. [CrossRef]
9. Pecorelli, N.; Carrara, G.; De Cobelli, F.; Cristel, G.; Damascelli, A.; Balzano, G. Effect of sarcopenia and visceral obesity on mortality and pancreatic fistula following pancreatic cancer surgery. *Br. J. Surg.* **2016**, *103*, 434–442. [CrossRef]
10. Joglekar, S.; Asghar, A.; Mott, S.L.; Johnson, B.E.; Button, A.M.; Clark, E. Sarcopenia is an independent predictor of complications following pancreatectomy for adenocarcinoma. *J. Surg. Oncol.* **2015**, *111*, 771–775. [CrossRef]
11. Kazemi-Bajestani, S.M.R.; Mazurak, V.C.; Baracos, V. Computed tomography-defined muscle and fat wasting are associated with cancer clinical outcomes. *Semin. Cell Dev. Biol.* **2016**, *54*, 2–10. [CrossRef]
12. Okumura, S.; Kaido, T.; Hamaguchi, Y.; Fujimoto, Y.; Kobayashi, A.; Iida, T. Impact of the preoperative quantity and quality of skeletal muscle on outcomes after resection of extrahepatic biliary malignancies. *Surgery* **2016**, *159*, 821–833. [CrossRef]
13. Okumura, S.; Kaido, T.; Hamaguchi, Y.; Fujimoto, Y.; Masui, T.; Mizumoto, M. Impact of preoperative quality as well as quantity of skeletal muscle on survival after resection of pancreatic cancer. *Surgery* **2015**, *157*, 1088–1098. [CrossRef]
14. Sabel, M.S.; Lee, J.; Cai, S.; Englesbe, M.J.; Holcombe, S.; Wang, S. Sarcopenia as a prognostic factor among patients with stage III melanoma. *Ann. Surg. Oncol.* **2011**, *18*, 3579–3585. [CrossRef]
15. Antoun, S.; Lanoy, E.; Iacovelli, R.; Albiges-Sauvin, L.; Loriot, Y.; Merad-Taoufik, M. Skeletal muscle density predicts prognosis in patients with metastatic renal cell carcinoma treated with targeted therapies. *Cancer* **2013**, *119*, 3377–3384. [CrossRef]
16. Arnold, M.; Rutherford, M.J.; Bardot, A.; Ferlay, J.; Andersson, T.M.L.; Myklebust, T.Å. Progress in cancer survival, mortality, and incidence in seven high-income countries 1995–2014 (ICBP SURVMARK-2): A population-based study. *Lancet Oncol.* **2019**, *20*, 1493–1505. [CrossRef]
17. Chong, E.; Ratnayake, B.; Lee, S.; French, J.J.; Wilson, C.; Roberts, K.J. Systematic review and meta-analysis of risk factors of postoperative pancreatic fistula after distal pancreatectomy in the era of 2016 International Study Group Pancreatic Fistula definition. *HPB* **2021**. [CrossRef]
18. DeOliveira, M.L.; Winter, J.M.; Schafer, M.; Cunningham, S.C.; Cameron, J.L.; Yeo, C.J. Assessment of complications after pancreatic surgery: A novel grading system applied to 633 patients undergoing pancreaticoduodenectomy. *Ann. Surg.* **2006**, *244*, 931–937. [CrossRef]
19. Bundred, J.; Kamarajah, S.K.; Roberts, K.J. Body composition assessment and sarcopenia in patients with pancreatic cancer: A systematic review and meta-analysis. *HPB* **2019**, *21*, 1603–1612. [CrossRef]
20. Joglekar, S.; Nau, P.N.; Mezhir, J.J. The impact of sarcopenia on survival and complications in surgical oncology: A review of the current literature. *J. Surg. Oncol.* **2018**, *112*, 503–509. [CrossRef]
21. Wagner, D. Role of frailty and sarcopenia in predicting outcomes among patients undergoing gastrointestinal surgery. *World J. Gastrointest Surg.* **2016**, *8*, 27. [CrossRef]
22. Siegel, R.L.; Miller, K.D.; Jemal, A. Cancer statistics, 2020. *CA Cancer J. Clin.* **2020**, *70*, 7–30. [CrossRef] [PubMed]
23. Roeland, E.J.; Ma, J.D.; Nelson, S.H.; Seibert, T.; Heavey, S.; Revta, C. Weight loss versus muscle loss: Re-evaluating inclusion criteria for future cancer cachexia interventional trials. *Support Care Cancer* **2017**, *25*, 365–369. [CrossRef] [PubMed]
24. Mourtzakis, M.; Prado, C.M.M.; Lieffers, J.R.; Reiman, T.; McCargar, L.J.; Baracos, V.E. A practical and precise approach to quantification of body composition in cancer patients using computed tomography images acquired during routine care. *Appl. Physiol. Nutr. Metab.* **2008**, *33*, 997–1006. [CrossRef]
25. Tan, B.H.L.; Birdsell, L.A.; Martin, L.; Baracos, V.E.; Fearon, K.C.H. Sarcopenia in an overweight or obese patient is an adverse prognostic factor in pancreatic cancer. *Clin. Cancer Res.* **2009**, *15*, 6973–6979. [CrossRef]
26. Prado, C.M.; Lieffers, J.R.; McCargar, L.J.; Reiman, T.; Sawyer, M.B.; Martin, L. Prevalence and clinical implications of sarcopenic obesity in patients with solid tumours of the respiratory and gastrointestinal tracts: A population-based study. *Lancet Oncol.* **2008**, *9*, 629–635. [CrossRef]

27. Martin, L.; Birdsell, L.; MacDonald, N.; Reiman, T.; Clandinin, M.T.; McCargar, L.J. Cancer cachexia in the age of obesity: Skeletal muscle depletion is a powerful prognostic factor, independent of body mass index. *J. Clin. Oncol.* **2013**, *31*, 1539–1547. [CrossRef]
28. Moher, D.; Liberati, A.; Tetzlaff, J.; Altman, D.G. Preferred reporting items for systematic reviews and meta-analyses: The PRISMA statement. *J. Clin. Epidemiol.* **2009**, *62*, 1006–1012. [CrossRef]
29. Dindo, D.; Demartines, N.; Clavien, P.-A. Classification of surgical complications: A new proposal with evaluation in a cohort of 6336 patients and results of a survey. *Ann. Surg.* **2004**, *240*, 205–213. [CrossRef]
30. Baumgartner, R.N. Body composition in healthy aging. *Ann. N. Y. Acad. Sci.* **2000**, *904*, 437–448. [CrossRef]
31. Peng, P.; Hyder, O.; Firoozmand, A.; Kneuertz, P.; Schulick, R.D.; Huang, D. Impact of Sarcopenia on Outcomes Following Resection of Pancreatic Adenocarcinoma. *J. Gastrointest Surg.* **2012**, *16*, 1478–1486. [CrossRef]
32. Amini, N.; Spolverato, G.; Gupta, R.; Margonis, G.A.; Kim, Y.; Wagner, D. Impact Total Psoas Volume on Short- and Long-Term Outcomes in Patients Undergoing Curative Resection for Pancreatic Adenocarcinoma: A New Tool to Assess Sarcopenia. *J. Gastrointest Surg.* **2015**, *19*, 1593–1602. [CrossRef]
33. Clark, W.; Swaid, F.; Luberice, K.; Bowman, T.A.; Downs, D.; Ross, S.B. Can pancreatic cancer behavior be predicted based on computed tomography measurements of fat and muscle mass? *Int. J. Surg. Oncol.* **2016**, *1*, e04. [CrossRef]
34. Delitto, D.; Judge, S.M.; George, T.J.; Sarosi, G.A.; Thomas, R.M.; Behrns, K.E. A clinically applicable muscular index predicts long-term survival in resectable pancreatic cancer. *Surgery* **2017**, *161*, 930–938. [CrossRef]
35. Okumura, S.; Kaido, T.; Hamaguchi, Y.; Kobayashi, A.; Shirai, H.; Yao, S. Visceral Adiposity and Sarcopenic Visceral Obesity are Associated with Poor Prognosis After Resection of Pancreatic Cancer. *Ann. Surg. Oncol.* **2017**, *24*, 3732–3740. [CrossRef]
36. Ninomiya, G.; Fujii, T.; Yamada, S.; Yabusaki, N.; Suzuki, K.; Iwata, N. Clinical impact of sarcopenia on prognosis in pancreatic ductal adenocarcinoma: A retrospective cohort study. *Int. J. Surg.* **2017**, *39*, 45–51. [CrossRef]
37. Sugimoto, M.; Farnell, M.B.; Nagorney, D.M.; Kendrick, M.L.; Truty, M.J.; Smoot, R.L. Decreased Skeletal Muscle Volume Is a Predictive Factor for Poorer Survival in Patients Undergoing Surgical Resection for Pancreatic Ductal Adenocarcinoma. *J. Gastrointest Surg.* **2018**, *22*, 831–839. [CrossRef]
38. Choi, M.H.; Yoon, S.B.; Lee, K.; Song, M.; Lee, I.S.; Lee, M.A. Preoperative sarcopenia and post-operative accelerated muscle loss negatively impact survival after resection of pancreatic cancer. *J. Cachexia Sarcopenia Muscle* **2018**, *9*, 326–334. [CrossRef]
39. Gruber Id, E.S.; Id, G.J.; Tamandl, D.; Gnant, M.; Schindl, M.; Sahora, K. Sarcopenia and sarcopenic obesity are independent adverse prognostic factors in resectable pancreatic ductal adenocarcinoma. *PLoS ONE* **2019**, *14*, e0215915. [CrossRef]
40. Peng, Y.C.; Wu, C.W.; Tien, Y.W.; Lu, T.P.; Wang, Y.H.; Chen, B.B. Preoperative sarcopenia is associated with poor overall survival in pancreatic cancer patients following pancreaticoduodenectomy. *Eur. Radiol.* **2020**, *31*, 2472–2481. [CrossRef]
41. Choi, Y.; Oh, D.Y.; Kim, T.Y.; Lee, K.H.; Han, S.W.; Im, S.A. Skeletal muscle depletion predicts the prognosis of patients with advanced pancreatic cancer undergoing palliative chemotherapy, independent of body mass index. *PLoS ONE* **2015**, *10*, e0139749. [CrossRef]
42. Clarke, M.; Horton, R. Bringing it all together: Lancet-Cochrane collaborate on systematic reviews. *Lancet* **2001**, *357*, 1728. [CrossRef]
43. Stroup, D.F.; Berlin, J.A.; Morton, S.C.; Olkin, I.; Williamson, G.D.; Rennie, D. Meta-analysis of observational studies in epidemiology: A proposal for reporting. *J. Am. Med. Assoc.* **2000**, *283*, 2008–2012. [CrossRef]
44. Hozo, S.P.; Djulbegovic, B.; Hozo, I. Estimating the mean and variance from the median, range, and the size of a sample. *BMC Med. Res. Methodol.* **2005**, *5*, 1–10. [CrossRef] [PubMed]
45. Higgins, J.P.T.; Thompson, S.G. Quantifying heterogeneity in a meta-analysis. *Stat. Med.* **2002**, *21*, 1539–1558. [CrossRef] [PubMed]
46. Nathan, M.; William, H. Statistical aspects of the analysis of data from retrospective studies of disease. *J. Natl. Cancer Inst.* **1959**, *22*, 719–748. [CrossRef]
47. R Core Team. *R: A Language and Environment for Statistical Computing*; R Foundation for Statistical Computing: Vienna, Austria, 2013.
48. Bauer, J.; Morley, J.E.; Schols, A.M.W.J.; Ferrucci, L.; Cruz-Jentoft, A.J.; Dent, E. Sarcopenia: A Time for Action. An SCWD Position Paper. *J. Cachexia Sarcopenia Muscle* **2019**, *10*, 956–961. [CrossRef]
49. Baracos, V.E.; Martin, L.; Korc, M.; Guttridge, D.C.; Fearon, K.C.H. Cancer-associated cachexia. *Nat. Rev. Dis. Prim.* **2018**, *4*, 1–18. [CrossRef]
50. Neoptolemos, J.P.; Kleeff, J.; Michl, P.; Costello, E.; Greenhalf, W.; Palmer, D.H. Therapeutic developments in pancreatic cancer: Current and future perspectives. *Nat. Rev. Gastroenterol. Hepatol.* **2018**, *15*, 333–348. [CrossRef]
51. Byun, Y.; Choi, Y.J.; Han, Y.; Kang, J.S.; Kim, H.; Kwon, W. Outcomes of 5,000 pancreatectomies in Korean single referral center and literature reviews. *J. Hepatobiliary Pancreat Sci.* **2021**. Online ahead of print.
52. Cooper, C.; Dere, W.; Evans, W.; Kanis, J.A.; Rizzoli, R.; Sayer, A.A. Frailty and sarcopenia: Definitions and outcome parameters. *Osteoporos. Int.* **2012**, *23*, 1839–1848. [CrossRef]
53. Stretch, C.; Aubin, J.M.; Mickiewicz, B.; Leugner, D.; Al-manasra, T.; Tobola, E. Sarcopenia and myosteatosis are accompanied by distinct biological profiles in patients with pancreatic and periampullary adenocarcinomas. *PLoS ONE* **2018**, *13*, e0196235. [CrossRef]
54. Peng, P.D.; Van Vledder, M.G.; Tsai, S.; De Jong, M.C.; Makary, M.; Ng, J. Sarcopenia negatively impacts short-term outcomes in patients undergoing hepatic resection for colorectal liver metastasis. *HPB* **2011**, *13*, 439–446. [CrossRef]

55. Ratnayake, C.B.; Loveday, B.P.; Shrikhande, S.V.; Windsor, J.A.; Pandanaboyana, S. Impact of preoperative sarcopenia on postoperative outcomes following pancreatic resection: A systematic review and meta-analysis. *Pancreatology* **2018**, *18*, 996–1004. [CrossRef]
56. Akahori, T.; Sho, M.; Kinoshita, S.; Nagai, M.; Nishiwada, S.; Tanaka, T. Prognostic Significance of Muscle Attenuation in Pancreatic Cancer Patients Treated with Neoadjuvant Chemoradiotherapy. *World J. Surg.* **2015**, *39*, 2975–2982. [CrossRef]
57. Rollins, K.E.; Tewari, N.; Ackner, A.; Awwad, A.; Madhusudan, S.; Macdonald, I.A. The impact of sarcopenia and myosteatosis on outcomes of unresectable pancreatic cancer or distal cholangiocarcinoma. *Clin. Nutr.* **2016**, *35*, 1103–1109. [CrossRef]

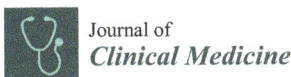

Article

The Clinical Significance of PIWIL3 and PIWIL4 Expression in Pancreatic Cancer

Weiyao Li [1,†], Javier Martinez-Useros [1,*,†], Nuria Garcia-Carbonero [1], Maria J. Fernandez-Aceñero [2], Alberto Orta [1], Luis Ortega-Medina [3], Sandra Garcia-Botella [4], Elia Perez-Aguirre [4], Luis Diez-Valladares [4], Angel Celdran [5] and Jesús García-Foncillas [1,*]

1. Translational Oncology Division, OncoHealth Institute, Fundacion Jimenez Diaz University Hospital, Av. Reyes Católicos 2, 28040 Madrid, Spain
2. Pathology Department, University Hospital Gregorio Marañon, C/del Dr. Esquerdo 46, 28007 Madrid, Spain
3. Pathology Department, Clinico San Carlos University Hospital, C/Profesor Martin Lagos, 28040 Madrid, Spain
4. Surgery Department (Pancreatobiliary Unit), Hospital Clínico San Carlos, C/Profesor Martin Lagos, 28040 Madrid, Spain
5. Hepatobiliary and Pancreatic Surgery Unit, General and Digestive Tract Surgery Department, Fundacion Jimenez Diaz University Hospital, Av. Reyes Católicos 2, 28040 Madrid, Spain
* Correspondence: javier.museros@oncohealth.eu (J.M.-U.); jesus.garciafoncillas@oncohealth.eu (J.G.-F.); Tel.:+34-915-504-800 (J.M.-U. & J.G.-F.)
† Both authors contributed equally to this work.

Received: 26 March 2020; Accepted: 23 April 2020; Published: 26 April 2020

Abstract: P-element-induced wimpy testis (PIWI) proteins have been described in several cancers. PIWIL1 and PIWIL2 have been recently evaluated in pancreatic cancer, and elevated expression of PIWIL2 conferred longer survival to patients. However, PIWIL3's and PIWIL4's role in carcinogenesis is rather controversial, and their clinical implication in pancreatic cancer has not yet been investigated. In the present study, we evaluated PIWIL1, PIWIL2, PIWIL3 and PIWIL4 expression in pancreatic cancer-derived cell lines and in one non-tumor cell line as healthy control. Here, we show a differential expression in tumor and non-tumor cell lines of PIWIL3 and PIWIL4. Subsequently, functional experiments with PIWIL3 and/or PIWIL4 knockdown revealed a decrease in the motility ratio of tumor and non-tumor cell lines through downregulation of mesenchymal factors in pro of epithelial factors. We also observed that PIWIL3 and/or PIWIL4 silencing impaired undifferentiated phenotype and enhanced drug toxicity in both tumor- and non-tumor-derived cell lines. Finally, PIWIL3 and PIWIL4 evaluation in human pancreatic cancer samples showed that patients with low levels of PIWIL4 protein expression presented poor prognosis. Therefore, PIWIL3 and PIWIL4 proteins may play crucial roles to keep pancreatic cell homeostasis not only in tumors but also in healthy tissues.

Keywords: PIWI proteins; PIWIL3; PIWIL4; pancreatic cancer; EMT; chemoresistance; motility; HNF4A; survival

1. Introduction

Pancreatic cancer (PC) has arisen as one of the tumors with higher incidence in developed countries. Indeed, the incidence of PC is expected to be higher than breast, prostate or colorectal cancers and to reach the second cause of cancer-related death by 2030 [1]. The 5-year survival rate is 50% when tumors are <2 cm in size and close to 100% for tumors <1 cm [2]; unfortunately, PC is normally asymptomatic, and it is often diagnosed when the tumor has metastasized to distant organs [3]. Adjuvant treatment for complete resected patients (R0) is usually based on Gemcitabine [4], or 5-fluorouracil for six months [5]. Regimens based on Gemcitabine in combination with Nanoalbumin bound-Paclitaxel (Nab-Paclitaxel) is recommended to patients with advanced disease [6]. Nevertheless, PC develops multi-pathways chemoresistance as a result of the interaction between tumor cells, cancer stem cells and the tumor microenvironment [7].

P-element-induced wimpy testis (PIWI) proteins belong to the Argonaute (AGO) family and have been firstly discovered in germline cells [8]. Based on their protein sequence, eight members of the Argonaute family have been classified into two subfamilies: the PIWI subfamily (PIWIL1, PIWIL2, PIWIL3 and PIWIL4) and the AGO subfamily (AGO1, AGO2, AGO3 and AGO4) [9]. The AGO family regulates gene expression through complementary recognition and guidance of short RNAs against their target genes [10]. Recently, it has been reported how PIWI proteins are expressed during the epigenetic remodeling and meiosis of the germline [11]. They also recognize and bind a unique type of non-coding small RNAs called piRNAs (PIWI-interacting RNAs), which constitutes the so-called piRNA-induced silencing complex (piRISC). PIWI proteins have an important role in epigenetic regulation, silencing of transposable elements, protection of genome integrity, gametogenesis and piRNA biogenesis [12]. Indeed, the expression of PIWI proteins promotes some of the hallmarks of cancer such as cell proliferation, genomic integrity, apoptosis, invasion and metastasis [13]. Therefore, an increasing number of studies report their differential expression patterns between healthy and tumor samples and how their modulation affects the behavior of tumor cells. PIWIL1 downregulation drastically reduces the proliferation, invasion and migration of hepatocellular carcinoma cells [14]. Other studies describe how PIWIL1 downregulation in sarcoma inhibits cell growth and allows cell differentiation and support the idea that PIWIL1 tumorigenic activity is due to its ability to regulate DNA hypermethylation [15]. Downregulation of PIWIL1 suppresses cell proliferation, migration and invasion of gastric cancer and lung cancer cells [16–18]. These studies sustain the oncogenic features of PIWIL1 and support the idea that PIWIL1 could be used as a target for anticancer therapies. In contrast, other reports showed that overexpression of PIWIL1 decreases proliferation and migration of chronic myeloid leukemia cells through inhibition of expression of matrix metalloproteinase-2 and -9 [19]. Our group has recently described the prognostic role of PIWIL1 and PIWIL2 protein expression in PC, especially PIWIL2 protein, which exhibited higher prognostic potential to predict longer progression-free survival ($p = 0.029$) and longer overall survival ($p = 0.025$). Furthermore, we provided new insight into the link between PIWIL1 and PIWIL2 with the progenitor molecular subtype of PC [20].

PIWIL3 is expressed in stage III epithelial ovarian cancer in both primary tumor and metastatic tissues compared with their adjacent normal tissues ($p < 0.01$), and the expression is higher in the metastatic foci [21]. PIWIL3 is also considered a prognostic biomarker of breast cancer since its upregulation was significantly associated to a short progression-free survival ($p = 0.01$) and a poor overall survival ($p = 0.02$) [22]. Furthermore, PIWIL3 seems to play a crucial role in melanoma progression, and its expression is higher with the higher tumor stage [23]. In gastrointestinal cancers, expression of PIWIL3 was also higher in tumors compared with their paired untransformed tissues [24]. Furthermore, upregulation of PIWIL3 increases proliferation, migration and invasion of gastric cancer cells [24]. In contrast, PIWIL3 seems to play a protective effect due to its overexpression-reduced proliferation, migration and invasion of glioma cells in vitro and decreased tumor size in vivo [25].

The role of PIWIL4 involves chromatin modifications in human somatic cells [26], and it is able to process precursor hairpins to generate several miRNAs in the absence of the endoribonuclease DICER [27]. The lack of PIWIL4 could derive to the development of type 2 diabetes since its downregulation in pancreatic beta cells resulted in defective insulin secretion [28]. However, its function in tumorigenesis is rather controversial. On the one hand, high expression of PIWIL4 is found in tumor tissues of colorectal cancer [29], cervical cancer [30], gastric cancer [31] and primary and metastatic foci of ovarian cancer [21] compared with their adjacent tissues. Its downregulation not only enhanced significantly the apoptotic effect of treatment in Leydig cell tumor [32] but also apoptosis, migration and invasion of breast cancer cells in vitro [33,34]. In hepatocellular carcinoma, the nuclear expression of PIWIL4 together with PIWIL2 has been found to confer worse outcome [35]. On the other hand, other studies have reported that low PIWIL4 expression was significantly associated with a worse prognosis in hepatocellular carcinoma [36], soft tissue sarcoma [37], non-small cell lung cancer [38] and renal cell carcinoma [39]. Low levels of PIWIL4 were also found in hepatocellular carcinoma tissues [36] and in other tumors like breast tumors [22] and non-small cell lung cancer [38] compared to the non-cancerous tissues. Moreover, the lack of PIWIL4 expression caused by CpG island hypermethylation has also been found in testicular tumors [40].

Since PIWIL3 and PIWIL4 expression has not been studied in PC and the functions of PIWI proteins in cancer seem to be rather controversial, we have evaluated the role of PIWIL3 and PIWIL4 expression in pancreatic cells and dissect their prognostic potential in PC.

2. Experimental Section

2.1. Cell Lines and Cell Culture

The human PC-derived cell lines PANC 04.03(ATCC ref: CRL-2555), PL45(ATCC ref: CRL-2558), BxPC-3(ATCC ref: CRL-1687) and one non-tumor human pancreatic ductal epithelial cell line hTERT-HPNE (ATCC ref: CRL-4023) were purchased and cultured under American Type Culture Collection (ATCC) recommendations. RWP1 and PANC-1 were kindly provided by Dr. Fatima Gebauer (CRG, Barcelona, Spain). RWP1, PANC-1 cells were routinely grown in RPMI supplemented with 10% fetal bovine serum (FBS) and 1% Penicillin-Streptomycin (P/S). All cell lines were maintained at 37 °C in a humidified atmosphere with 5% CO_2.

2.2. Patient Samples

We evaluated the prognostic potential of PIWIL3 and PIWIL4 in a training set and in a validation set of PC samples with tissue microarrays (TMA). TMA of the training set was performed with 44 formalin-fixed, paraffin-embedded tumor samples from BioBank of University Hospital Fundacion Jimenez Diaz—Universidad Autonoma de Madrid (PT13/0010/0012), and the TMA for validation set was constructed with 182 available formalin-fixed and paraffin-embedded tumor samples from BioBank of University Hospital Clinico San Carlos (B.0000725; PT17/0015/0040; ISCIII-FEDER). (Detailed descriptions of all experimental procedures are provided in Supplementary Information 1: Materials and Methods)

3. Results

3.1. PIWIL3 and PIWIL4 Are Overexpressed in Non-Tumor and Tumor-Derived Cell Lines

All human PIWI proteins were evaluated by Western blot and by immunohistochemistry (IHC) in a panel of five PC-derived cell lines: four from duct-adenocarcinoma differentiation (BxPC-3, Panc04.03, PL45 and RWP1), and one from epithelioid-carcinoma differentiation (PANC-1). Moreover, PIWI proteins were determined in one non-tumor cell line developed from human pancreatic duct transduced with a retroviral expression vector containing the human *TERT* gene (hTERT-HPNE) (Figure 1A,B).

Protein expression was compared with the expression of human testis as positive control. PIWIL1 and PIWIL2 showed very scarce expression in all pancreatic cell lines, not only in the tumor-derived but also in the non-tumor cell lines. PIWIL1 expression in all cell lines was not detected by WB (Figure 1A), although it could be visualized in some cells of BxPc-3 or Panc04.03 by IHC (Figure 1B). Expression levels of PIWIL2 were unnoticeable by both techniques (Figure 1A,B). In contrast, PIWIL3 and PIWIL4 showed overexpression in almost all tumor-derived cell lines, and in the non-tumor pancreatic cell line compared to control (Figure 1A,B). Both PIWIL3 and PIWIL4 exhibited a clear cytoplasmic expression pattern with some nuclear staining (Figure 1B). Panc04.03 was the only PC-derived cell line with the lowest expression levels of PIWIL3 or PIWIL4 (Figure 1A,B). Since PIWIL3 and PIWIL4 are expressed in the immortalized non-tumor pancreatic cell line, we cannot conclude that PIWIL3 or PIWIL4 could act as an oncogene. Then, we wondered whether PIWIL3 or

PIWIL4 take part in other mechanisms and which is the response of cells after PIWIL3 or PIWIL4 downregulation in the absence of PIWIL1 and PIWIL2. To this aim, we downregulated PIWIL3 and/or PIWIL4 with two different validated siRNA sequences. The highest expression levels have been shown in two pancreatic ductal adenocarcinoma-derived cell lines (PL45 and RWP1) (Figure 1C,D) and the non-tumor pancreatic cell line (hTERT-HPNE) (Figure 1E). As PL45 showed almost five-fold PIWIL3 expression levels compared with control, and two independent combinations with two different siRNA were necessary to downregulate PIWIL3 (Figure 1C). We also decided to evaluate PIWIL3 or PIWIL4 downregulation on hTERT-HPNE by IHC rather than by Western blot due to the low cellularity that exhibited this cell line. Here, we found that maximum PIWIL3 or PIWIL4 downregulation was achieved later in both tumor cell lines than in non-tumor cell line. Higher PIWIL3 or PIWIL4 downregulation in both tumor cell lines was achieved between the fifth/sixth days (Figure 1C,D) compared with the second day obtained in the non-tumor cell line (Figure 1E).

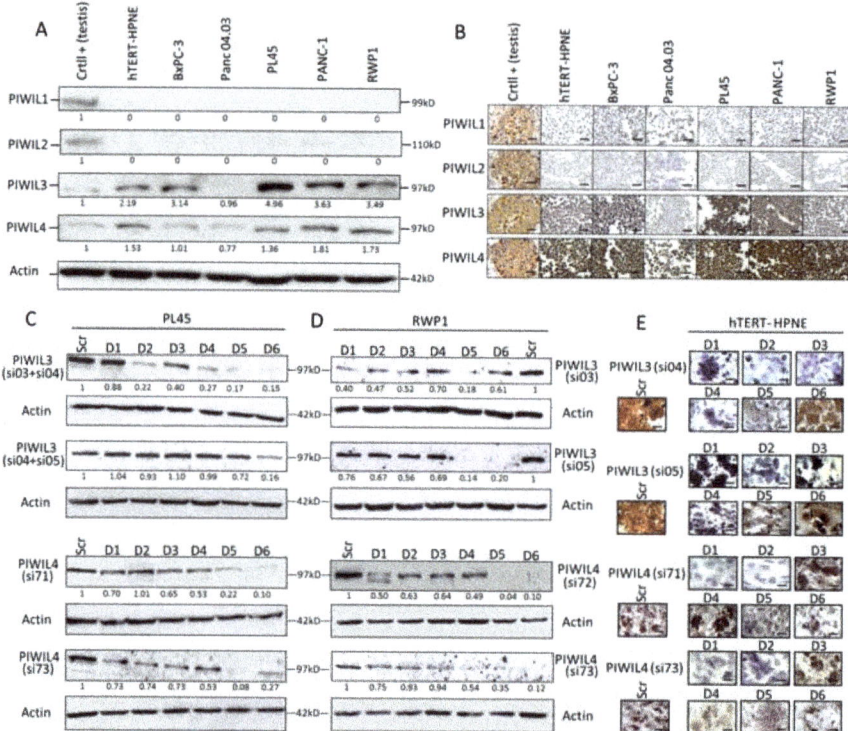

Figure 1. P-element-induced wimpy testis (PIWI) proteins present differential expression in pancreatic cancer (PC), and a late downregulation of PIWIL3 or PIWIL4 in tumor cell lines was found compared to non-tumor cell line. (**A**) Western blot analysis, and (**B**) representative micrographs of immunohistochemical staining of a panel of five human PC-derived cell lines and one non-tumor pancreatic cell line (hTERT-HPNE). A human testis tissue was used as positive control. Two independent downregulations of PIWIL3 (top) and PIWIL4 (bottom) were performed to carry out functional experiments with PL45 (**C**), RWP1 (**D**) and hTERT-HPNE (**E**). Crtl: control. kDa: kilodalton. Scr: Scramble. D1–6: Days 1–6. PIWIL3/Actin or PIWIL4/Actin ratio is represented under each protein band. Scale bar: 50 μm.

3.2. PIWIL3 and/or PIWIL4 Are Necessary for Cell Motility of Both Non-Tumor and Tumor-Derived Cell Lines

Since one of the characteristics of PC is its ability to migrate and metastasize to distant organs, we evaluated the role of PIWIL3 or PIWIL4 in cell motility. Here, we performed functional experiments with two different tumor-derived cell lines and one non-tumor cell line. Interestingly, wound healing assay showed a delay in the motility ratio in all cell lines, normal and tumoral, after PIWIL3 and/or PIWIL4 silencing (Figure 2A).

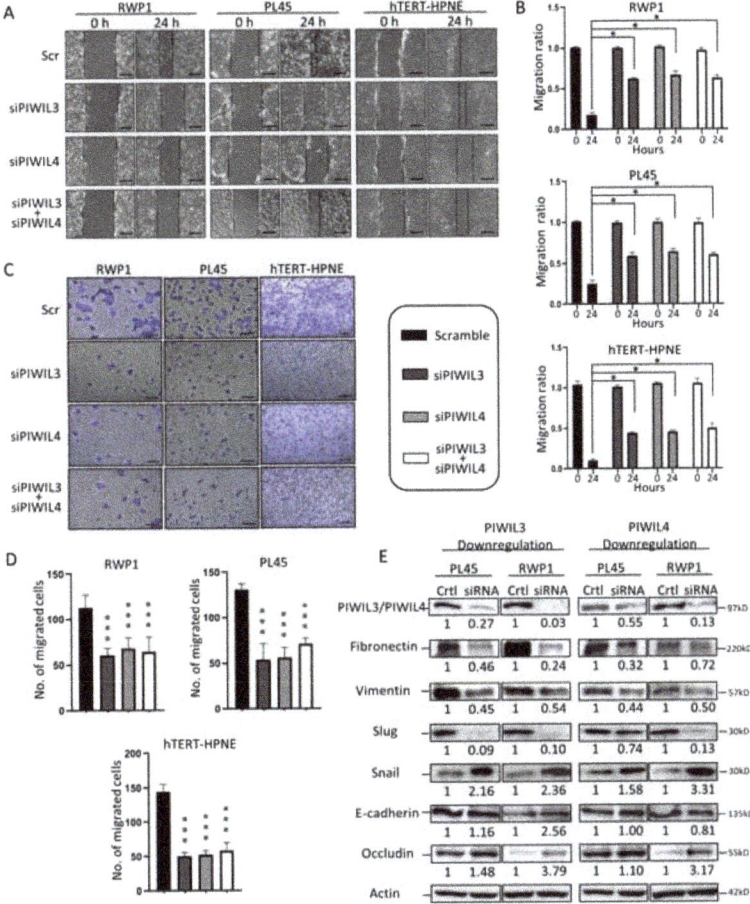

Figure 2. Downregulation of PIWIL3 and/or PIWIL4 decreased motility of PC and non-tumor cell lines through regulation of epithelial-to-mesenchymal transition (EMT). (**A**) Micrographs of wound healing assay showed reduced cell motility after PIWIL3 and/or PIWIL4 silencing in both PC-derived cell lines and in the non-tumor pancreatic-derived cell line. Representative images have been taken at 0 and 24 h after scratching. Broken lines indicate migration heads. (**B**) Statistical analyses of the motility ratio for each cell line according to PIWIL3 and/or PIWIL4 silencing. (**C**) Representative images from Boyden chamber assay of different cell lines taken at 24 h after seeding. (**D**) Statistical analyses of the number of migrated cells for each cell line according to PIWIL3 and/or PIWIL4 silencing. (**E**) Western blot for the expression of PIWIL3 (left) or PIWIL4 (right), Fibronectin, Vimentin, Slug, E-Cadherin and Occludin in PL45 and RWP1 after PIWIL3 or PIWIL4 silencing. The ratio of each protein/Actin ratio is represented under each protein band. Color-coding for each protein downregulation is indicated in the legend box. kDa: kilodalton. Scale bar: 50 μm. *$p < 0.05$; ***$p < 0.001$.

Statistical analyses compared to control revealed a significant reduction in the motility ratio of all cell lines downregulated for PIWIL3 or PIWIL4 individually or in combination ($p < 0.05$) (Figure 2B). To verify our previous results, a Boyden chamber assay was performed as previously described by Chen [41]. Although all cell lines and scrambles were cultured with the same chemotactic agent (20% FBS), the number of migrating cells decreased significantly after individual PIWIL3 and/or PIWIL4 knockdown alone or in combination compared to scramble ($p < 0.001$) (Figure 2C,D). Interestingly, this fact was not only observed in tumor cell lines but also in the normal cell line, which also decreased its motility after PIWIL3 and/or PIWIL4 downregulation. These results suggest that PIWIL3 and PIWIL4 not only modulate invasiveness of tumor cells but also motility of normal cells, which could impair wound healing processes of adult healthy tissues.

To further study how PIWIL3 and PIWIL4 affect cell motility, we evaluated the expression of different markers involved in epithelial-to-mesenchymal transition (EMT). Interestingly, the mesenchymal proteins Fibronectin and Vimentin reduced their expression after PIWIL3 or PIWIL4 downregulation (Figure 2E). Transition factor Slug highly reduced its protein level after PIWIL3 or PIWIL4 downregulation (Figure 2E). Moreover, epithelial markers like Occludin increased its expression after PIWIL3 or PIWIL4 knockdown in both cell lines, while E-Cadherin raised its protein levels only after PIWIL3 silencing (Figure 2E). These results highlight the role of PIWIL3/PIWIL4 in cell motility and wound healing of pancreatic cells through regulation of EMT factors. Taking into consideration that downregulation of PIWIL3 or PIWIL4 reverses EMT of normal cell line, the modulation of these two proteins could affect adult tissue reconstruction after trauma, toxic treatments or inflammatory processes.

3.3. Downregulation of PIWIL3 and/or PIWIL4 Impairs Undifferentiated Phenotype

Following with functional experiments with PIWIL3 and/or PIWIL4 downregulation, we evaluated the ability of both tumor and non-tumor pancreatic derived cell lines to form pancreatic spheres in stem cell enrichment culture media (Figure 3A).

PL45 was not able to dedifferentiate, and to the best of our knowledge, no detailed research reached PL45 dedifferentiation. The spheres observed from scramble controls ranged from 2 to 4 µm of diameter and formed between 10 and 20 spheres per 10,000 seeded cells. Non-tumor cell line presented the lowest number of spheres and the lowest sphere diameter in control conditions. Remarkably, we observed that PIWIL3 and/or PIWIL4 knockdown dropped drastically the number and diameter of spheres of tumor cell line RWP1 ($p < 0.001$) (Figure 3B). However, the same effect was observed on the non-tumor cell line, hTERT-HPNE, not only in the number of spheres ($p < 0.001$) but also in their diameter ($p < 0.05$) (Figure 3C). These results suggest the role of PIWIL3 and PIWIL4 in the maintenance of undifferentiated phenotype of pancreatic cells; however, it seems not to be only necessary for neoplastic cells, but also for normal cells differentiation. These results hamper the clinical use of PIWIL3 or PIWIL4 modulation in PC patients because it may disrupt the dedifferentiation mechanism not only of tumor cells but also of other healthy tissues and could lead to a severe medical condition for patients.

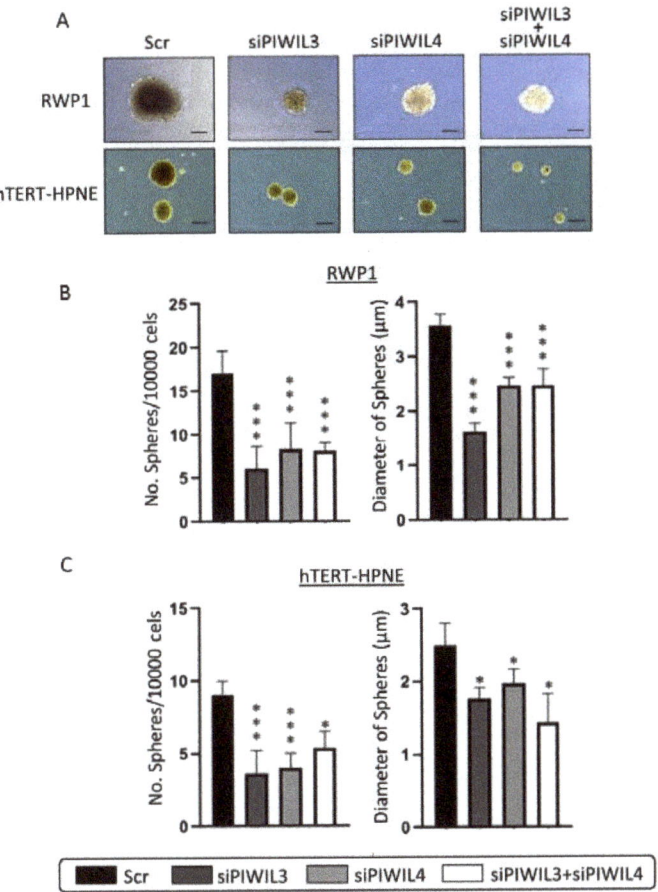

Figure 3. PIWIL3 and PIWIL4 impair undifferentiated phenotype. (**A**) Representative micrographs of undifferentiated pancreatic spheres derived from RWP1 and hTERT-HPNE transfected with siRNA for PIWIL3 (siPIWIL3) or PIWIL4 (siPIWIL4) downregulation individually or in combination. (**B**) Statistical analyses of number and diameter of spheres according to PIWIL3 and/or PIWIL4 downregulation of RWP1 cell line. (**C**) Statistical analyses of number and diameter of spheres according to PIWIL3 and/or PIWIL4 downregulation of the non-tumor hTERT-HPNE cell line. Color-coding for each protein downregulation is indicated in the legend box. Scr: scramble. Scale bar: 50 μm. * $p < 0.05$; *** $p < 0.001$.

3.4. PIWIL3 and PIWIL4 Downregulation Potentiate the Cytotoxic Effect of Chemotherapies

Gemcitabine is one of the gold standard adjuvant treatments for PC management, alone or in combination with Nab-Paclitaxel. Therefore, we wondered whether PIWIL3 and/or PIWIL4 regulate response to these chemotherapies. To evaluate the cytotoxicity of these two factors, tumor and normal cell lines were treated with Gemcitabine or Nab-Paclitaxel individually or in combination after PIWIL3 and/or PIWIL4 knockdown. Then, logarithmically growing tumor-derived cell lines, RWP1 and PL45, and normal cell line, hTERT-HPNE, were treated with previously determined IC_{50} doses of Gemcitabine or Nab-Paclitaxel (Supplementary file). To determine doses for treatment combination for each cell line, IC_{25} dose of Nab-Paclitaxel was set due to its high toxicity, and different concentrations of Gemcitabine were tested to achieve 50% of cell death as previously reported by Awasthi N. et al. [42]. Individual protein downregulation was not enough to achieve an effect, and PIWIL3 and PIWIL4 double downregulation were necessary to decrease significantly cell viability of RWP1 after single treatments ($p = 0.023$ for Gemcitabine; $p = 0.038$ for Nab-Paclitaxel). PIWIL4 downregulation per se achieved a significant effect on the combined treatment ($p = 0.038$); although, double downregulation achieved the maximum effect ($p = 0.001$) (Figure 4A). In contrast, neither PIWIL3 nor PIWIL4 knockdown affected cytotoxicity of PL45 cell line, neither with individual treatments nor in combination (Figure 4B).

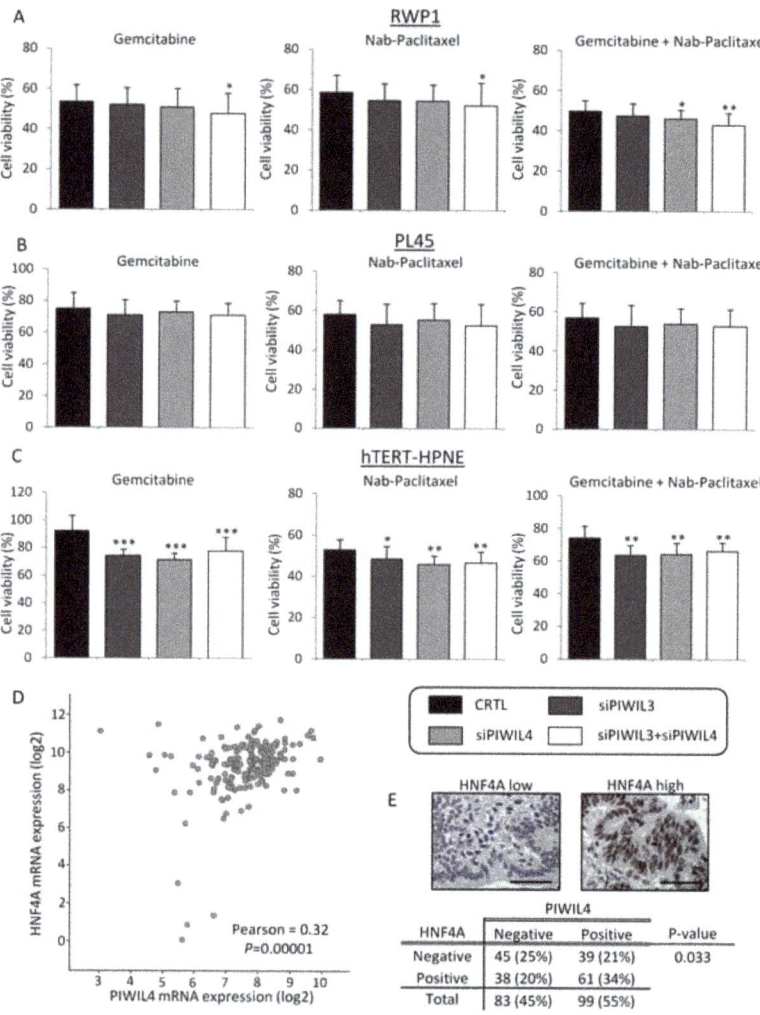

Figure 4. PIWIL3 and PIWIL4 downregulation potentiates the cytotoxic effect of chemotherapy. (**A**) Cell viability analyses after PIWIL3 and/or PIWIL4 silencing according to Gemcitabine (left) or Nab-Paclitaxel (center) individual treatments or in combination (right) of RWP1 cell line, PL45 (**B**) and hTERT-HPNE (**C**) cell lines. (**D**) Scatterplot and statistical analysis of HNF4A mRNA expression (y axis) and PIWIL4 mRNA expression (x axis) of 178 patient cohort from The Cancer Genome Atlas (TCGA). (**E**) Representative micrographs of HNF4A low expression (top-left) and high expression top-right). Statistical association between HNF4A and PIWIL4 protein expression of 182 PC samples (bottom). Color-coding for each protein downregulation is indicated in the legend box. Scale bars: 50 μm. * $p < 0.05$; ** $p < 0.01$; *** $p < 0.001$.

On the other hand, non-tumor cell line hTERT-HPNE initially presented a complete resistance to Gemcitabine; then, functional experiments were performed with the highest concentration of Gemcitabine tested (250 µM). This concentration was 42,000 times higher than IC_{50} concentration of Gemcitabine for RWP1 and 700 times higher than IC_{50} concentration of Gemcitabine for PL45. Furthermore, IC_{50} dose of Nab-Paclitaxel for non-tumor cell line (235 µM), which was 21 times higher than IC_{50} dose of Nab-Paclitaxel for RWP1 and 1.6 times higher than for PL45. Interestingly, the highest effect of all treatments was observed in the non-tumor derived cell line. Indeed, PIWIL3 and/or PIWIL4 silencing overcame Gemcitabine resistance of the non-tumor cell line ($p < 0.001$), and significantly increased the other treatment effects ($p = 0.003$ for Nab-Paclitaxel; $p = 0.001$ for Gemcitabine + Nab-Paclitaxel) (Figure 4C). Therefore, these results support PIWIL3 and PIWIL4 as crucial factors in chemoresistance of PC tumor cells and in the toxicity of normal cells. However, from a clinical point of view, depletion of PIWIL3 or PIWIL4 proteins with target therapies should be done with great care due to the potential high toxicity and adverse events that they could bring to PC patients.

In order to dissect one of the underlying mechanisms whereby PIWIL3 or PIWIL4 expression confers chemoresistance, we evaluated the link between these two proteins and hENT1, which is responsible for Gemcitabine uptake and effect on cells [43]. For this, we used 178 available expression profile data from a 186-patient dataset from The Cancer Genome Atlas (TCGA, Firehose Legacy), and statistical correlation was assessed using cBioPortal [44,45]. In this first attempt, piwil3 or piwil4 showed no correlation with hEnt1 at mRNA level ($p = 0.26$ and $p = 0.19$, respectively). Another factor that drives cytotoxicity of tumor cells is HNF4A. It has been previously described to be a negative regulator of hENT1 and necessary for cell proliferation and drug resistance in PC [46]. Then, we assessed the correlation between piwil3 or piwil4 and hnf4a; however, piwil3 mRNA expression did not show any connection with hnf4a at the mRNA level ($p = 0.36$). Interestingly, mRNA analysis showed a moderate positive correlation between piwil4 and hnf4a ($r = 0.32$; $p = 0.00001$) (Figure 4D). To validate this result, we stained by IHC 182 PC patient samples with anti-HNF4A antibody. HNF4A exhibited a clear nuclear staining and a marked differential expression pattern between samples (Figure 4E, top). The statistical analysis revealed a link between PIWIL4 and HNF4A at the protein level in patient samples ($p = 0.033$)(Figure 4E, bottom). We also assessed an association between PIWIL3 and HNF4A at the protein level. Although no association was found, statistical analysis revealed a high trend towards significance ($p = 0.080$). These results highlight a connection between PIWIL3 and PIWIL4 with HNF4A factor, which could explain a feasible mechanism of chemoresistance of PC cells and cytotoxicity of normal cells.

3.5. Low Expression of PIWIL4 Is a Poor Prognosis Factor of Pancreatic Cancer Patients

To study the prognostic potential of PIWIL3 or PIWIL4 in PC, we evaluated their protein expression levels in a cohort composed of 44 patients from Fundacion Jimenez Diaz Hospital. To assess the survival analysis all samples with positive margins of resection (R1) were excluded from the study ($n = 7$ patients) (Table 1).

Immunohistochemical staining of patient samples showed differential expression levels of PIWIL3 and PIWIL4. All the samples that stained positively for PIWIL3 exhibited a cytoplasmic localization, especially in those cases with high PIWIL3 expression (Figure 5A). The expression pattern of PIWIL4 was limited to cytoplasm and cell membrane of tumor cells, and no positive nuclear staining was found (Figure 5B). Survival analyses were assessed with this data set. Nevertheless, neither PIWIL3 nor PIWIL4 associated significantly with progression-free or overall survival of PC patients (Figure 5C,D). However, although statistical analyses revealed no significant association between these PIWI proteins and prognosis, we found that patients with low expression levels of PIWIL3 or PIWIL4 presented shorter progression-free and overall survival than high levels of both proteins. The mean progression-free survival of patients with low PIWIL3 expression was 17 months (95% CI = 7–27 months), while the mean time-to-progression of high PIWIL3 expression was 30 months (95% CI = 6–54 months) (Figure 5C, top). Concerning overall survival, patients with low PIWIL3 expression exhibited a mean survival of

37 months (95% CI = 22–53 months), and those with high PIWIL3 expression lived a mean of 62 months (95% CI = 33–90 months) (Figure 5C, bottom). Similarly, low PIWIL4 expression presented shorter mean progression-free and overall survival than high-expression patients. The mean progression-free survival of patients with low PIWIL4 expression was 19 months (95% CI = 6–31 months), while the mean time-to-progression of high PIWIL4 expression was 23 months (95% CI = 8–39 months) (Figure 5D, top). Furthermore, patients with low PIWIL4 expression presented shorter overall survival (mean = 39 months; 95% CI = 23–56 months) than patients with high PIWIL4 expression (mean = 56 months; 95% CI = 30–82 months) (Figure 5D, bottom).

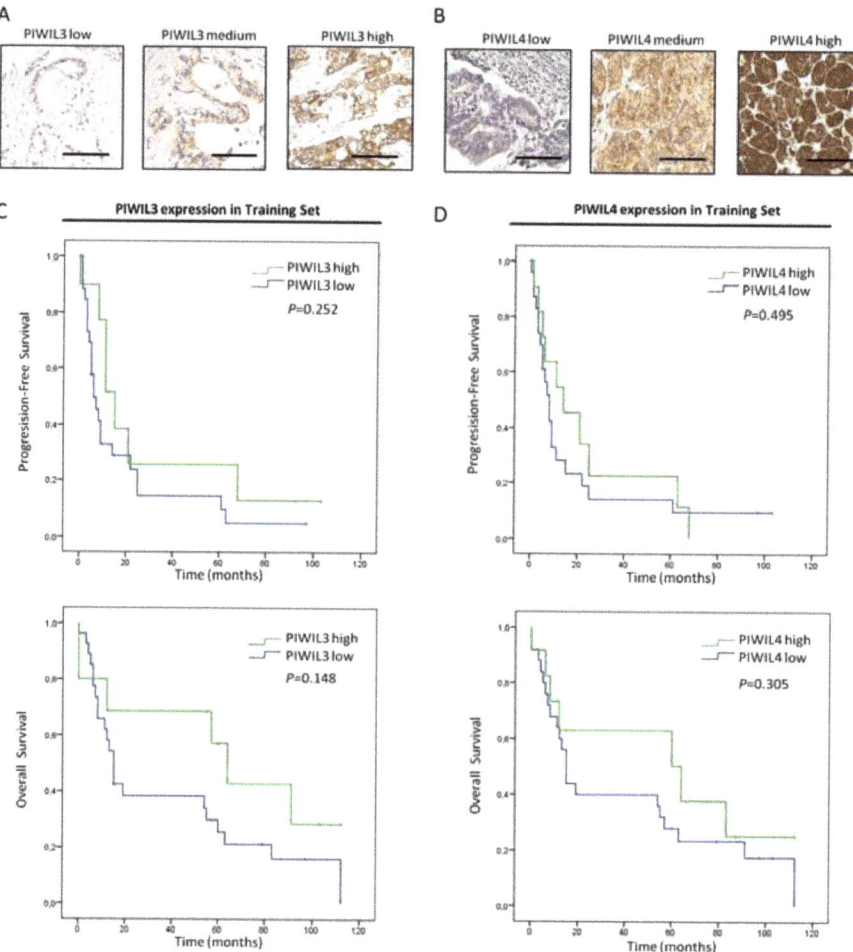

Figure 5. Prognostic impact of PIWIL3 or PIWIL4 in PC patients from the training set. (**A**) Representative micrographs of tumors with low (left), intermediate (middle) and high PIWIL3 expression (right). (**B**) Representative micrographs of tumors with low (left), intermediate (middle) and high PIWIL4 expression levels (right). (**C**) Kaplan–Meier curves according to PIWIL3 protein expression for both progression-free (top) and overall survival (bottom). (**D**) Kaplan–Meier curves according to PIWIL4 protein expression for both progression-free (top) and overall survival (bottom). *p*-values were obtained by log-rank test. Scale bars: 50 µm.

Table 1. Clinico-pathologic characteristics of completed resected R0 pancreatic cancer patients from the training set.

Clinical Characteristics	N	%	Clinical Characteristics	N	%
Age			Neural invasion		
<65 years	16	43	No	12	32
>65 years	21	57	Yes	25	68
Gender			Lymph nodes involved		
Male	21	57	N0	14	38
Female	16	43	N1	23	62
Size			Adjuvant treatment		
<2 cm	20	54	No	21	57
>2 cm	17	46	Yes	14	38
Stage			N/A	2	5
I	9	24	pT		
II	28	76	T1	6	16
Grade			T2	5	14
High	30	81	T3	26	70
Low	7	19	N/A	3	2
Vascular invasion					
No	12	32	Total	37	100
Yes	25	68			

N: number of patients; N/A: not available; cm: centimeters.

One of the possible reasons that may justify the lack of statistical significance of these analyses could be the limited sample size of the study. Therefore, we evaluated the expression of PIWIL3 and PIWIL4 in a larger cohort composed of 182 patients samples from Clinico San Carlos Hospital. As before, all samples with positive margins of resection were excluded from the study ($n = 54$ patients) (Table 2).

Table 2. Clinico-pathologic characteristics of complete resected R0 pancreatic cancer patients from the validation set.

Clinical Characteristics	N	%	Clinical Characteristics	N	%
Age			Grade		
<65 years	25	20	High	19	15
>65 years	103	80	Low	105	82
Gender			N/A	4	3
Male	63	49	Vascular invasion		
Female	65	51	No	75	59
Diabetes Mellitus			Yes	43	33
No	88	69	N/A	10	8
Yes	33	26	Neural invasion		
N/A	7	5	No	47	37
Adjuvant treatment			Yes	71	55
No	75	58	N/A	10	8
Yes	24	19	pT		
N/A	29	23	T1	30	23
Size			T2	44	35
<2 cm	31	24	T3	51	40
>2 cm	69	54	N/A	3	2
N/A	28	22	Lymph nodes involved		
Stage			N0	70	55
I	46	36	N1	51	40
II	74	58	N/A	7	5
N/A	8	6	Total	128	100

N: number of patients; N/A: not available; cm: centimeters.

We assessed survival analyses with patients with available data of progression-free survival ($n = 113$) or overall survival ($n = 118$). Here, PIWIL3 expression did not associate either with progression-free survival ($p = 0.214$) or overall survival ($p = 0.337$) (Figure 6A,B). Thus, these results led us to exclude PIWIL3 expression as a prognostic biomarker for PC. Interestingly, those PC patients with low expression of PIWIL4 presented not only a shorter progression-free survival ($p = 0.002$) but also a shorter overall survival ($p < 0.001$) than patients with high expression levels (Figure 6C,D). Here, patients with low PIWIL4 expression showed a mean progression-free survival of 31 months (95% CI = 20–41 months), while patients with high PIWIL4 expression presented a mean progression-free survival of 75 months (95% CI = 54–96 months) (Figure 6C). Overall survival of patients with low PIWIL4 expression presented a mean of 29 months (95% CI = 21–37 months), while that of patients with high PIWIL4 expression was significantly longer with a mean of 68 months (95% CI = 46–89 months) (Figure 6D).

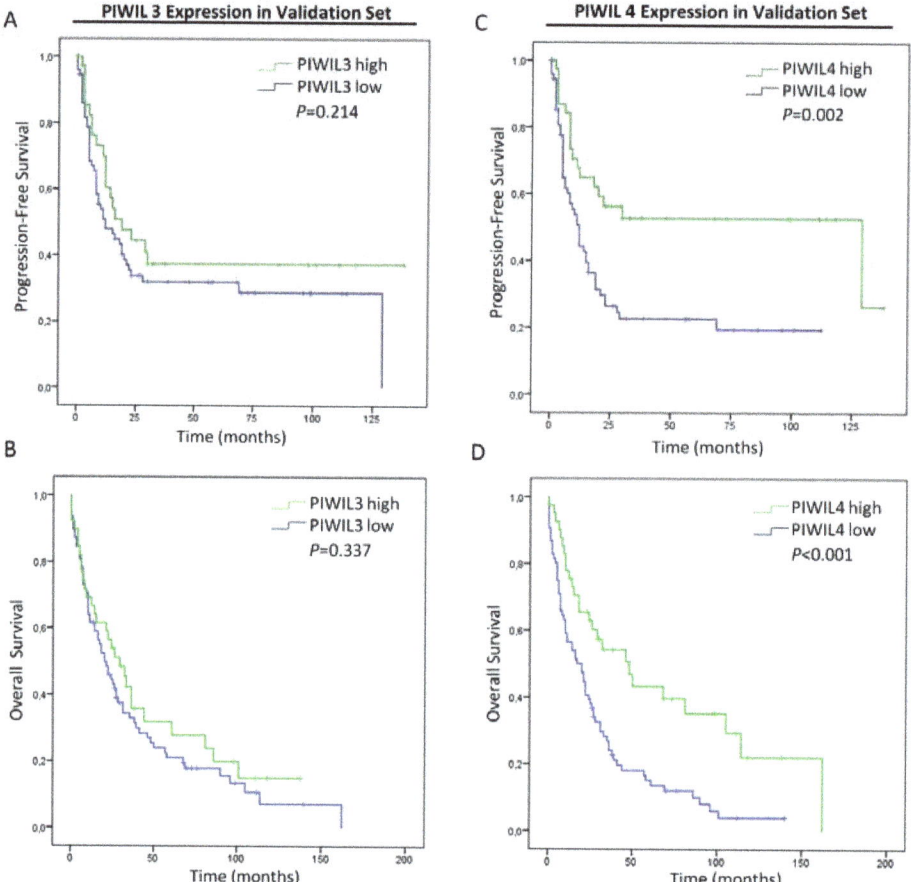

Figure 6. Prognostic impact of PIWIL3 or PIWIL4 in PC patients from the validation set. (**A**) Kaplan–Meier curves according to PIWIL3 protein expression for progression-free survival. (**B**) Kaplan–Meier curves according to PIWIL3 protein expression for overall survival. (**C**) Kaplan–Meier curves according to PIWIL4 protein expression for progression-free survival. (**D**) Kaplan–Meier curves according to PIWIL4 protein expression for overall survival. *p*-values were obtained by log-rank test.

In order to validate the prognosis potential of PIWIL4 expression with respect to other clinico-pathological characteristics, we performed a Cox proportional hazards model for both progression-free and overall survival of patients (Table 3). The univariate analysis for progression-free survival revealed that patients with a low expression of PIWIL4 showed a higher risk of recurrence after surgery compared with patients with high expression (hazard ratio (HR) = 1.979; 95% CI: 1.178–3.325; p = 0.010). As survival curves confirmed previously, PIWIL3 did not raise significance to predict progression-free survival (p = 0.227). Other pathological characteristics that associated significantly with high risk of progression in the univariate analysis were tumor size (HR = 3.023; 95% CI: 1.413–6.465; p = 0.004), T stage (HR = 1.682; 95% CI: 1.033–2.738; p = 0.037), tumor stage (HR = 1.866; 95% CI: 1.105–3.151; p = 0.020) and neural invasion (HR = 1.757; 95% CI: 1.027–3.007; p = 0.040). In the multivariate analysis, low PIWIL4 expression remained statistically significant for a higher risk of progression (HR = 2.036; 95% CI: 1.025–4.044; p = 0.042) together with tumor size (HR = 3.095; 95% CI: 1.237–7.744; p = 0.016). Univariate analyses for overall survival also revealed low expression of PIWIL4 as a high risk factor (HR = 2.093; 95% CI: 1.344–3.260; p = 0.001). Other clinico-pathologic characteristics that associated significantly with shorter overall survival were T stage (HR = 1.679; 95% CI: 1.110–2.540; p = 0.014), tumor stage (HR = 1.795; 95% CI: 1.148–2.807; p = 0.010), lymph nodes positive (HR = 1.573; 95% CI: 1.025–2.414; p = 0.038) and neural invasion (HR = 1.658; 95% CI: 1.060–2.593; p = 0.027). However, the only clinical variable that associated significantly with reduced overall survival in the multivariate analysis was low PIWIL4 expression (HR = 2.185; 95% CI: 1.313–3.636; p = 0.003) (Table S3). Thus, these results highlight the detrimental role of low expression of PIWIL4 and allow the identification of two different risk subgroups of PC patients to be managed with differential treatment strategies to improve survival.

Table 3. Uni- and multivariate proportional hazards model for progression-free and overall survival of patients from the validation cohort.

	Univariate PFS (95% CI)				Univariate OS (95% CI)			
	HR	Lower	Upper	p	HR	Lower	Upper	p
Age (< 65 years vs. > 65 years)	1.060	0.604	1.860	0.840	1.198	0.723	1.986	0.484
Gender (Male vs. Female)	1.494	0.920	2.425	0.104	1.182	0.785	1.778	0.423
Diabetes Mellitus (No vs. Yes)	1.070	0.614	1.864	0.811	1.113	0.694	1.784	0.658
Adjuvant treatment (Yes vs. No)	1.016	0.556	1.857	0.959	1.226	0.781	2.094	0.456
Size (<2 cm vs. >2 cm)	3.023	1.413	6.465	0.004	1.255	0.754	2.087	0.382
pT (I / II vs. III)	1.682	1.033	2.738	0.037	1.679	1.110	2.540	0.014
Stage (I vs. II)	1.866	1.105	3.151	0.020	1.795	1.148	2.807	0.010
Grade (low vs. high)	1.406	0.695	2.845	0.343	1.221	0.664	2.245	0.522
Lymph nodes involved (No vs. Yes)	1.548	0.943	2.540	0.084	1.573	1.025	2.414	0.038
Vascular invasion (No vs. Yes)	1.348	0.807	2.252	0.254	1.481	0.959	2.287	0.077
Neural invasion (No vs. Yes)	1.757	1.027	3.007	0.040	1.658	1.060	2.593	0.027
PIWIL3 (high vs. low)	1.380	0.819	2.327	0.227	1.237	0.798	1.917	0.342
PIWIL4 (high vs. low)	1.979	1.178	3.325	0.010	2.093	1.344	3.260	0.001
	Multivariate PFS (95% CI)				Multivariate OS (95% CI)			
Size (<2 cm vs. > 2 cm)	3.095	1.237	7.744	0.016				
pT (I / II vs. III)	1.339	0.609	2.944	0.467	1.178	0.608	2.284	0.627
Stage (I vs. II)	1.596	0.655	3.890	0.304	1.691	0.683	4.188	0.256
Lymph nodes involved (No vs. Yes)					1.084	0.549	2.141	0.817
Neural invasion	1.232	0.620	2.449	0.551	1.229	0.761	1.985	0.398
PIWIL4 (high vs. low)	2.036	1.025	4.044	0.042	2.185	1.313	3.636	0.003

PFS: progression-free survival; OS: Overall survival; HR: hazard ratio; CI: confidence interval; vs.: versus; cm: centimeters.

In view of these results, we verified whether PIWIL3 or PIWIL4 could be related to any of the pathological characteristics registered in our study (Table S4). In this analysis, low levels of PIWIL3 associated significantly with neural invasion (p = 0.050). Low PIWIL4 expression associated significantly with female patients ($p = 0.050$). Furthermore, a higher percentage of patients with T3 tumors associated significantly with low PIWIL4 expression ($p = 0.020$); the same occurred with neural invasion and low PIWIL4 expression ($p = 0.019$) (Table 4). These results suggest the lack of PIWIL4 expression as a deleterious effect in PC and support previous survival results.

Table 4. Statistical association between PIWIL3 and PIWIL4 protein expression with clinico-pathological characteristics.

Parameters	PIWIL3 Low N (%)	PIWIL3 High N (%)	p-Value	PIWIL4 Low N (%)	PIWIL4 High N (%)	p-Value
Gender			0.946			0.050
Male	43 (34%)	20 (16%)		34 (26%)	29 (23%)	
Female	44 (34%)	21 (16%)		46 (36%)	19 (15%)	
Age			0.630			0.227
<65 years	18 (14%)	7 (5%)		13 (10%)	12 (9%)	
>65 years	69 (54%)	34 (27%)		67 (53%)	36 (28%)	
Diabetes Mellitus			0.724			0.939
No	59 (49%)	29 (24%)		54 (45%)	34 (28%)	
Yes	21 (17%)	12 (10%)		20 (16%)	13 (11%)	
Stage			0.791			0.204
I	30 (25%)	16 (13%)		26 (22%)	20 (16%)	
II	50 (42%)	24 (20%)		49 (41%)	25 (21%)	
pT			0.503			0.020
I/II	48 (38%)	26 (21%)		40 (32%)	34 (27%)	
III	36 (29%)	15 (12%)		38 (31%)	13 (10%)	
Adjuvant treatment			0.704			0.085
No	50 (51%)	25 (25%)		52 (53%)	23 (23%)	
Yes	17 (17%)	7 (7%)		12 (12%)	12 (12%)	
Size			0.264			0.705
<2 cm	19 (19%)	12 (12%)		19 (19%)	12 (12%)	
>2 cm	50 (50%)	19 (19%)		45 (45%)	24 (24%)	
Lymph nodes involved			0.956			0.713
No	47 (39%)	23 (19%)		43 (36%)	27 (22%)	
Yes	34 (28%)	17 (14%)		33 (27%)	18 (15%)	
Vascular Invasion			0.950			0.875
No	51 (43%)	24 (20%)		46 (34%)	29 (30%)	
Yes	29 (25%)	14 (12%)		27 (25%)	16 (11%)	
Neural Invasion			0.050			0.019
No	27 (23%)	20 (17%)		23 (20%)	24 (20%)	
Yes	53 (45%)	18 (15%)		50 (42%)	21 (18%)	
Grade			0.095			0.917
Low	68 (55%)	37 (30%)		65 (52%)	40 (32%)	
High	16 (13%)	3 (2%)		12 (10%)	7 (6%)	

N: Number of patients; cm: centimeters.

4. Discussion

PC is an extremely lethal malignancy, in which an early diagnosis is crucial to increase patient survival. Therefore, molecular biomarkers will play an important role in the future management of this neoplasm. To date, the only biomarkers approved by the Food and Drug Administration (FDA) for PC are preoperative levels of CA19-9; however, the applicability of this biomarker has been questioned due to the fact that the biliary obstruction can also increase CA19-9 levels, not to mention that up to 10% of the population cannot synthesize this antigen [47]. Therefore, new biomarkers that combine high sensitivity and specificity are needed in the clinical management of PC. Recently, novel proteins called

PIWI have been discovered, and their expression was found in several types of tumors; thus, these factors may provide new perspectives in the clinical practice of PC [12]. In the present study, we have evaluated the expression of the four members of the PIWI family in PC-derived cell lines and one normal pancreatic cell line used as control. Interestingly, both PIWIL1 and PIWIL2 presented nearly undetectable expression levels in all cell lines. Indeed, this fact could be explained by the presence of CpG islands in the promoter region of *PIWIL1* [48] and *PIWIL2* [49]. It has been reported that downregulation of PIWIL1 and PIWIL2 by promoter CpG island hypermethylation has been observed in other types of tumors like testicular or non-small cell lung cancer [38]. It has also been described how PIWIL1 downregulation regulates migration of Schwann cells for peripheral nerve regeneration after injury [50]. Since we found low levels of PIWIL1 and PIWIL2 in a pancreatic normal cell line, this event seems not to be exclusive of tumor cells. In fact, these genes play crucial roles in spermatogenesis, and their downregulation impairs germ cell development that might associate with male infertility [51].

On the other hand, PIWIL3 and PIWIL4 showed higher protein levels and a differential expression pattern throughout cell lines, which includes a non-tumor cell line. This first attempt implied that PIWIL3 and PIWIL4 might not act as an oncogene in PC. Nevertheless, the role of PIWIL3 and PIWIL4 in tumorigenesis is rather controversial. For this, we decided to evaluate their role with functional experiments in tumor cell lines and a non-tumor cell line as normal control. Some studies have reported the expression of these proteins with oncogenic features; e.g., one study described how cancer cells re-express PIWIL3 to promote cancer cell growth [52]. Other research highlighted that PIWIL3 and PIWIL4 presented oncogenic potential in several types of cancers [13]. In contrast, PIWIL3 exhibited a protective effect in glioma cells [25], and low expression of PIWIL4 has been found in tumor cells from hepatocellular carcinoma [36], breast cancer [22] and non-small cell lung cancer [38]. Therefore, the role of PIWIL3 and PIWIL4 in tumor initiation and development remains still unclear. In our functional experiments, we were able to evaluate cell response to PIWIL3 and/or PIWIL4 downregulation. Moreover, the inclusion of a non-tumor cell line in these experiments led us to discern between a true oncogenic role and a normal cell function. Our experiments, designed to evaluate cell motility, chemoresistance and undifferentiated phenotype, revealed that the effect observed after PIWIL3 and/or PIWIL4 downregulation in tumor cells were also shown by the non-tumor cell line. Here, we observed how PIWIL3 and PIWIL4 knockdown decreased motility of both tumor and normal cells through a mesenchymal arrest in favor of the epithelial phenotype. This reduction of the cell motility by PIWIL4 downregulation has previously been described in breast cancer cells through an impairment of Vimentin and N-Cadherin [33]. However, this study only provided evidence of migration delay in MCF-7 tumor cell line but not in a non-tumor cell line. Then, it is still unknown whether PIWIL4 downregulation exclusively affects cell motility of breast cancer cells or also impairs motility of normal cells. For this concern, it has been reported how PIWIL2 regulates invasion abilities of prostate cancer cells through modulation of EMT protein expression [53]. HPV16 is also able to increase PIWIL2 levels to increase proliferation and invasion of cervical cancer cells [54]. However, not only do PIWI proteins play a role as invasion promoting factors, but also their associated piRNAs. It has been described how downregulation of piRNA-36712 promotes invasion and migration of tumor cells; thus, it is considered a potential tumor suppressor in breast cancer [55]. Another study supports the tumor-suppressive properties of piR-823 because its upregulation inhibits tumor cell growth in gastric cancer models [56]. In addition, piR-823 downregulation suppressed cell proliferation of colorectal cancer cells by a direct modulation of the transcriptional activity of HSF1 [57]. Other functional experiments have demonstrated that piR-651 promotes tumor formation in non-small cell lung cancer mediated by Cyclin D1 and CDK4 [58]. To the best of our knowledge, we have described for the first time the implication of PIWIL3 and PIWIL4 in cell motility through EMT modulation of tumor and non-tumor pancreatic cells. From a clinical point of view, this connection between PIWIL3/PIWIL4 and EMT should be managed carefully since EMT is the most critical mechanism by which adult tissues, including pancreatic β-cells, are repaired after inflammatory, toxic or trauma injuries [59–61].

Many works have reported that PIWI proteins have the ability to regulate transposable elements to maintain genomic stability of stem cells [62]. In our functional studies, we observed a diminished undifferentiated phenotype of pancreatic cells, and we found a decrease in the number and size of pancreatic stem-cell-like spheres after PIWIL3 and/or PIWIL4 downregulation. This result supports the role of PIWIL3/PIWIL4 in the maintenance of undifferentiated phenotype both in tumor and in normal cells, as was previously observed in normal spermatogenesis of mammals [63]. Moreover, downregulation of PIWIL2 decreased proliferation and survival of breast cancer stem cells through a decrease in the protein levels of STAT3, BCL-XL and Cyclin D1 [64]. This link between PIWI proteins and undifferentiated phenotype has also been demonstrated when downregulation of PIWI proteins impaired whole-body regeneration of certain marine organisms [65]. Hence, the role of PIWIL3/PIWIL4 seems not to be exclusive of tumorigenesis and suggests a crucial function in fundamental tissue maintenance.

Since expression of PIWI proteins increased resistance to drugs in cervical cancer [66] and in non-small cell lung cancer [67], we decided to evaluate whether PIWIL3 or PIWIL4 were able to modulate chemoresistance of PC. Here, we described how PIWIL3 and PIWIL4 downregulation increases the effect of the gold standard chemotherapies against PC. Surprisingly, PL45 cell line showed no effect after individual or combined downregulation. However, the lack of effect in PL45 could be explained not only by its mutations in *KRAS*, *TP53* or *DPC4*, which are commonly found in PC, but also by its mutation in *BRCA2* gene, which could confer chemoresistance in PC as recently described by Wang et al. [68]. As we observed and as previously reported in the literature, non-tumor cell line hTERT-HPNE showed Gemcitabine resistance [69]. Nevertheless, it reverted completely its chemoresistance after PIWIL3 and/or PIWIL4 knockdown and significantly increased the effect of Gemcitabine alone or in combination with Nab-Paclitaxel. However, this statistically significant drug response exhibited after double downregulation achieved neither additive nor synergic effect compared with individual protein downregulation in the presence of single treatment or combination. The fact that PIWIL3 and/or PIWIL4 downregulation increased considerably drug response on the normal cell line does not make modulation of PIWIL3 or PIWIL4 suitable for future drug design against PC. This effect on normal cells could imply higher toxicity and adverse events, which could compromise tolerability and safety of patients. In order to explain the link between these two PIWI proteins and chemoresistance, we explored factors related to Gemcitabine or Nab-Paclitaxel resistance in PC. Hepatocyte Nuclear Factor Alpha (HNF4A) appeared rapidly as a potential factor that may account for this finding. HNF4A is overexpressed in hepatocytes, enterocytes and pancreatic β-cells. It also ensures expression of intermediary genes required for metabolism of glucose and lipids, and it is necessary for cell differentiation [70]. In PC, high expression levels of HNF4A have been correlated with poor prognosis. HNF4A has been described as conferring chemoresistance in other types of tumors like breast cancer, where it has been the most upregulated gene after hypoxic conditions and led to a higher Doxorubicin resistance [71]. Indeed, a synthetic HNF4A antagonist is under investigation to selectively eradicate cancer cells [72]. Moreover, the mechanism of HNF4A to confer chemoresistance to Gemcitabine is through (a) direct regulation of hENT1, which is responsible for Gemcitabine uptake of tumor cells [46]. At first glance, neither PIWIL3 nor PIWIL4 exhibited a correlation with hENT1. Nevertheless, a high trend towards significance was found between PIWIL3 and HNF4A at the protein level, and a statistically significant correlation was found between PIWIL4 and HNF4A both at mRNA and at the protein level. Therefore, these results support the role of these PIWI proteins as crucial factors for regulation of chemotherapy uptake of cells.

Finally, we assessed survival analyses by staining PIWIL3 or PIWIL4 in PC samples. We were struck in particular by the fact that PIWIL3 and PIWIL4 were expressed in pancreatic normal tissues [73,74]; consequently, our hypothesis as oncogenes was found baseless and was simply discarded. Furthermore, survival analyses revealed that low expression of PIWIL4 associated significantly with both shorter progression-free and overall survival. These results suggested a deleterious effect of low levels of PIWIL4. Since PC is a deadly disease and survival of patients is rather limited, our findings allow the identification of two different risk subgroups of PC patients that can be clinically managed independently to improve survival. Only tumor size higher than 2 cm emerged as statistically significant together with low PIWIL4 expression in Cox multivariate analysis for progression-free survival. This result could be expected, since tumor size at diagnostic is closely related to survival. It has been reported that the 5-year survival rate is around 50% when tumors are below 2 cm [75] and close to 100% when tumors are below 1 cm [76]. Moreover, we found that a higher percentage of patients with low PIWIL4 expression exhibited a link with T3 tumors and neural invasion compared with those with high PIWIL4 expression.

On the other hand, the fact that low levels of PIWIL4 are related to reduced cell motility seemed to go against our results that suggest it as a poor prognostic biomarker of PC. However, our results suggest that the lack of PIWIL4 could increase treatment toxicity and adverse events to patients, an impaired tissue repair driven by a delay in cell motility through EMT reversion, and a default on cell differentiation. All these mechanisms could retard the healing process of PC patients and lead to shorter progression-free and overall survival.

5. Conclusions

In our study, we have compiled some functional experiments and survival analysis according to PIWIL3 or PIWIL4 expression to dissect the role of these proteins in PC. Our findings support PIWIL3 and PIWIL4 as crucial factors in the regulation of cell motility, stem cell maintenance and drug resistance both in tumor and healthy pancreatic cells. Moreover, low PIWIL4 expression is able to predict shorter survival of PC patients. These results provide new insights into the knowledge of PIWI proteins functions and their controversial role in tumorigenesis.

Supplementary Materials: The following are available online at http://www.mdpi.com/2077-0383/9/5/1252/s1, Supplementary file: Materials and Methods.

Author Contributions: J.M.-U. and J.G.-F. designed the study. L.O.-M., S.G.-B., E.P.-A., L.D.-V. and A.C. collected clinical samples and elaborated the database. W.L. and N.G.-C. performed the experiments. J.M.-U., W.L., A.O. and N.G.-C. analyzed the data of the in vitro experiments. M.J.F.-A. and L.O.-M. evaluated and scored immunohistochemical stainings. J.M.-U. wrote the paper. J.M.-U., W.L., A.O., and N.G.-C. critically revised the manuscript. J.G.-F. provided funding. All authors have read and agreed to the published version of the manuscript.

Funding: This research was funded by Spanish Health Research Project Funds (PI16/01468) from Instituto de Salud Carlos III -FEDER (J.G.-F.) of the Spanish Ministry of Economy, Industry, and Competitiveness.

Acknowledgments: We thank Oliver Shaw (FIIS-FJD) for editing the manuscript for English usage, clarity, and style; Elena Molina from the BioBank of University Hospital Clinico San Carlos (B.0000725; PT17/0015/0040; ISCIII-FEDER), Biobank of Fundacion Jimenez Diaz Hospital (PT13/0010/0012), and all Lab. Technicians from both institutions for providing technical support of priceless value. We also thank Fatima Gebauer from the Centre for Genomic Regulation of Barcelona for kindly providing RWP1 and PANC-1 cell lines and Eva Castillo-Bazan from the Pharmacology Department of Fundacion Jimenez Diaz Hospital for providing all drugs used in this study.

Conflicts of Interest: The authors declare that they have no competing interests.

References

1. Rahib, L.; Smith, B.D.; Aizenberg, R.; Rosenzweig, A.B.; Fleshman, J.M.; Matrisian, L.M. Projecting cancer incidence and deaths to 2030: The unexpected burden of thyroid, liver, and pancreas cancers in the United States. *Cancer Res.* **2014**, *74*, 2913–2921. [CrossRef] [PubMed]
2. Tamm, E.P.; Bhosale, P.R.; Vikram, R.; de Almeida Marcal, L.P.; Balachandran, A. Imaging of pancreatic ductal adenocarcinoma: State of the art. *World J. Radiol.* **2013**, *5*, 98–105. [CrossRef] [PubMed]
3. Kelsen, D.P.; Portenoy, R.; Thaler, H.; Tao, Y.; Brennan, M. Pain as a predictor of outcome in patients with operable pancreatic carcinoma. *Surgery* **1997**, *122*, 53–59. [CrossRef]
4. Oettle, H.; Post, S.; Neuhaus, P.; Gellert, K.; Langrehr, J.; Ridwelski, K.; Schramm, H.; Fahlke, J.; Zuelke, C.; Riess, H.; et al. Adjuvant chemotherapy with gemcitabine vs observation in patients undergoing curative-intent resection of pancreatic cancer: A randomized controlled trial. *JAMA* **2007**, *297*, 267–277. [CrossRef] [PubMed]

5. Neoptolemos, J.P.; Stocken, D.D.; Bassi, C.; Ghaneh, P.; Cunningham, D.; Goldstein, D.; Valle, J.W.; Palmer, D.H.; Mckay, C.J.; Doi, R.; et al. Adjuvant chemotherapy with fluorouracil plus folinic acid vs gemcitabine following pancreatic cancer resection: A randomized controlled trial. *JAMA* **2010**, *304*, 1073–1081. [CrossRef] [PubMed]
6. Vera, R.; Dotor, E.; Feliu, J.; González, E.; Laquente, B.; Macarulla, T.; Maurel, J. SEOM Clinical Guideline for the treatment of pancreatic cancer (2016). *Clin. Trans. Oncol.* **2016**, *18*, 1172–1178. [CrossRef] [PubMed]
7. Zeng, S.; Pöttler, M.; Lan, B.; Grützmann, R.; Pilarsky, C.; Yang, H. Chemoresistance in Pancreatic Cancer. *Int. J. Mol. Sci.* **2019**, *20*, 4504. [CrossRef]
8. Vagin, V.V.; Sigova, A.; Li, C.; Seitz, H.; Gvozdev, V.; Zamore, P.D. A distinct small RNA pathway silences selfish genetic elements in the germline. *Science* **2006**, *313*, 320–324. [CrossRef]
9. Sasaki, T.; Shiohama, A.; Minoshima, S.; Shimizu, N. Identification of eight members of the Argonaute family in the human genome. *Genomics* **2003**, *82*, 323–330. [CrossRef]
10. Farazi, T.A.; Juranek, S.A.; Tuschl, T. The growing catalog of small RNAs and their association with distinct Argonaute/Piwi family members. *Development* **2008**, *135*, 1201–1214. [CrossRef]
11. Gomes Fernandes, M.; He, N.; Wang, F.; Van Iperen, L.; Eguizabal, C.; Matorras, R.; Roelen, B.A.J. Human-specific subcellular compartmentalization of P-element induced wimpy testis-like (PIWIL) granules during germ cell development and spermatogenesis. *Hum. Reprod.* **2018**, *33*, 258–269. [CrossRef] [PubMed]
12. Siomi, M.C.; Sato, K.; Pezic, D.; Aravin, A.A. PIWI-interacting small RNAs: The vanguard of genome defence. *Nat. Rev. Mol. Cell Biol.* **2011**, *12*, 246–258. [CrossRef] [PubMed]
13. Han, Y.-N.; Li, Y.; Xia, S.-Q.; Zhang, Y.-Y.; Zheng, J.-H.; Li, W. PIWI Proteins and PIWI-Interacting RNA: Emerging Roles in Cancer. *Cell Physiol. Biochem.* **2017**, *44*, 1–20. [CrossRef] [PubMed]
14. Xie, Y.; Yang, Y.; Ji, D.; Zhang, D.; Yao, X.; Zhang, X. Hiwi downregulation, mediated by shRNA, reduces the proliferation and migration of human hepatocellular carcinoma cells. *Mol. Med. Rep.* **2015**, *11*, 1455–1461. [CrossRef] [PubMed]
15. Siddiqi, S.; Terry, M.; Matushansky, I. Hiwi Mediated Tumorigenesis Is Associated with DNA Hypermethylation. *PLoS ONE* **2012**, *7*, e33711. [CrossRef] [PubMed]
16. Gao, C.; Sun, R.; Li, D.; Gong, F. PIWI-like protein 1 upregulation promotes gastric cancer invasion and metastasis. *Onco Targets Ther.* **2018**, *11*, 8783–8789. [CrossRef]
17. Xie, K.; Zhang, K.; Kong, J.; Wang, C.; Gu, Y.; Liang, C.; Qin, N.; Liu, M.; Ma, H.; Dai, J.; et al. Cancer-testis gene PIWIL1 promotes cell proliferation, migration, and invasion in lung adenocarcinoma. *Cancer Med.* **2017**, *7*, 157–166. [CrossRef]
18. Wang, Y.; Liu, J.; Wu, G.; Yang, F. Manipulations in HIWI level exerts influence on the proliferation of human non-small cell lung cancer cells. *Exp. Ther. Med.* **2016**, *11*, 1971–1976. [CrossRef]
19. Wang, Y.; Jiang, Y.; Ma, N.; Sang, B.; Hu, X.; Cong, X. Overexpression of Hiwi Inhibits the Growth and Migration of Chronic Myeloid Leukemia Cells. *Cell Biochem. Biophys.* **2015**, *73*, 117–124. [CrossRef]
20. Li, W.; Martinez-Useros, J.; Garcia-Carbonero, N.; Fernandez-Aceñero, M.J.; Ortega-Medina, L.; Garcia-Botella, S. The Prognosis Value of PIWIL1 and PIWIL2 Expression in Pancreatic Cancer. *J. Clin. Med.* **2019**, *8*, 1275. [CrossRef]
21. Chen, C.; Liu, J.; Xu, G. Overexpression of PIWI proteins in human stage III epithelial ovarian cancer with lymph node metastasis. *Cancer Biomark.* **2013**, *13*, 315–321. [CrossRef] [PubMed]
22. Krishnan, P.; Ghosh, S.; Graham, K.; Mackey, J.R.; Kovalchuk, O.; Damaraju, S. Piwi-interacting RNAs and PIWI genes as novel prognostic markers for breast cancer. *Oncotarget* **2016**, *7*, 37944–37956. [CrossRef] [PubMed]
23. Gambichler, T.; Kohsik, C.; Höh, A.-K.; Lang, K.; Käfferlein, H.U.; Brüning, T. Expression of PIWIL3 in primary and metastatic melanoma. *J. Cancer Res. Clin. Oncol.* **2017**, *143*, 433–437. [CrossRef] [PubMed]
24. Jiang, L.; Wang, W.-J.; Li, Z.-W.; Wang, X.-Z. Downregulation of Piwil3 suppresses cell proliferation, migration and invasion in gastric cancer. *Cancer Biomark.* **2017**, *20*, 499–509. [CrossRef] [PubMed]
25. Liu, X.; Zheng, J.; Xue, Y.; Yu, H.; Gong, W.; Wang, P.; Li, Z. PIWIL3/OIP5-AS1/miR-367-3p/CEBPA feedback loop regulates the biological behavior of glioma cells. *Theranostics* **2018**, *8*, 1084–1105. [CrossRef] [PubMed]
26. Sugimoto, K.; Kage, H.; Aki, N.; Sano, A.; Kitagawa, H.; Nagase, T. The induction of H3K9 methylation by PIWIL4 at the p16Ink4a locus. *Biochem. Biophys. Res. Commun.* **2007**, *359*, 497–502. [CrossRef]
27. Coley, W.; Van Duyne, R.; Carpio, L.; Guendel, I.; Kehn-Hall, K.; Chevalier, S. Absence of DICER in monocytes and its regulation by HIV-1. *J. Biol. Chem.* **2010**, *285*, 31930–31943. [CrossRef]

28. Henaoui, I.S.; Jacovetti, C.; Guerra Mollet, I.; Guay, C.; Sobel, J.; Eliasson, L. PIWI-interacting RNAs as novel regulators of pancreatic beta cell function. *Diabetologia* **2017**, *60*, 1977–1986. [CrossRef]
29. Li, L.; Yu, C.; Gao, H.; Li, Y. Argonaute proteins: Potential biomarkers for human colon cancer. *BMC Cancer* **2010**, *10*, 38. [CrossRef]
30. Su, C.; Ren, Z.-J.; Wang, F.; Liu, M.; Li, X.; Tang, H. PIWIL4 regulates cervical cancer cell line growth and is involved in down-regulating the expression of p14ARF and p53. *FEBS Lett.* **2012**, *586*, 1356–1362. [CrossRef]
31. Wang, Y.; Liu, Y.; Shen, X.; Zhang, X.; Chen, X.; Yang, C.; Chen, X.M. The PIWI protein acts as a predictive marker for human gastric cancer. *Int. J. Clin. Exp. Pathol.* **2012**, *5*, 315–325. [PubMed]
32. Wang, Q.; Hao, J.; Pu, J.; Zhao, L.; Lü, Z.; Hu, J. Icariin induces apoptosis in mouse MLTC-10 Leydig tumor cells through activation of the mitochondrial pathway and down-regulation of the expression of piwil4. *Int. J. Oncol.* **2011**, *39*, 973–980. [PubMed]
33. Heng, Z.S.L.; Lee, J.Y.; Subhramanyam, C.S.; Wang, C.; Thanga, L.Z.; Hu, Q. The role of 17β-estradiol-induced upregulation of Piwi-like 4 in modulating gene expression and motility in breast cancer cells. *Oncol. Rep.* **2018**, *40*, 2525–2535. [CrossRef] [PubMed]
34. Wang, Z.; Liu, N.; Shi, S.; Liu, S.; Lin, H. The Role of PIWIL4, an Argonaute Family Protein, in Breast Cancer. *J. Biol. Chem.* **2016**, *291*, 10646–10658. [CrossRef]
35. Zeng, G.; Zhang, D.; Liu, X.; Kang, Q.; Fu, Y.; Tang, B.; Guo, W.; Zhang, Y.; Wei, G.; He, D.; et al. Co-expression of Piwil2/Piwil4 in nucleus indicates poor prognosis of hepatocellular carcinoma. *Oncotarget* **2017**, *8*, 4607–4617. [CrossRef]
36. Kitagawa, N.; Ojima, H.; Shirakihara, T.; Shimizu, H.; Kokubu, A.; Urushidate, T. Downregulation of the microRNA biogenesis components and its association with poor prognosis in hepatocellular carcinoma. *Cancer Sci.* **2013**, *104*, 543–551. [CrossRef]
37. Greither, T.; Koser, F.; Kappler, M.; Bache, M.; Lautenschläger, C.; Göbel, S. Expression of human Piwi-like genes is associated with prognosis for soft tissue sarcoma patients. *BMC Cancer* **2012**, *12*, 272. [CrossRef]
38. Navarro, A.; Tejero, R.; Viñolas, N.; Cordeiro, A.; Marrades, R.M.; Fuster, D.; Caritg, O.; Molins, L. The significance of PIWI family expression in human lung embryogenesis and non-small cell lung cancer. *Oncotarget* **2015**, *6*, 31544–31556. [CrossRef]
39. Iliev, R.; Stanik, M.; Fedorko, M.; Poprach, A.; Vychytilova-Faltejskova, P.; Slaba, K. Decreased expression levels of PIWIL1, PIWIL2, and PIWIL4 are associated with worse survival in renal cell carcinoma patients. *Onco Targets Ther.* **2016**, *9*, 217–222.
40. Ferreira, H.J.; Heyn, H.; Garcia del Muro, X.; Vidal, A.; Larriba, S.; Muñoz, C. Epigenetic loss of the PIWI/piRNA machinery in human testicular tumorigenesis. *Epigenetics* **2014**, *9*, 113–118. [CrossRef]
41. Chen, H.-C. Boyden Chamber Assay. *Methods Mol. Biol.* **2005**, *294*, 15–22. [PubMed]
42. Awasthi, N.; Zhang, C.; Schwarz, A.M.; Hinz, S.; Wang, C.; Williams, N.S.; Schwarz, M.N.; Schwarz, R.E. Comparative benefits of Nab-paclitaxel over gemcitabine or polysorbate-based docetaxel in experimental pancreatic cancer. *Carcinogenesis* **2013**, *34*, 2361–2369. [CrossRef] [PubMed]
43. Spratlin, J.; Sangha, R.; Glubrecht, D.; Dabbagh, L.; Young, J.D.; Dumontet, C. The absence of human equilibrative nucleoside transporter 1 is associated with reduced survival in patients with gemcitabine-treated pancreas adenocarcinoma. *Clin. Cancer Res.* **2004**, *10*, 6956–6961. [CrossRef] [PubMed]
44. Gao, J.; Aksoy, B.A.; Dogrusoz, U.; Dresdner, G.; Gross, B.; Sumer, S.O.; Sinha, R. Integrative analysis of complex cancer genomics and clinical profiles using the cBioPortal. *Sci. Signal* **2013**, *6*, pl1. [CrossRef] [PubMed]
45. Cerami, E.; Gao, J.; Dogrusoz, U.; Gross, B.E.; Sumer, S.O.; Aksoy, B.A. The cBio cancer genomics portal: An open platform for exploring multidimensional cancer genomics data. *Cancer Discov.* **2012**, *2*, 401–404. [CrossRef]
46. Sun, Q.; Xu, W.; Ji, S.; Qin, Y.; Liu, W.; Hu, Q.; Zhang, Z.; Liu, M.; Yu, X.; Xu, X.; et al. Role of hepatocyte nuclear factor 4 alpha in cell proliferation and gemcitabine resistance in pancreatic adenocarcinoma. *Cancer Cell Int.* **2019**, *19*, 49. [CrossRef]
47. Martinez-Useros, J.; Garcia-Foncillas, J. Can Molecular Biomarkers Change the Paradigm of Pancreatic Cancer Prognosis? *Biomed. Res. Int.* **2016**, *2016*, 4873089. [CrossRef]

48. Human hg38 chr12:130329199-130381325 UCSC Genome Browser v396. Available online: https://genome.ucsc.edu/cgi-bin/hgTracks?db=hg38&lastVirtModeType=default&lastVirtModeExtraState=&virtModeType=default&virtMode=0&nonVirtPosition=&position=chr12%3A130329199%2D130381325&hgsid=823730117_z8PjbiTzqWd3ZdNvqbZjD0RPpY1I (accessed on 6 March 2020).
49. Human hg38 chr8:22275316-22357568 UCSC Genome Browser v395. Available online: https://genome.ucsc.edu/cgi-bin/hgTracks?db=hg38&lastVirtModeType=default&lastVirtModeExtraState=&virtModeType=default&virtMode=0&nonVirtPosition=&position=chr8%3A22275316%2D22357568&hgsid=813260055_s97A3RqtBxTmk9YMuex2A8Ay0wgb (accessed on 6 March 2020).
50. Sohn, E.J.; Jo, Y.R.; Park, H.T. Downregulation MIWI-piRNA regulates the migration of Schwann cells in peripheral nerve injury. *Biochem. Biophys. Res. Commun.* **2019**, *519*, 605–612. [CrossRef]
51. Heyn, H.; Ferreira, H.J.; Bassas, L.; Bonache, S.; Sayols, S.; Sandoval, J. Epigenetic Disruption of the PIWI Pathway in Human Spermatogenic Disorders. *PLoS ONE* **2012**, *7*, e47892. [CrossRef]
52. Abell, N.S.; Mercado, M.; Cañeque, T.; Rodriguez, R.; Xhemalce, B. Click Quantitative Mass Spectrometry Identifies PIWIL3 as a Mechanistic Target of RNA Interference Activator Enoxacin in Cancer Cells. *J. Am. Chem. Soc.* **2017**, *139*, 1400–1403. [CrossRef]
53. Yang, Y.; Zhang, X.; Song, D.; Wei, J. Piwil2 modulates the invasion and metastasis of prostate cancer by regulating the expression of matrix metalloproteinase-9 and epithelial-mesenchymal transitions. *Oncol. Lett.* **2015**, *10*, 1735–1740. [CrossRef] [PubMed]
54. Ling, W.; Zhigang, H.; Tian, H.; Bin, Z.; Xiaolin, X.; Hongxiu, Z. HPV 16 infection up-regulates Piwil2, which affects cell proliferation and invasion in cervical cancer by regulating MMP-9 via the MAPK pathway. *Eur. J. Gynaecol. Oncol.* **2015**, *36*, 647–654. [PubMed]
55. Tan, L.; Mai, D.; Zhang, B.; Jiang, X.; Zhang, J.; Bai, R.; Zhao, Q.; Li, X.X.; Yang, J.; Li, D.X.; et al. PIWI-interacting RNA-36712 restrains breast cancer progression and chemoresistance by interaction with SEPW1 pseudogene SEPW1P RNA. *Mol. Cancer* **2019**, *18*, 9. [CrossRef]
56. Cheng, J.; Deng, H.; Xiao, B.; Zhou, H.; Zhou, F.; Shen, Z. piR-823, a novel non-coding small RNA, demonstrates in vitro and in vivo tumor suppressive activity in human gastric cancer cells. *Cancer Lett.* **2012**, *315*, 12–17. [CrossRef] [PubMed]
57. Yin, J.; Jiang, X.; Qi, W.; Ji, C.; Xie, X.; Zhang, D. piR-823 contributes to colorectal tumorigenesis by enhancing the transcriptional activity of HSF1. *Cancer Sci.* **2017**, *108*, 1746–1756. [CrossRef] [PubMed]
58. Li, D.; Luo, Y.; Gao, Y.; Yang, Y.; Wang, Y.; Xu, Y.; Tan, S.; Zhang, Y.; Duan, J.; Yang, Y. piR-651 promotes tumor formation in non-small cell lung carcinoma through the upregulation of cyclin D1 and CDK4. *Int. J. Mol. Med.* **2016**, *38*, 927–936. [CrossRef] [PubMed]
59. Kalluri, R.; Neilson, E.G. Epithelial-mesenchymal transition and its implications for fibrosis. *J. Clin. Investig.* **2003**, *112*, 1776–1784. [CrossRef] [PubMed]
60. López-Novoa, J.M.; Nieto, M.A. Inflammation and EMT: An alliance towards organ fibrosis and cancer progression. *EMBO Mol. Med.* **2009**, *1*, 303–314. [CrossRef]
61. Joglekar, M.V.; Hardikar, A. Epithelial-to-mesenchymal transition in pancreatic islet β cells. *Cell Cycle* **2010**, *9*, 4077–4079. [CrossRef]
62. Klattenhoff, C.; Theurkauf, W. Biogenesis and germline functions of piRNAs. *Development* **2008**, *135*, 3–9. [CrossRef]
63. Rojas-Ríos, P.; Simonelig, M. piRNAs and PIWI proteins: Regulators of gene expression in development and stem cells. *Development* **2018**, *145*, 1–13. [CrossRef] [PubMed]
64. Lee, J.H.; Jung, C.; Javadian-Elyaderani, P.; Schweyer, S.; Schütte, D.; Shoukier, M.; Navernia, K. Pathways of Proliferation and Antiapoptosis Driven in Breast Cancer Stem Cells by Stem Cell Protein Piwil2. *Cancer Res.* **2010**, *70*, 4569–4579. [CrossRef] [PubMed]
65. Rinkevich, Y.; Voskoboynik, A.; Rosner, A.; Rabinowitz, C.; Paz, G.; Oren, M. Repeated, long-term cycling of putative stem cells between niches in a basal chordate. *Dev. Cell* **2013**, *24*, 76–88. [CrossRef] [PubMed]
66. Liu, W.; Gao, Q.; Chen, K.; Xue, X.; Li, M.; Chen, Q.; Zhu, G.; Gao, Y. Hiwi facilitates chemoresistance as a cancer stem cell marker in cervical cancer. *Oncol. Rep.* **2014**, *32*, 1853–1860. [CrossRef]
67. Wang, Y.; Gable, T.; Ma, M.Z.; Clark, D.; Zhao, J.; Zhang, Y. A piRNA-like Small RNA Induces Chemoresistance to Cisplatin-Based Therapy by Inhibiting Apoptosis in Lung Squamous Cell Carcinoma. *Mol. Ther. Nucleic Acids* **2017**, *6*, 269–278. [CrossRef]

68. Wang, H.; Mao, C.; Li, N.; Sun, L.; Zheng, Y.; Xu, N. A case report of a dramatic response to olaparib in a patient with metastatic pancreatic cancer harboring a germline BRCA2 mutation. *Medicine* **2019**, *98*, e17443. [CrossRef]
69. Wang, H.; Word, B.R.; Lyn-Cook, B.D. Enhanced Efficacy of Gemcitabine by Indole-3-carbinol in Pancreatic Cell Lines: The Role of Human Equilibrative Nucleoside Transporter 1. *Anticancer. Res.* **2011**, *31*, 3171–3180.
70. Stoffel, M.; Duncan, S.A. The maturity-onset diabetes of the young (MODY1) transcription factor HNF4alpha regulates expression of genes required for glucose transport and metabolism. *Proc. Natl. Acad. Sci. USA* **1997**, *94*, 13209–13214. [CrossRef]
71. Hamdan, F.H.; Zihlif, M.A. Gene expression alterations in chronic hypoxic MCF7 breast cancer cell line. *Genomics* **2014**, *104*, 477–481. [CrossRef]
72. Kiselyuk, A.; Lee, S.-H.; Farber-Katz, S.; Zhang, M.; Athavankar, S.; Cohen, T. HNF4α antagonists discovered by a high-throughput screen for modulators of the human insulin promoter. *Chem. Biol.* **2012**, *19*, 806–818. [CrossRef]
73. Tissue Expression of PIWIL3—Staining in Pancreas—The Human Protein Atlas version 19.3. Available online: https://www.proteinatlas.org/ENSG00000184571-PIWIL3/tissue/pancreas (accessed on 6 March 2020).
74. Tissue Expression of PIWIL4—Staining in Pancreas—The Human Protein Atlas version 19.3. Available online: https://www.proteinatlas.org/ENSG00000134627-PIWIL4/tissue/pancreas (accessed on 6 March 2020).
75. Egawa, S.; Takeda, K.; Fukuyama, S.; Motoi, F.; Sunamura, M.; Matsuno, S. Clinicopathological Aspects of Small Pancreatic Cancer. *Pancreas* **2004**, *28*, 235–240. [CrossRef] [PubMed]
76. Ariyama, J.; Suyama, M.; Satoh, K.; Sai, J. Imaging of Small Pancreatic Ductal Adenocarcinoma. *Pancreas* **1998**, *16*, 396–401. [CrossRef] [PubMed]

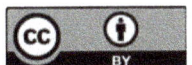

© 2020 by the authors. Licensee MDPI, Basel, Switzerland. This article is an open access article distributed under the terms and conditions of the Creative Commons Attribution (CC BY) license (http://creativecommons.org/licenses/by/4.0/).

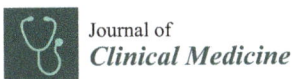

Article

Serotonin-Secreting Neuroendocrine Tumours of the Pancreas

Anna Caterina Milanetto [1,*], Matteo Fassan [2], Alina David [1] and Claudio Pasquali [1]

1. Pancreatic and Endocrine Digestive Surgical Unit, Department of Surgery, Oncology and Gastroenterology, University of Padua, via Giustiniani, 2-35128 Padua, Italy; alina.david@studenti.unipd.it (A.D.); claudio.pasquali@unipd.it (C.P.)
2. Surgical Pathology Unit, Department of Medicine, University of Padua, via Giustiniani, 2-35128 Padua, Italy; matteo.fassan@unipd.it
* Correspondence: acmilanetto@unipd.it; Tel.: +39-0498-218-831

Received: 3 April 2020; Accepted: 2 May 2020; Published: 6 May 2020

Abstract: Background: Serotonin-secreting pancreatic neuroendocrine tumours (5-HT-secreting pNETs) are very rare, and characterised by high urinary 5-hydroxyindole-acetic acid (5-HIAA) levels (or high serum 5-HT levels). Methods: Patients with 5-HT-secreting pancreatic neoplasms observed in our unit (1986–2015) were included. Diagnosis was based on urinary 5-HIAA or serum 5-HT levels. Results: Seven patients were enrolled (4 M/3 F), with a median age of 64 (range 38–69) years. Two patients had a carcinoid syndrome. Serum 5-HT was elevated in four patients. Urinary 5-HIAA levels were positive in six patients. The median tumour size was 4.0 (range 2.5–10) cm. All patients showed liver metastases at diagnosis. None underwent resective surgery; lymph node/liver biopsies were taken. Six lesions were well-differentiated tumours and one a poorly differentiated carcinoma (Ki67 range 3.4–70%). All but one patient received chemotherapy. Four patients received somatostatin analogues; three patients underwent ablation of liver metastases. One patient is alive with disease 117 months after observation. All the others died from disease progression after a follow-up within 158 months. Conclusions: Primary 5-HT-secreting pNETs are mostly metastatic to the liver; patients are not amenable to resective surgery. Despite high 5-HIAA urinary levels, few patients present with carcinoid syndrome. A five-year survival rate of 42.9% may be achieved with multimodal treatment.

Keywords: pancreatic neuroendocrine neoplasm; primary pancreatic carcinoid; serotonin-secreting pancreatic tumour; serotonin-producing pancreatic tumour

1. Introduction

"Carcinoid tumours" were originally classified into foregut (including those arising in the pancreas), midgut and hindgut tumours, according to their embryologic origin [1]. The term "carcinoid" has been used for a long time to indicate midgut or small intestinal neuroendocrine tumours (NETs), which produce serotonin (5-HT), and cause the typical "carcinoid syndrome". These NETs can be identified by twenty-four-hour measurement of urinary 5-hydroxyindole-acetic acid (5-HIAA), which has an 88% specificity for 5-HT-producing NETs [2].

Pancreatic NETs (pNETs) may show positive immunostaining for hormones, neuropeptides and amines, including 5-HT [3,4], and about 4–8% of small pNETs can show a variable portion of cells staining for 5-HT [5,6], even if they are non-functioning (in which case the patient will not complain of symptoms related to hormonal hypersecretion). Recently, small pNETs with a positive 5-HT staining have been called "serotoninomas" [7], while La Rosa [6] in 2011 proposed the term "5-HT-producing EC cell tumours of the pancreas".

In the literature, there are different definitions of "pancreatic carcinoids", and it is not always clear whether reports refer to 5-HT-secreting, or 5-HT-staining pancreatic tumours. The term "foregut carcinoid", used before the year 2000, includes pNETs with normal levels of 5-HT and urinary 5-HIAA [8], and some pancreatic adenocarcinomas with neuroendocrine differentiation and carcinoid-like symptoms [9,10]. Therefore, it is difficult to estimate the actual incidence and prevalence of 5-HT-secreting tumours of the pancreas.

The aim of the present study is to focus on pancreatic NETs secreting 5-HT, rare entities that may be defined as "5-HT-secreting pNETs" and diagnosed in the presence of a pancreatic mass, an increased urinary 5-HIAA level above the upper limit of normal, and/or an increased serum 5-HT level. The experience of a single high-volume pancreatic and referral centre for NETs is analysed, and the clinic-pathological features, treatment and prognosis of these patients are discussed.

2. Methods

Clinical records of patients who were observed for a 5-HT-secreting pNET from January 1986 to December 2015 in our unit were retrieved. The diagnosis of 5-HT-secreting pNET was made in the presence of a pancreatic mass assessed by imaging studies, an increased urinary 5-HIAA level above the upper limit of normal, and/or an increased serum 5-HT level. Patients with only a positive 5-HT immunostaining should be defined as having a non-functioning 5-HT-staining pNET, and were not included in the present study. Patients were diagnosed with a pNET using the following imaging studies: computed tomography-CT scan, magnetic resonance imaging-MRI, 111In-Scintigraphy and/or 18F-FDG positron emission tomography (PET)/CT. Patients presenting with a pNET and a concomitant small intestinal NET, or who had previously been operated on for a small intestinal NET, were not included in the present study. At the time of initial evaluation, plasma and urine samples of the patients were assayed for 5-HT and 5-HIAA, respectively, which since 1992 has been carried out using high-pressure liquid chromatography. Serotonin levels were measured in serum after separation of platelets, apart from the first patient (case n.1), for whom an old radiometric method was used.

The following data were analysed: age, gender, medical history and clinical presentation, blood and urinary tests (serum 5-HT, 24-h urinary 5-HIAA, and other serum tumour markers and gastrointestinal hormones), tumour location in the pancreas, and type of surgery or tumour biopsy. The diagnosis and grading of pancreatic neuroendocrine neoplasms were carried out according to the World Health Organization (WHO) 2019 Classification of Digestive System Tumours [11] and the European Neuroendocrine Tumor Society (ENETS) TNM classification [12]. In particular, tumour size (cm), lymph node metastases (Nx, N0, N1), distant metastases (Mx, M0, M1) and tumour grade (G1, G2 and G3, assessed by mitotic index and Ki67 labelling index) were evaluated. Immunohistochemical analysis was performed for synaptophysin, chromogranin A (CgA) and neuron-specific enolase (NSE), and for expression of other hormones and neuroendocrine markers (insulin, glucagon, somatostatin, pancreatic polypeptide, 5-HT, gastrin, vasoactive intestinal peptide and calcitonin).

All the patients had a regular follow-up, with clinical evaluation, blood and urinary tests (in particular, serum 5-HT and urinary 5-HIAA) and imaging studies as above (including ^{68}Ga-DOTA-peptide PET/CT) to define the extent of the tumour and detect any tumour progression. Other non-surgical treatments, liver metastases embolisation or ablation treatments were recorded. Overall survival (OS) was evaluated in all patients, based on death certificates, or if still living either using a telephone interview or at the last follow-up visit. Follow-up closed in December 2019. Survival curves were estimated using the Kaplan–Meier method. The research was conducted ethically in accordance with the World Medical Association Declaration of Helsinki. Subjects have given their written informed consent to data processing anonymously for research purposes. The ethics committee of the Azienda Ospedaliera di Padova approved the present study (project code: 2872p).

3. Results

3.1. Patient Characteristics and Laboratory Diagnosis

Among 239 patients with a histologically confirmed pNET observed in our unit during the study period, seven (2.9%) patients had a 5-HT-secreting pNET. The study population consisted of four men and three women, with a median age of 64 (range 38–69) years. Only two patients had symptoms related to a carcinoid syndrome with flushing and diarrhoea (Figure 1); all the others presented with a non-functioning pNET. The leading presenting symptom was weight loss in three (43%) patients, and two (29%) patients complained about abdominal pain (Figure 2). One patient had a cervical lymphadenopathy, and another presented with jaundice and ascites due to portal vein thrombosis (Figure 3).

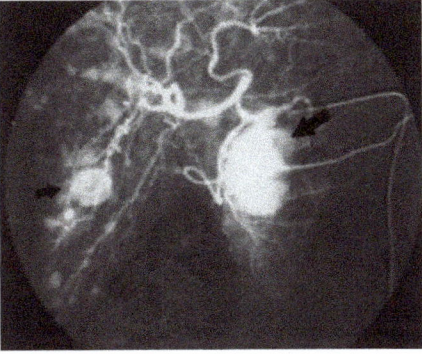

Figure 1. Angiography of the celiac trunk showing a mass in the pancreatic head (big arrow) and multiple liver metastases (small arrow) in a patient with carcinoid syndrome (case n.1).

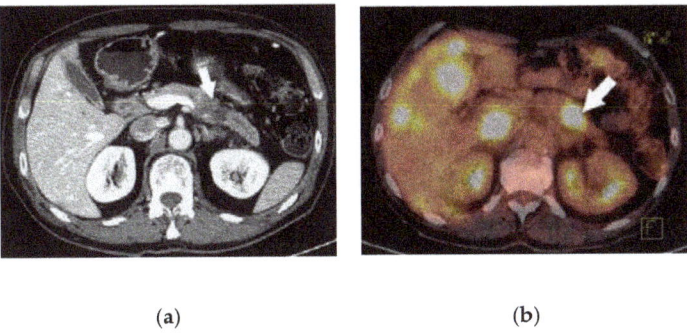

(a)   (b)

Figure 2. Computed tomography scan 2 (a) and ^{18}F-FDG positron emission tomography/CT 2 (b) showing a pancreatic neuroendocrine tumor in the body of the pancreas (white arrow) with multiple liver metastases (case n.7).

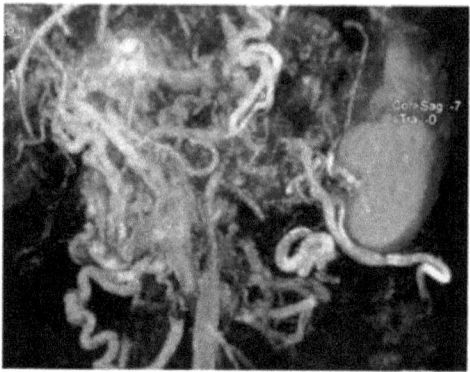

Figure 3. Abdominal magnetic resonance imaging showing several huge mesenteric and left gastric vein compensation collateral circles due to portal vein thrombosis and portal hypertension (case n.6).

Six patients had increased urinary 5-HIAA levels (up to 18x the upper limit of normal), and four patients had an increased serum 5-HT (up to 5x the upper limit of normal). Notably, four patients with high urinary 5-HIAA levels, two of them also with increased serum 5-HT levels, had no symptoms related to a carcinoid syndrome. Some patients showed a co-secretion of other peptides: four patients had an increased serum CgA, and three had raised calcitonin levels (Table 1).

Table 1. Clinical presentation and laboratory tests at diagnosis in patients with serotonin-secreting pancreatic NETs.

No.	Obs	Gender/Age	Clinical Presentation	Carcinoid Syndrome	24-h Urinary 5-HIAA *	Serum 5-HT *	Other Serum NE Markers and GI Hormones	
							normal	elevated
1	1986	F/67	Abdominal pain	Yes (flushing, diarrhoea)	n.a.	5.1x	Gastrin, Glucagon, Calcitonin	NSE
2	1995	M/64	Asymptomatic	No	12.3x	3.8x	Gastrin	NSE, Calcitonin
3	1999	M/69	n.a.	n.a.	5.2x	n.a.	NSE, Insulin, Gastrin, Calcitonin	no
4	2002	M/44	Weight loss, dyspepsia	No diarrhoea	1.8x	n.a.	NSE, Gastrin	CgA, Glucagon, Calcitonin
5	2004	F/44	Cervical lymphadenopathy	No	6.7x	n.a.	NSE, Insulin	CgA
6	2010	F/38	Weight loss, jaundice, portal vein thrombosis, ascites, fatigue	Yes (flushing, diarrhoea)	17.4x	1.3x	NSE, SS, VIP, Calcitonin	CgA, Gastrin
7	2011	M/68	Abdominal pain, weight loss, fatigue	No diarrhoea	4.5x	2.1x	Gastrin	CgA, NSE, Calcitonin

Obs year of observation, F female, M male, n.a. not applicable, 5-HIAA 5-hydroxyndoleacetic acid, 5-HT 5-hydroxytryptamine, NE neuroendocrine, GI gastrointestinal, NSE neuron specific enolase, SS somatostatin, VIP vasoactive intestinal peptide, CgA chromogranin A. * Expressed as "times the upper limit of normal".

3.2. Histology and Immunohistochemical Features

The median primary tumour size was 4.0 (range 2.5–10) cm, and the primary tumour was located in the pancreatic body in four out of seven cases. Despite all patients showing bilobar liver metastases at diagnosis, only two presented with a carcinoid syndrome. None of the patients underwent a pancreatic resection. Therefore, final diagnosis of pNET was made in five patients after a liver biopsy and in the others by lymph node biopsies. Tumour grading (used since 1998) was available in three cases, two G2 NETs (3.4% and 16%) and one G3 NET (70%). Of the other four cases, three were well-differentiated NETs and one was a poorly differentiated large cell neuroendocrine carcinoma (NEC). In particular, the NEC was characterised by a solid growth pattern, large areas of necrosis and large polygonal cells having amphophilic cytoplasm, vesicular chromatin and prominent nucleoli. Data on immunohistochemical analysis were available in five cases, all of them showing a positivity for CgA; in addition, two patients had a positive 5-HT staining (Figure 4). Unfortunately, no remaining tissue was available to perform 5-HT staining, or to detect the other peptides secreted by the tumour.

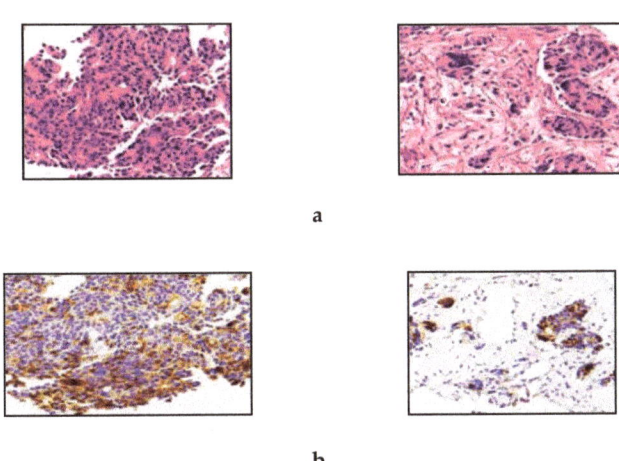

Figure 4. Representative hematoxylin and eosin stain 4 (**a**) and serotonin immunostaining 4 (**b**) of case n.7. The neoplasia was characterized by a trabecular pattern of growth, high mitotic activity (MIB1-labelling index > 70%), areas of necrosis, and high-grade cytonuclear pleomorphism. A final diagnosis of G3 neuroendocrine tumour (NET G3) was reached. The lesion showed a heterogeneous serotonin pattern of staining, which was positive in most neoplastic cells (original magnifications, 20×).

3.3. Prognosis and Follow-Up

All the patients were evaluated in terms of OS, after a median follow-up of 29 (range 5–158) months. Four patients were treated with somatostatin analogues (SS-A), two of whom had a carcinoid syndrome and showed an improvement of symptoms. Three patients also underwent a local ablation of liver metastases (trans-arterial (chemo)-embolisation, microwave ablation), and all but one patient received polychemotherapy regimens. Multimodal treatment with chemotherapy, SS-A and/or loco-regional liver ablation was performed in all the patients, and they demonstrated, occasionally, a long survival (up to 158 months). One patient is still alive with the disease at late evaluation 117 months after diagnosis. All the others died due to disease progression after a median follow-up of 22.5 (range 5–158) months Table 2. Disease-related survival at 1, 3 and 5 years was 71.4%, 42.9% and 42.9%, respectively (Table 2).

Table 2. Pathological findings and follow-up in patients with serotonin-secreting pancreatic NETs.

No.	Pancreatic Site Size (cm)	Distant Metastases	Biopsy	TNM Stage [12]	NET/NEC Ki67	Immunohistochemistry Positive	Immunohistochemistry Negative	Other Therapies	Follow-Up (Months)	Status
1	Head 4.0	Bilobar liver	Liver	T2 Nx M1 IV	NET n.a.	5-HT 20–20–30% Grimelius	Insulin, Gastrin, PP	SS-A, CT [a]	158	DOD
2	Tail 2.5	Bilobar liver	Liver	T2 Nx M1 IV	NET n.a.	CgA	n.a.	TACE	12	DOD
3	Body 4.0	Bilobar liver, mediastinal LN	Liver	T2 N1 M1 IV	NET n.a.	CgA, Grimelius	n.a.	CT [b]	29	DOD
4	Tail 6.0	Bilobar liver	Abdominal LN	T3 N1 M1 IV	NET 3.4%	CgA, Syn, NSE	5-HT, Insulin, Gastrin, Glucagon, SS, PP, Calcitonin	SS-A, CT [b], TAE, PRRT	96	DOD
5	Body 10.0	Bilobar liver, cervical LN	Cervical LN	T4 N1 M1 IV	NEC n.a.	n.a.	n.a.	SS-A, CT [c]	16	DOD
6	Body 4.0	Bilobar liver	Liver	T2 N1 M1 IV	NET 16%	CgA, Syn	n.a.	Biliary stent SS-A, CT [d] Liver MW Everolimus	117	AWD
7	Body 3.6	Bilobar liver	Liver	T2 Nx M1 IV	NET 70%	5-HT, CgA, Syn, Calcitonin	NSE, Insulin, Gastrin, Glucagon, SS, PP, VIP	CT [e]	5	DOD

LN lymph node, NET neuroendocrine tumour, NEC neuroendocrine carcinoma, n.a. not applicable, 5-HT 5-hydroxytryptamine, CgA chromogranin A, Syn synaptophysin, NSE neuron specific enolase, PP pancreatic polypeptide, SS somatostatin, VIP vasoactive intestinal peptide, SS-A somatostatin analogue, CT chemotherapy, TACE transarterial chemoembolisation, TAE transarterial embolisation, PRRT peptide receptor radionuclide therapy, MW microwave, DOD died of disease, AWD alive with disease. [a] Dacarbazine. [b] not available. [c] First line: paclitaxel, cisplatin, and gemcitabine; second line: doxorubicin and streptozotocin. [d] First line: 5-fluorouracil, dacarbazine, and epirubicin; second line: capecitabine. [e] Epirubicin, 5-fluorouracil and dacarbazine.

4. Discussion

The old term "pancreatic carcinoids", corresponding to 5-HT-producing pNETs, accounts for 0.58% to 1.4% of two large series of "carcinoids" [13,14], but it is difficult to estimate the actual incidence of 5-HT-secreting pNETs, because pNETs causing a clinically evident carcinoid syndrome are very rare [6]. In fact, in a large series of so-called "pancreatic carcinoids", Soga et al. [14] observed only 23% of patients complaining of a carcinoid syndrome.

Currently, 5-HT staining and urinary 5-HIAA measurement are not routinely tested or recommended in pNETs [6,7,15]; it is likely that the true incidence and prevalence of 5-HT-producing/secreting pNETs may be underestimated. In our experience, the systematic measurement of urinary 5-HIAA or serum 5-HT in patients with a pNET (although asymptomatic) allowed the selection of a subset of primary pNETs with an excess of 5-HT secretion in the bloodstream, revealed by the excretion of its urinary metabolite 5-HIAA.

In our series, patients were affected by large pNETs (median size 4 cm, up to 10 cm in size), with multiple liver metastases at presentation. A similar rate of liver metastases (95%) in 22 patients with 5-HT-secreting pNETs has been reported by Zandee et al. [16]. Despite liver metastases and urinary 5-HIAA levels increasing to up to 18 times the upper limit of normal, in our series only two out of seven patients presented with a carcinoid syndrome. Maurer et al. [8] showed similar results in a review of 29 cases of 5-HT-secreting "pancreatic carcinoids"; in these patients, no complete typical carcinoid syndrome occurred, despite the evidence of distant metastases in 69%, and elevated urinary 5-HIAA levels in 85% of cases.

We can only speculate on the reasons why a high tumour burden and high levels of 5-HT metabolite (and thus of 5-HT secretion) are not always associated with the carcinoid syndrome: (1) no (or not enough, or with low affinity) 5-HT receptors are available in the target tissues (thus limiting its effects); (2) a hyperactivation of 5-HT clearance in specific tissue prevents any secondary effects of 5-HT. Moreover, some of the several factors and substances involved in the development of carcinoid syndrome may be lacking or inactive. In fact, diarrhoea and flushing in carcinoid syndrome may be due to a variety of tumour substances released, including 5-HT, tachykinins (substance P, neurokinin A and neuropeptide K) and prostaglandins [17], and several hypotheses have been proposed to explain the pathophysiology of these symptoms [18–20]. In our series, almost all patients showed a co-secretion of other hormones and substances detected in the serum, mostly CgA, NSE, calcitonin and gastrin. Zandee et al. [16] reported about 78% of patients with 5-HT-secreting pNETs with a serum CgA of more than 20 times the upper limit of normal, reflecting high tumour burden and a poor prognosis [16]. In addition, co-secretion of other ectopic hormones (i.e., calcitonin, gastrin and 5-HT) from an endocrine neoplasm may suggest a de-differentiation usually related to a more aggressive behaviour.

Multihormonal immunostaining (including 5-HT) has been found in one third of all pNETs [21]; thus, it is a common finding without prognostic significance. In our series, even a G3 NET demonstrated positive immunostaining for 5-HT, chromogranin and also for calcitonin. Unfortunately, due to the small amount of tissue in biopsy samples in our series of unresectable tumours, we were unable to perform a complete immunohistochemical analysis in all patients, selecting those studies useful to define the neuroendocrine origin and the grade of the tumour. Serotonin-secreting pNETs may originate as de-differentiated tumours with a mixed cellularity, showing a co-secretion of other substances/hormones (i.e., 5-HT, calcitonin, gastrin, substance P, neurokinins, etc.), or from pancreatic enterochromaffin cells well differentiated in 5-HT production. In fact, small numbers of EC cells producing substance P, neurokinins, and 5-HT have been found in the human pancreas, scattered in the pancreatic duct and acini [22], and even the β-cells, as well as some other islet cell types, express all the genes required to synthesise, package, and secrete 5-HT [23]. This is in line with our findings, where all but one patient had a well-differentiated pNET.

Non-functioning pNETs may show positive immunostaining for hormones, neuropeptides and amines, including 5-HT [3,4]. Serotonin-secreting pNETs have a very different prognosis from 5-HT-staining pNETs. The former (with or without associated carcinoid syndrome) are usually of large size at diagnosis and metastatic in up to 88% of cases [24], whereas 5-HT-staining pNETs are usually small, and patients can undergo surgery, providing the chance of a complete histologic and immunostaining study. In our series, no patient underwent a pancreatic resection, and all but one died from disease progression after a median time of 22.5 (range 5–158) months.

Recently, using data from the SEER database, Dasari et al. [25] reported a median OS of 3.6 years for pancreatic NETs. Notably, G1–G2 pNETs with distant metastases diagnosed between 2000 and 2012 showed a median survival of 60 months, and 3- and 5-year survival rates were 62% and 50%, respectively [25]. In the present study, after multimodal treatment consisting mainly of chemotherapy, SS-A and/or ablation of liver metastases, patients demonstrated a 5-year disease-related survival rate of 42.9%, with an occasional long survival (up to 158 months). Zandee et al. [16] observed a 5-year survival rate of 46% in patients with 5-HT-secreting pNETs. Whether high levels of urinary 5-HIAA are related to a worse prognosis in pNETs or not is unknown, and the same topic is still a matter of debate in the more frequent small intestinal NETs [26]. It has been reported that the presence of a carcinoid syndrome is associated with a worse prognosis in pNETs [6]. In our experience, the two patients presenting with a carcinoid syndrome had the longest OS; one died of disease 158 months after diagnosis and another is still alive 117 months after diagnosis.

In conclusion, 5-HT-secreting pancreatic NETs are rare entities, which include those tumours able to secrete high levels of 5-HT in the bloodstream, and consequently have high excretion of their urinary metabolite 5-HIAA. Although presenting with large pancreatic masses with liver metastases not amenable to resective surgery, patients complain of carcinoid syndrome in a minority of cases. This subset of pNETs are not associated with a worse prognosis than other stage IV pNETs reported in the literature; in fact, a five-year disease-related survival of 42.9% can be achieved with multimodal treatment.

Author Contributions: Conceptualization, A.C.M. and C.P.; Data curation, A.C.M., M.F. and A.D.; Writing—original draft, A.C.M.; Writing—review & editing, M.F. and C.P. All authors have read and agreed to the published version of the manuscript.

Funding: This research received no external funding.

Conflicts of Interest: The authors declare no conflict of interest.

References

1. Williams, E.D.; Sanders, M. The classification of carcinoid tumors. *Lancet* **1963**, *1*, 238–239. [CrossRef]
2. Gustafsson, B.I. Small Intestinal Neuroendocrine Tumours. In *A Century of Advances in Neuroendocrine Tumour Biology and Treatment*; Modlin, I.M., Ed.; Felsenstein C.C.C.P.: Hannover, Germany, 2008; p. 103.
3. Öberg, K. Non-Functioning Pancreatic Endocrine Tumour. In *A Century of Advances in Neuroendocrine Tumour Biology and Treatment*; Modlin, I.M., Ed.; Felsenstein C.C.C.P.: Hannover, Germany, 2008; p. 87.
4. Wilson, R.W.; Gal, A.A.; Cohen, C.; DeRose, P.B.; Millikan, W.J. Serotonin immunoreactivity in pancreatic endocrine neoplasms (carcinoid tumors). *Mod. Pathol.* **1991**, *4*, 727–732. [PubMed]
5. Bilimoria, K.Y.; Tomlinson, J.S.; Merkow, R.P.; Stewart, A.K.; Ko, C.Y.; Talamonti, M.S.; Bentrem, D.J. Clinicopathologic features and treatment trends of pancreatic neuroendocrine tumors: Analysis of 9,821 patients. *J. Gastrointest. Surg.* **2007**, *11*, 1460–1467. [CrossRef] [PubMed]
6. La Rosa, S.; Franzi, F.; Albarello, L.; Schmitt, A.; Bernasconi, B.; Tibiletti, M.G.; Finzi, G.; Placidi, C.; Perren, A.; Capella, C. Serotonin-producing enterochromaffin cell tumors of the pancreas: Clinicopathologic study of 15 cases and comparison with intestinal enterochromaffin cell tumors. *Pancreas* **2011**, *40*, 883–895. [CrossRef]
7. Massironi, S.; Partelli, S.; Petrone, M.C.; Zilli, A.; Conte, D.; Falconi, M.; Arcidiacono, P.G. Endoscopic ultrasound appearance of pancreatic serotonin-staining neuroendocrine neoplasms. *Pancreatology* **2018**, *18*, 792–798. [CrossRef]
8. Maurer, C.A.; Baer, H.U.; Dyong, T.H.; Mueller-Garamvoelgyi, E.; Friess, H.; Ruchti, C.; Reubi, J.C.; Büchler, M.W. Carcinoid of the pancreas: Clinical characteristics and morphological features. *Eur. J. Cancer* **1996**, *32*, 1109–1116. [CrossRef]
9. Dollinger, M.R.; Ratner, L.H.; Shamoian, C.A.; Blackboume, B.D. Carcinoid syndrome associated with pancreatic tumors. *Arch. Int. Med.* **1967**, *120*, 575–580. [CrossRef]
10. Eusebi, V.; Capella, C.; Bondi, A.; Sessa, F.; Vezzadini, P.; Mancini, A.M. Endocrine-paracrine cells in pancreatic exocrine carcinomas. *Histopathology* **1981**, *5*, 599–613. [CrossRef]
11. Digestive System Tumours. *WHO Classification of Tumours*, 5th ed.; WHO Classification of Tumours Editorial Board, Ed.; International Agency for Research on Cancer (IARC): Lyon, France, 2019.
12. Rindi, G.; Klöppel, G.; Alhman, X.; Caplin, M.; Couvelard, A.; De Herder, W.W.; Erikssson, B.; Falchetti, A.; Falconi, M.; Komminoth, P.; et al. TNM staging of foregut (neuro)endocrine tumors: A consensus proposal including a grading system. *Virchows Arch* **2006**, *449*, 395–401. [CrossRef]
13. Modlin, I.M.; Lye, K.D.; Kidd, M. A 5-decade analysis of 13,715 carcinoid tumors. *Cancer* **2003**, *97*, 934–959. [CrossRef]
14. Soga, J. Carcinoids of the pancreas: An analysis of 156 cases. *Cancer* **2005**, *104*, 1180–1187. [CrossRef] [PubMed]
15. Falconi, M.; Eriksson, B.; Kaltsas, G.; Bartsch, D.K.; Capdevila, J.; Caplin, M.; Kos-Kudla, B.; Kwekkeboom, D.; Rindi, G.; Klöppel, G.; et al. ENETS consensus guidelines update for the management of patients with functional pancreatic neuroendocrine tumors and non-functional pancreatic neuroendocrine tumors. *Neuroendocrinology* **2016**, *103*, 153–171. [CrossRef] [PubMed]
16. Zandee, W.T.; van Adrichem, R.C.; Kamp, K.; Feelders, R.A.; van Velthuysen, M.F.; de Herder, W.W. Incidence and prognostic value of serotonin secretion in pancreatic neuroendocrine tumours. *Clin. Endocrinol. (Oxf.)* **2017**, *87*, 165–170. [CrossRef] [PubMed]
17. Osamura, R.Y. Serotonin-secreting tumours. In *Pathology and Genetics of Tumours of Endocrine Organs. World Health Organization Classification of Tumours*, 3rd ed.; DeLellis, R.A., Ed.; IARC Press: Lyon, France, 2004; p. 198.

18. Yeo, C.J.; Couse, N.F.; Zinner, M.J. Serotonin and substance P stimulate intestinal secretion in the isolated perfused ileum. *Surgery* **1989**, *105*, 86–92.
19. von der Ohe, M.R.; Camilleri, M.; Kvols, L.K.; Thomforde, G.M. Motor dysfunction of the small bowel and colon in patients with the carcinoid syndrome and diarrhea. *N. Engl. J. Med.* **1993**, *329*, 1073–1078. [CrossRef]
20. Vinik, A.I.; Gonin, J.; England, B.G.; Jackson, T.; McLeod, M.K.; Cho, K. Plasma substance-P in neuroendocrine tumors and idiopathic flushing: The value of pentagastrin stimulation tests and the effects of somatostatin analog. *J. Clin. Endocrinol. Metab.* **1990**, *70*, 1702–1709. [CrossRef]
21. Kapran, Y.; Bauersfeld, J.; Anlauf, M.; Sipos, B.; Klöppel, G. Multihormonality and entrapment of islets in pancreatic endocrine tumors. *Virchows Arch* **2006**, *448*, 394–398. [CrossRef]
22. Rindi, G. Classification of neuroendocrine tumours. In *Handbook of Gastroenteropancreatic and Thoracic Neuroendocrine Tumours*, 1st ed.; Caplin, M., Ed.; BioScientifica: Bristol, UK, 2011; p. 35.
23. Ohta, Y.; Kosaka, Y.; Kishimoto, N.; Wang, J.; Smith, S.B.; Honig, G.; Kim, H.; Gasa, R.M.; Neubauer, N.; Liou, A.; et al. Convergence of the insulin and serotonin programs in the pancreatic β-cell. *Diabetes* **2011**, *60*, 3208–3216. [CrossRef]
24. Mao, C.; el Attar, A.; Domenico, D.R.; Kim, K.; Howard, J.M. Carcinoid tumors of the pancreas. Status report based on two cases and review of the world's literature. *Int. J. Pancreatol.* **1998**, *23*, 153–164. [CrossRef]
25. Dasari, A.; Shen, C.; Halperin, D.; Zhao, B.; Zhou, S.; Xu, Y.; Shih, T.; Yao, J.C. Trends in the incidence, prevalence, and survival oucomes in patients with neuroendocrine tumors in the United States. *JAMA Oncol.* **2017**, *3*, 1335–1342. [CrossRef]
26. Zandee, W.T.; Kamp, K.; van Adrichem, R.C.; Feelders, R.A.; de Herder, W.W. Limited value for urinary 5-HIAA excretion as prognostic marker in gastrointestinal neuroendocrine tumours. *Eur. J. Endocrinol.* **2016**, *175*, 361–366. [CrossRef] [PubMed]

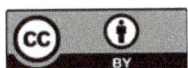

© 2020 by the authors. Licensee MDPI, Basel, Switzerland. This article is an open access article distributed under the terms and conditions of the Creative Commons Attribution (CC BY) license (http://creativecommons.org/licenses/by/4.0/).

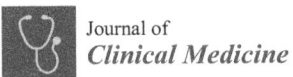

Article

Reduced and Normalized Carbohydrate Antigen 19-9 Concentrations after Neoadjuvant Chemotherapy Have Comparable Prognostic Performance in Patients with Borderline Resectable and Locally Advanced Pancreatic Cancer

Woohyung Lee [1], Yejong Park [1], Jae Woo Kwon [1], Eunsung Jun [1], Ki Byung Song [1], Jae Hoon Lee [1], Dae Wook Hwang [1], Changhoon Yoo [2], Kyu-pyo Kim [2], Jae Ho Jeong [2], Heung-Moon Chang [2], Baek-Yeol Ryoo [2], Seo Young Park [3] and Song Cheol Kim [1,*]

[1] Division of Hepatobiliary and Pancreatic Surgery, Department of Surgery, University of Ulsan College of Medicine, Asan Medical Center, Seoul 05505, Korea; ywhnet@amc.seoul.kr (W.L.); blackpig856@gmail.com (Y.P.); skunlvup@naver.com (J.W.K.); jeongo1040@gmail.com (E.J.); mtsong21c@naver.com (K.B.S.); hbpsurgeon@gmail.com (J.H.L.); dwhwang@amc.seoul.kr (D.W.H.)

[2] Department of Oncology, Asan Medical Center, University of Ulsan College of Medicine, Asan Medical Center, Seoul 05505, Korea; cyoo.amc@gmail.com (C.Y.); kkp1122@gmail.com (K.-p.K.); imdrho@gmail.com (J.H.J.); changhm@amc.seoul.kr (H.-M.C.); ryooby@amc.seoul.kr (B.-Y.R.)

[3] Department of Clinical Epidemiology and Biostatistics, University of Ulsan College of Medicine, Asan Medical Center, Seoul 05505, Korea; biostat81@amc.seoul.kr

* Correspondence: drksc@amc.seoul.kr; Tel.: +82-2-3010-3936; Fax: +82-2-3010-6701

Received: 22 April 2020; Accepted: 13 May 2020; Published: 14 May 2020

Abstract: Background: The association between optimal carbohydrate antigen (CA) 19-9 concentration after neoadjuvant chemotherapy (NACT) and prognosis has not been confirmed in patients with borderline resectable (BRPC) and locally advanced pancreatic cancer (LAPC). Methods: This retrospective study included 122 patients with BRPC and 103 with LAPC who underwent surgery after NACT between 2012 and 2019 in a tertiary referral center. Prognostic models were established based on relative difference of the CA 19-9 (RDC), with their prognostic performance compared using C-index and Akaike information criterion (AIC). Results: CA 19-9 concentrations of 37–1000 U/mL before NACT showed prognostic significance in patients with BRPC and LAPC (hazard ratio [HR]: 0.262; 95% confidence interval [CI]: 0.092–0.748; $p = 0.012$). Prognostic models in this subgroup showed that RDC was independently prognostic of better overall survival (HR: 0.262; 95% CI: 0.093–0.739; $p = 0.011$) and recurrence free survival (HR: 0.299; 95% CI: 0.140–0.642; $p = 0.002$). The prognostic performances of RDC (C-index: 0.653; AIC: 227.243), normalization of CA 19-9 after NACT (C-index: 0.625; AIC: 230.897) and surgery (C-index: 0.613; AIC: 233.114) showed no significant differences. Conclusion: RDC was independently associated with better prognosis after NACT in patients with BRPC or LAPC. Decreased CA19-9 after NACT was a prognostic indicator of better survival and recurrence, as was normalization of CA 19-9 after both NACT and surgery.

Keywords: pancreatic cancer; neoadjuvant chemotherapy; response; carbohydrate antigen 19-9

1. Introduction

Pancreatic ductal adenocarcinoma (PDAC) is a rare gastrointestinal cancer, with patients having a dismal prognosis. Surgical treatment is the mainstay for curative treatment. However, only 15–20% of diagnosed patients have resectable disease, and only 30% have borderline resectable disease [1]. Radical surgery, including vascular reconstruction, has been reported as technically feasible, expanding surgical indications for PDAC [2]. Moreover, recent studies showed that patients with borderline resectable (BRPC) or locally advanced pancreatic cancer (LAPC) who underwent surgery after neoadjuvant chemotherapy (NACT) had better survival outcomes than those who underwent upfront surgery [3–6].

Although the optimal NACT regimen has not yet been determined, a recent meta-analysis found that FOLFIRINOX-based NACT yielded better oncologic outcomes than gemcitabine-based NACT, despite the former having greater toxicity [1,7]. The resection rate after NACT was 65.3%, with 57.4% of the patients who underwent surgery achieving R0 resection [7]. However, prognostic markers for responders to NACT have not yet been identified except circulating tumor cell or DNA [8]. Although several studies found that normalization of carbohydrate antigen (CA) 19-9 concentration is associated with better patient prognosis [9], 5–10% of patients with PDAC have normal CA 19-9 at diagnosis because of a Lewis-negative phenotype, and waiting until normalization of CA 19-9 is difficult in real-world practice [10,11]. This study investigated the ability of reduced CA 19-9 rather than normalized CA 19-9 after NACT to predict oncologic outcomes in patients with BRPC or LAPC. The present study also compared the prognostic ability of reduced and normalized CA 19-9 to evaluate response after NACT in patients with BRPC and LAPC.

2. Methods

2.1. Patients and Study Design

The present study included patients with BRPC and LAPC who underwent surgery following NACT at a tertiary referral center between July 2012 and August 2019. BRPC was defined as a tumor in contact with the common hepatic artery without extension to the celiac axis or hepatic artery bifurcation; a tumor in contact with ≤180° of the circumference of the superior mesenteric artery; a tumor in contact with >180° of the circumference of the superior mesenteric vein or portal vein; and a tumor in contact with ≤180° of the circumference of either vein and with a contour irregularity or thrombosis of the vein but with possible reconstruction [12]. Patients who underwent upfront surgery were excluded.

NACT was administered based on each patient's general condition, and concurrent radiotherapy was not used routinely. The patients were evaluated by serial abdominal computed tomography (CT) and positron emission tomography (PET), and by measuring CA 19-9 concentrations during NACT. CT was evaluated using modified Response Evaluation Criteria in Solid Tumors [13]. Surgery after NACT was evaluated by a multidisciplinary team based on regressive or stable tumor with possibility of resectability of involved vessels. Pathologic response after surgery was reported using the College of American pathologist regression grading system [14]. After operation, the patients were administered chemotherapy except those with complete resolution of PDAC. Radiotherapy was used in the patients with R1 resection. The response to chemotherapy after surgery was evaluated every 3 months for 2 years by means of abdominal CT and tumor markers. Recurrence was diagnosed based on serial imaging studies with changing tumor markers and biopsy if possible.

CA 19-9 concentrations were measured before and after NACT, and after surgery, with relative difference of the CA 19-9 (RDC) calculated as follows: [(CA19-9 after NACT) − (CA 19-9 before NACT)]/(CA 19-9 before NACT). The association between RDC and prognosis was investigated, and prognostic models were constructed for predicting overall survival (OS) and recurrence free survival (RFS). The abilities of normalized and reduced CA 19-9 concentrations to predict outcomes were compared.

Clinical data were obtained from patients' medical records. Recorded preoperative factors included age, sex, body mass index (BMI), American Society of Anesthesiologists (ASA) score, and imaging results before and after NACT, with tumor markers. Intraoperative factors included extent of resection, operation time, intraoperative transfusion, and estimated blood loss. Pathologic factors included tumor regression grade, node metastasis, the number of retrieved lymph nodes, and the presence of lympho-vascular or perineural invasion. Postoperative factors included length of hospital stay, postoperative complication based on Clavien-Dindo classification, 30-day mortality, recurrence, and survival. Informed consent was obtained from each patient before surgery. The study protocol was approved by the Institutional Review Board of Asan Medical Center (IRB No: 2018-1336).

2.2. Statistical Analyses

Continuous variables are reported as the mean (standard deviation) and are compared by Student's t-tests, and categorical variables are reported as numbers and percentages and are compared by χ^2 tests. Survival rates were estimated by the Kaplan–Meier method and compared by log-rank tests. A multivariable Cox proportional hazards model was used to identify factors prognostic of OS and RFS. These variables were selected based on their clinical significance and statistical significance in a univariate Cox model, with caution to avoid overfitting and to ensure generalizability. To compare three methods of parameterization of CA19-9 (RDC, normalization after NACT, and postoperative normalization of CA19-9), c-indices were calculated for the final Cox model: one with RDC, the same model with RDC replaced by post-NACT normalization of CA 19-9, and the same model with RDC replaced by postoperative normalization of CA19-9. To evaluate the statistical difference of these three c-indices and Akaike information criterion (AIC), their standard errors were determined using 500 bootstrap samples, and their p-values were calculated. All statistical analyses were performed using SPSS® version 22.0 (SPSS Corp., Chicago, IL, USA) and R 3.5.1 (R Foundation for Statistical Computing, Vienna, Austria) software, with two-sided p-values <0.05 considered statistically significant.

3. Results

3.1. Patient Characteristics

Gemcitabine or FOLFIRINOX based NACT were administered to 816 patients. Of these, 225 (27.5%) patients underwent curative intent surgery after NACT. A review of the medical records at our institution identified 225 eligible patients of mean age 59.7 years, including 115 (51.1%) men and 110 (48.9%) women. Their mean CA 19-9 concentrations before and after NACT were 676.5 U/mL and 188.4 U/mL, respectively, and their median RDC was 0.62 (with interquartile range: 0.21–0.85). Of these patients, 122 (54.2%) had BRPC and 103 (45.8%) had LAPC, with 96 (42.7%), 27 (12%), and 95 (42.3%) found to have invasion of the adjacent vein, artery, and both, respectively. The NACT regimen consisted of FOLFIRINOX-based chemotherapy in 167 (74.2%) patients and gemcitabine-based chemotherapy in 58 (25.8%), with 7 (3.1%) patients receiving concurrent radiotherapy. Surgery consisted of pancreaticoduodenectomy in 138 (61.3%) patients, distal pancreatectomy in 67 (29.8%), total pancreatectomy in 16 (7.1%), and palliative surgery in 4 (1.7%) depending on the tumor site, with 122 (54.2%) patients also undergoing adjacent vessel resection and 173 (76.9 %) undergoing R0 resection (Table 1).

3.2. Prognostic Implications of RDC Based on CA19-9 Concentration before NACT

Of 225 patients, 30 (13.3%) patients showed increased CA19-9 after NACT, which means RDC < 0, and 188 (83.6 %) patients showed decreased or similar CA19-9 after NACT, which means RDC ≥ 0. We compared oncologic outcomes between RDC ≥ 0 and RDC < 0 groups. The patients with RDC ≥ 0 showed better median recurrence free period compared with RDC < 0 significantly (10.9 vs. 6.8 months, p = 0.016; Figure 1). There was no significant difference in median survival period between RDC ≥ 0 and RDC < 0 groups (37.1 vs. 26.3 months, p = 0.293; Figure 2). Perioperative variables were compared between two groups. The patients with RDC < 0 showed higher nodal stage than RDC ≥ 0 group (p = 0.037). Otherwise, there were no significant differences between the two groups (Supplementary Table S1). We investigated the effect of prognosis based on CA 19-9 concentration before NACT and the degree of reduction during NACT. Normal and high CA 19-9 concentrations were defined as < 37 U/mL and >1000 U/mL, respectively, with concentrations of 37–1000 U/mL classified as intermediate [15]. Neither the 62 patients with CA19-9 < 37 U/mL nor the 26 patients with CA 19-9 >1000 U/mL before NACT showed significant improvements in OS and RFS during NACT. However, the 133 patients with CA 19-9 37–1000 U/mL before NACT showed better OS (hazard ratio [HR]: 0.262; 95% confidence interval [CI]: 0.092–0.748; $p = 0.012$) and RFS (HR: 0.290; 95% CI: 0.134–0.628; $p = 0.002$) after NACT. Because these CA 19-9 concentrations before NACT were prognostically significant of survival outcomes after NACT, we established prognostic models and compared their prognostic performance in this patient subgroup (Table 2).

Table 1. Patient characteristics ($n = 225$).

	n (%) or Mean ± SD
Age (years)	59.7 ± 8.6
Sex (M/F)	115 (51.1)/110 (48.9)
ASA score (I/II/III)	15 (6.7)/189 (84)/19 (8.4)
BRPC/LAPC	122 (54.2)/103 (45.8)
Invasion (SMV/SMA/Both)	96 (42.7)/27 (12)/95 (42.3)
NACT regimen	
Gemcitabine based	58 (25.8)
FOLFIRINOX based	167 (74.2)
NACT cycle	6.5 ± 3.3
Concurrent neoadjuvant radiotherapy	7 (3.1)
CA19-9 before NACT (U/mL)	676.5 ± 3142.3
CA19-9 after NACT (U/mL)	188.4 ± 522.1
Median relative change of CA19-9 during NACT	0.62 (interquartile range: 0.21–0.85)
CA19-9 7 days after surgery (U/mL)	166.0 ± 1500.4
Preoperative response on CT (PR/SD)	67 (29.8)/158 (70.2)
Operation time	315.2 ± 97.4
Operation (PD/DP/TP/Palliative surgery)	138 (61.3)/67 (29.8)/16 (7.1)/4 (1.7)
Intraoperative transfusion	37 (16.4)
Vessel resection (vein/artery)	95 (57.8)/41 (18.2)
Adjacent organ resection	19 (8.4)
Postoperative complication	44 (19.6)
Differentiation (CR/WD/MD/PD/UD)	5 (2.2)/26 (11.6)/172 (76.4)/16 (7.1)/2 (0.9)
T-stage (CR/1/2/3/4), AJCC 8th	5 (2.2)/63 (28.0)/124 (55.1)/29 (12.9)/4 (1.8)
N-stage (0/1/2), AJCC 8th	122 (54.2)/80 (35.6)/23 (10.2)
Resection margin (R0/R1)	173 (76.9)/48 (21.3)

SD, standard deviation; ASA, American Society of Anesthesiologists; BRPC, borderline resectable pancreatic cancer; LAPC, locally advanced pancreatic cancer; NACT, neoadjuvant chemotherapy; FOLFIRINOX, 5-fluorouracil, irinotecan, and oxaliplatin; CA 19-9, carbohydrate antigen 19-9; CT, computed tomography; PR, partial response; SD, stable disease; PD, pancreaticoduodenectomy; DP, distal pancreatectomy; TP, total pancreatectomy; CR, complete regression; WD, well differentiated; MD, moderately differentiated; PD, poorly differentiated; UD, undifferentiated; AJCC, American Joint Committee on Cancer.

Table 2. Prognostic effects of carbohydrate antigen 19-9 concentration before neoadjuvant chemotherapy on overall survival and recurrence free survival.

	CA19-9 before NACT	HR	95% CI	p-Value
Overall survival	<37 U/mL ($n = 62$)	0.851	0.100–7.241	0.882
	37–1000 U/m ($n = 133$)	0.262	0.092–0.748	0.012
	>1000 U/mL ($n = 26$)	8.075	0.163–399.699	0.294
Recurrence free survival	<37 U/mL ($n = 62$)	0.708	0.222–2.257	0.560
	37–1000 U/mL ($n = 133$)	0.290	0.134–0.628	0.002
	>1000 U/mL ($n = 26$)	1.016	0.211–4.888	0.985

HR, hazard ratio; CI, confidence interval; CA19-9, carbohydrate antigen 19-9; NACT, neoadjuvant chemotherapy.

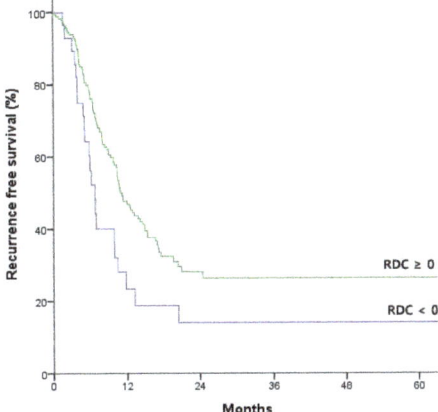

Figure 1. Kaplan-Meier analysis of recurrence free survival in patients with relative difference of carbohydrate antigen 19-9 (RDC) ≥ 0 and < 0. Median recurrence free survival was significantly longer in patients with RDC ≥ 0 than in those with RDC < 0 (10.9 vs. 6.8 months; $p = 0.016$ by log-rank test).

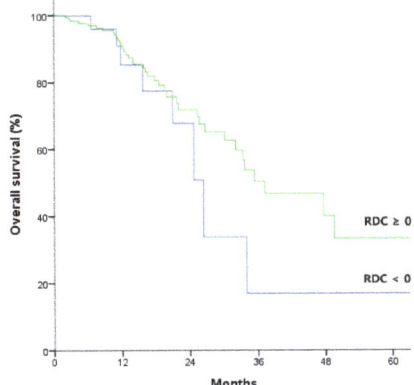

Figure 2. Kaplan-Meier analysis of overall survival in patients relative difference of carbohydrate antigen 19-9 (RDC) ≥ 0 and < 0. Median overall survival showed no significant difference between patients with RDC ≥ 0 and RDC < 0 (37.1 vs. 26.3 months; $p = 0.293$ by log-rank test).

3.3. Establishment of Prognostic Model for Survival and Recurrence in Patients with pre-NACT 37–1000 U/mL

The 3-year OS and RFS rates were 43.7% and 24.8%, respectively. Univariate analysis showed that adjacent vein resection (HR: 2.121; 95% CI: 1.028–4.377; $p = 0.042$), low RDC as a continuous variable (HR: 0.262; 95% CI: 0.092–0.748; $p = 0.012$), and intraoperative transfusion (HR: 2.172; 95% CI: 1.022–4.619; $p = 0.044$) were significantly associated with worse OS. Multivariate analysis showed that low RDC was the independent prognostic factor for worse OS (HR: 0.262; 95% CI: 0.093–0.739; $p = 0.011$; Table 3). Univariate analysis of factors prognostic of RFS found that adjacent vein resection (HR: 1.687; 95% CI: 1.075–2.649; $p = 0.023$), advanced T-stage ($p = 0.013$), and low RDC (HR: 0.290; 95% CI: 0.134–0.628; $p = 0.002$), were significantly prognostic of reduced RFS. Multivariate analysis showed that low RDC (HR: 0.299; 95% CI: 0.140–0.642; $p = 0.002$) and adjacent vein resection (HR: 1.612; 95% CI: 1.021–2.545; $p = 0.040$) were independently prognostic of early recurrence (Table 4).

Table 3. Univariate and multivariate analyses of factors associated with overall survival in patients with pancreatic cancer and carbohydrate antigen 19-9 concentrations of 37–1000 U/mL before neoadjuvant chemotherapy.

Variables		Univariate Analysis			Multivariate Analysis		
		HR	95% CI	p-Value	HR	95% CI	p-Value
Age		1.019	0.978–1.062	0.368			
Sex		0.884	0.434–1.801	0.734			
Partial response on preoperative CT		1.076	0.792–1.460	0.640			
Adjacent vein resection		2.121	1.028–4.377	0.042	1.923	0.897–4.122	0.093
Cell differentiation	WD,MD/PD,UD	3.202	1.243–8.245	0.016			
T-stage (AJCC 8th)	1,2/3,4	1.124	0.500–2.524	0.777			
N-stage (AJCC 8th)	N0 (ref)	1		0.560			
	N1	1.144	0.524–2.496	0.736			
	N2	1.806	0.649–5.021	0.257			
Tumor regression grade	0,1/2,3	1.139	0.403–3.219	0.806			
Lympho-vascular invasion		1.637	0.802–3.342	0.175			
Perineural invasion		1.306	0.531–3.209	0.561			
RDC		0.262	0.092–0.748	0.012	0.262	0.093–0.739	0.011
R1 resection		1.366	0.621–3.004	0.437			
Intraoperative transfusion		2.172	1.022–4.619	0.044	1.977	0.910–4.296	0.085

HR, hazard ratio; CI, confidence interval; CT, computed tomography; WD, well differentiated; MD, moderately differentiated; PD, poorly differentiated; UD, undifferentiated; AJCC, American Joint Committee on Cancer; RDC, relative difference of CA19-9.

Table 4. Univariate and multivariate analyses of factors associated with recurrence free survival in patients with pancreatic cancer and carbohydrate antigen 19-9 concentrations of 37–1000 U/mL before neoadjuvant chemotherapy.

Variables		Univariate Analysis			MultivAriate Analysis		
		HR	95% CI	p-Value	HR	95% CI	p-Value
Age		0.987	0.965–1.010	0.263			
Sex		1.161	0.745–1.808	0.509			
Partial response on preoperative CT		0.873	0.600–1.270	0.478			
Adjacent vein resection		1.687	1.075–2.649	0.023	1.612	1.021–2.545	0.040
Cell differentiation	WD,MD/PD,UD	1.184	0.577–2.429	0.198			
Tumor regression grade	0,1/2,3	1.531	0.800–2.930	0.198			
Lympho-vascular invasion		1.337	0.847–2.110	0.212			
Perineural invasion		1.261	0.751–2.118	0.381			
T-stage (AJCC 8th)	1,2/3,4	0.923	0.568–1.501	0.747			
N-stage (AJCC 8th)	N0 (ref)			0.159			
	N1	1.550	0.208–11.553	0.669			
	N2	1.883	0.984–3.607	0.056			
RDC		0.290	0.134–0.628	0.002	0.299	0.140–0.642	0.002
R1 resection		1.459	0.873–2.437	0.150			
Intraoperative transfusion		1.171	0.667–2.056	0.583			

HR, hazard ratio; CI, confidence interval; CT, computed tomography; WD, well differentiated; MD, moderately differentiated; PD, poorly differentiated; UD, undifferentiated; AJCC, American Joint Committee on Cancer; RDC, relative difference of carbohydrate antigen 19-9.

3.4. Comparative Prognostic Performance of Reduced and Normalized CA 19-9 after NACT and after Surgery

We compared prognostic performance of model using factors related with prognosis in this study. Prognostic model for OS included adjacent vein resection, and intraoperative transfusion, Additionally, Model 1, 2, and 3 included RDC as a continuous variable, normalization of CA19-9 after NACT, and normalization of CA19-9 after surgery, respectively. Model 1, 2, and 3 had C-index values for OS of 0.653, 0.625, and 0.613, respectively. Although the C-index of model 1 was higher than those of models 2 and 3, the differences were not statistically significant ($p = 0.904$ and $p = 0.680$, respectively). The AIC values for OS of models 1, 2, and 3 were 227.243, 230.897, and 233.114, respectively, with no statistically significant differences between model 1 and models 2 ($p = 0.896$) and 3 ($p = 0.912$). Prognostic model for RFS included adjacent vein resection. Additionally, Model 1, 2, and 3 included RDC as a continuous variable, normalization of CA19-9 after NACT, and normalization of CA19-9 after surgery, respectively. The three models had C-index values for RFS of 0.604, 0.584, and 0.602, respectively, with no statistically significant differences between model 1 and models 2 ($p = 0.812$) and

3 ($p = 0.592$). The AIC values for RFS of models 1, 2, and 3 groups were 636.138, 640.246, and 638.247, respectively, with no statistically significant differences between model 1 and models 2 ($p = 0.900$) and 3 ($p = 0.924$). Thus, the prognostic performances of the three models for OS and RFS were similar (Table 5).

Table 5. Prognostic performance of models that included decreases and normalization of carbohydrate antigen 19-9 concentration after neoadjuvant chemotherapy and surgery on overall survival and recurrence free survival.

Outcome	Prognostic Model	C-Index	95% CI	p-Value (1 vs. 2)	p-Value (1 vs. 3)	AIC	95% CI	p-Value (1 vs. 2)	p-Value (1 vs. 3)
Overall survival	Model 1	0.653	0.530–0.784	0.904	0.680	227.243	142.091–297.964	0.896	0.912
	Model 2	0.625	0.501–0.767			230.897	145.695–303.928		
	Model 3	0.613	0.523–0.760			233.114	148.409–305.646		
Recurrence free survival	Model 1	0.604	0.534–0.676	0.812	0.592	636.138	546.638–726.578	0.900	0.924
	Model 2	0.584	0.532–0.654			640.246	548.808–727.833		
	Model 3	0.602	0.547–0.673			638.247	545.773–722.073		

CI, confidence interval; AIC, Akaike information criterion; Model 1, prognostic model including decreased carbohydrate antigen 19-9 concentration during neoadjuvant chemotherapy; Model 2, prognostic model including normalization of carbohydrate antigen 19-9 concentration after neoadjuvant chemotherapy; Model 3, prognostic model including normalization of carbohydrate antigen 19-9 concentration after surgery.

3.5. Prognostic Models in Patients with Borderline Resectable Pancreatic Cancer and Locally Advanced Pancreatic Cancer

We evaluated performance for the prognostic model in patients with CA19-9 concentration of 37–1000 U/mL before NACT for BRPC ($n = 73$) and LAPC ($n = 60$) subgroup. In BRPC subgroup, adjacent vein resection (HR: 2.806; 95% CI: 1.116–7.051; $p = 0.028$) and RDC (HR: 0.456; 95% CI: 0.211–0.986; $p = 0.046$) were independent prognostic factors for OS. RDC (HR: 0.279; 95% CI: 0.137–0.570; $p < 0.001$) was an independent prognostic factor for RFS. We evaluated prognostic performance among models including prognostic factors in BRPC subgroup. Model 1 (C-index; 0.680, AIC; 126.030), 2 (C-index; 0.693, AIC; 126.403), and 3 (C-index; 0.682, AIC; 128.347) for OS showed no statistical significance among groups. Prognostic model 1 (C-index; 0.624, AIC; 302.496), 2 (C-index; 0.647, AIC; 302.562), and 3 (C-index; 0.622, AIC; 314.809) for RFS showed similar results without statistical significance. In LAPC subgroup, Cell differentiation (HR: 86.399; 95% CI: 5.806–1285.760; $p = 0.001$) was an independent prognostic factor for OS. T stage (HR: 2.545; 95% CI: 1.060–6.110; $p = 0.037$), and RDC (HR: 0.634; 95% CI: 0.451–0.889; $p = 0.008$) were independent prognostic factors for RFS. Prognostic models for OS showed no statistical significance among model 1 (C-index; 0.919, AIC; 49.475), 2 (C-index; 0.907, AIC; 49.327), and 3 (C-index; 0.896, AIC; 49.476). Prognostic models for RFS showed no statistical significance among model 1 (C-index; 0.646, AIC; 193.838), 2 (C-index; 0.606, AIC; 199.314), and 3 (C-index; 0.661, AIC; 193.408) (Supplementary Table S2–S7).

4. Discussion

This study showed that a decrease in CA19-9 concentration after NACT was an indicator of better prognosis in patients with BRPC or LAPC. Furthermore, comparisons of three prognostic models of reduced and normalized CA 19-9 after NACT, and of normalized CA 19-9 after surgery, showed that the three models were similarly predictive of OS and RFS.

CA19-9 is a Lewis blood group oligosaccharide, also called sialyl Lewis A antigen, which is synthesized by exocrine epithelial cells. It has shown a 70–90% predictive value for diagnosing pancreatic cancer [16]. However, elevated CA 19-9 has also been associated with other gastrointestinal tumors, as well as with biliary tract inflammation. Moreover, 5–10% of patients with PDAC are Lewis antigen negative, with normal CA 19-9 concentrations [11]. CA 19-9 concentration after NACT may be a biologic marker in patients with BRPC and LAPC because normalized or reduced CA 19-9 concentration after NACT has been reported to be an important prognostic marker of better OS and RFS [17]. Compared with patients with RDC ≤ 0.5, those with RDC > 0.5 experienced better survival and higher resectability after NACT, suggesting that early surgery may benefit rapid responders [18]. However, 83% of responders had RDC > 0.5 after NACT; of these, 24% had resectable PDAC, suggesting they were biologically good responders. Although normalization of CA19-9 after NACT was found to be more prognostic of survival outcomes than reduced CA 19-9, that study included patients with CA 19-9 >1000 U/mL, with this subgroup showing higher CA19-9 and a lower normalization rate after NACT than patients with CA19-9 <1000 U/mL [9]. In addition, the evaluation of the relationship between RDC and OS in that study also included patients with high CA 19-9 concentrations. The present study found that RDC after NACT affected patient prognosis. High preoperative CA 19-9 was shown to be associated with early recurrence and lower resectability rates [16,19,20]. Patients with CA19-9 >1000 U/mL were classified as having BRPC, with NACT recommended even in patients with resectable tumors [15]. In the present study, only 14% of patients with high CA 19-9 before NACT achieved normalization after NACT, with survival outcomes being poorer than in patients with CA19-9 <1000 U/mL before NACT, although the differences were not statistically significant. Other markers are required to evaluate tumor response in this subgroup. By contrast, evaluation of response to NACT using CA19-9 is inadequate for patients with CA19-9 <37 U/mL. These patients may have a Lewis-negative phenotype, suggesting that other markers, such as CEA and CA125, are needed to check their biologic status [21]. However, CA 19-9 concentrations were found to be elevated in patients with pancreatic cancer, despite 27.4% of these patients being Lewis antigen negative, suggesting that CA19-9 may be helpful in diagnosing pancreatic cancer in Lewis-negative patients, except in those with extremely low CA19-9 ≤5 U/mL [10,21].

This study found that RDC was an independent prognostic factor and that survival outcomes were better in good responders. Similarly, a previous study showed that RDC > 0.5 was an independent predictor of OS and that RDC > 0.9 was associated with pathologic complete regression [18]. The present study also showed similar prognostic performances of reduced and normalized CA 19-9 after NACT. That is, prognosis was similar in patients with higher RDC after NACT and in patients with normalized CA 19-9 after NACT or surgery.

The present study also found that the change of CA 19-9 was unable to predict the need for resection of adjacent vessels, R0 resection, or tumor regression grade. RDC was not a biologic marker predictive of curative resection after NACT. Similarly, normalization of CA 19-9 was not associated with a histopathologic response, with a negative predictive value of 28% [22]. Furthermore, radiologic response was not related to histologic response [23–25]. Additional studies are needed to identify biomarkers of resectability after NACT [26,27].

This study had several limitations, including its retrospective design, which may have resulted in potential selection bias. Furthermore, the relatively small number of patients was another limitation. However, this disease entity is rare, indicating a need for multicenter studies to evaluate larger patient populations.

5. Conclusions

RDC was independently prognostic of better OS and RFS rates in patients with CA19-9 concentrations of 37–1000 U/mL prior to NACT. Although normalization of CA19-9 after NACT is an indicator of good patient prognosis, its prognostic performance was comparable to a decrease in CA 19-9 during NACT.

Supplementary Materials: The following are available online at http://www.mdpi.com/2077-0383/9/5/1477/s1, Table S1: Characteristics of patients with relative difference of CA19-9 < 0 and ≥ 0, Table S2: Prognostic factors associated with overall survival in patients with borderline resectable pancreatic cancer and carbohydrate antigen 19-9 concentrations of 37–1000 U/ml before neoadjuvant chemotherapy (N = 73), Table S3: Prognostic factors associated with recurrence free survival in patients with borderline resectable pancreatic cancer and carbohydrate antigen 19-9 concentrations of 37–1000 U/ml before neoadjuvant chemotherapy (N = 73), Table S4: Prognostic performance of models that included decreases and normalization of carbohydrate antigen 19-9 concentration after neoadjuvant chemotherapy and surgery on overall survival and recurrence free survival for borderline resectable pancreatic cancer, Table S5: Prognostic factors associated with overall survival in patients with locally advanced pancreatic cancer and carbohydrate antigen 19-9 concentrations of 37–1000 U/ml before neoadjuvant chemotherapy (N = 60), Table S6: Prognostic factors associated with recurrence free survival in patients with locally advanced pancreatic cancer and carbohydrate antigen 19-9 concentrations of 37–1000 U/ml before neoadjuvant chemotherapy (N = 60), Table S7. Prognostic performance of models that included decreases and normalization of carbohydrate antigen 19-9 concentration after neoadjuvant chemotherapy and surgery on overall survival and recurrence free survival for locally advanced pancreatic cancer.

Author Contributions: Conceptualization, W.L., and S.C.K.; Methodology, Y.P., and E.J.; Formal analysis, S.Y.P., J.H.L., K.-p.K., and D.W.H.; Resources, K.B.S., C.Y., and J.H.J.; Data curation, W.H.L., and J.W.K, H.-M.C.; Writing, W.H.L., and B.-Y.R.; Supervision, S.C.K. All authors have read and agreed to the published version of the manuscript.

Funding: This study was supported by a grant from the Korean Health Technology R&D Project, Ministry of Health & Welfare, Republic of Korea (No. HI14C2640).

Conflicts of Interest: The authors declare no conflict of interest.

References

1. Kaufmann, B.; Hartmann, D.; D'Haese, J.G.; Stupakov, P.; Radenkovic, D.; Gloor, B.; Friess, H. Neoadjuvant Treatment for Borderline Resectable Pancreatic Ductal Adenocarcinoma. *Dig. Surg.* **2019**, *36*, 455–461. [CrossRef] [PubMed]
2. Hoshimoto, S.; Hishinuma, S.; Shirakawa, H.; Tomikawa, M.; Ozawa, I.; Wakamatsu, S.; Hoshi, S.; Hoshi, N.; Hirabayashi, K.; Ogata, Y. Reassessment of the clinical significance of portal-superior mesenteric vein invasion in borderline resectable pancreatic cancer. *Eur. J. Surg. Oncol.* **2017**, *43*, 1068–1075. [CrossRef] [PubMed]
3. Yoo, C.; Shin, S.H.; Kim, K.P.; Jeong, J.H.; Chang, H.M.; Kang, J.H.; Lee, S.S.; Park, D.H.; Song, T.J.; Seo, D.W.; et al. Clinical Outcomes of Conversion Surgery after Neoadjuvant Chemotherapy in Patients with Borderline Resectable and Locally Advanced Unresectable Pancreatic Cancer: A Single-Center, Retrospective Analysis. *Cancers* **2019**, *11*, 278. [CrossRef] [PubMed]
4. Jang, J.Y.; Han, Y.; Lee, H.; Kim, S.W.; Kwon, W.; Lee, K.H.; Oh, D.Y.; Chie, E.K.; Lee, J.M.; Heo, J.S.; et al. Oncological Benefits of Neoadjuvant Chemoradiation with Gemcitabine Versus Upfront Surgery in Patients With Borderline Resectable Pancreatic Cancer: A Prospective, Randomized, Open-label, Multicenter Phase 2/3 Trial. *Ann. Surg.* **2018**, *268*, 215–222. [CrossRef]
5. Hackert, T.; Ulrich, A.; Buchler, M.W. Borderline resectable pancreatic cancer. *Cancer Lett.* **2016**, *375*, 231–237. [CrossRef]
6. Kieler, M.; Unseld, M.; Bianconi, D.; Schindl, M.; Kornek, G.V.; Scheithauer, W.; Prager, G.W. Impact of New Chemotherapy Regimens on the Treatment Landscape and Survival of Locally Advanced and Metastatic Pancreatic Cancer Patients. *J. Clin. Med.* **2020**, *9*, 648. [CrossRef]
7. Tang, K.; Lu, W.; Qin, W.; Wu, Y. Neoadjuvant therapy for patients with borderline resectable pancreatic cancer: A systematic review and meta-analysis of response and resection percentages. *Pancreatology* **2016**, *16*, 28–37. [CrossRef]
8. Aldakkak, M.; Christians, K.K.; Krepline, A.N.; George, B.; Ritch, P.S.; Erickson, B.A.; Johnston, F.M.; Evans, D.B.; Tsai, S. Pre-treatment carbohydrate antigen 19-9 does not predict the response to neoadjuvant therapy in patients with localized pancreatic cancer. *HPB (Oxf.)* **2015**, *17*, 942–952. [CrossRef]
9. Tsai, S.; George, B.; Wittmann, D.; Ritch, P.S.; Krepline, A.N.; Aldakkak, M.; Barnes, C.A.; Christians, K.K.; Dua, K.; Griffin, M.; et al. Importance of Normalization of CA19-9 Levels Following Neoadjuvant Therapy in Patients With Localized Pancreatic Cancer. *Ann. Surg.* **2020**, *271*, 740–747. [CrossRef]
10. Luo, G.; Fan, Z.; Cheng, H.; Jin, K.; Guo, M.; Lu, Y.; Yang, C.; Fan, K.; Huang, Q.; Long, J.; et al. New observations on the utility of CA19-9 as a biomarker in Lewis negative patients with pancreatic cancer. *Pancreatology* **2018**, *18*, 971–976. [CrossRef]
11. Parra-Robert, M.; Santos, V.M.; Canis, S.M.; Pla, X.F.; Fradera, J.M.A.; Porto, R.M. Relationship Between CA 19.9 and the Lewis Phenotype: Options to Improve Diagnostic Efficiency. *Anticancer. Res.* **2018**, *38*, 5883–5888. [CrossRef] [PubMed]
12. Tempero, M.A.; Malafa, M.P.; Al-Hawary, M.; Asbun, H.; Bain, A.; Behrman, S.W.; Benson, A.B., 3rd; Binder, E.; Cardin, D.B.; Cha, C.; et al. Pancreatic Adenocarcinoma, Version 2.2017, NCCN Clinical Practice Guidelines in Oncology. *J. Natl. Compr. Cancer Netw.* **2017**, *15*, 1028–1061. [CrossRef] [PubMed]

13. Eisenhauer, E.A.; Therasse, P.; Bogaerts, J.; Schwartz, L.H.; Sargent, D.; Ford, R.; Dancey, J.; Arbuck, S.; Gwyther, S.; Mooney, M.; et al. New response evaluation criteria in solid tumours: Revised RECIST guideline (version 1.1). *Eur. J. Cancer* **2009**, *45*, 228–247. [CrossRef] [PubMed]
14. S, N.K.; Serra, S.; Dhani, N.; Hafezi-Bakhtiari, S.; Szentgyorgyi, E.; Vajpeyi, R.; Chetty, R. Regression grading in neoadjuvant treated pancreatic cancer: An interobserver study. *J. Clin. Pathol.* **2017**, *70*, 237–243. [CrossRef]
15. Tzeng, C.W.; Fleming, J.B.; Lee, J.E.; Xiao, L.; Pisters, P.W.; Vauthey, J.N.; Abdalla, E.K.; Wolff, R.A.; Varadhachary, G.R.; Fogelman, D.R.; et al. Defined clinical classifications are associated with outcome of patients with anatomically resectable pancreatic adenocarcinoma treated with neoadjuvant therapy. *Ann. Surg. Oncol.* **2012**, *19*, 2045–2053. [CrossRef]
16. Hartwig, W.; Strobel, O.; Hinz, U.; Fritz, S.; Hackert, T.; Roth, C.; Buchler, M.W.; Werner, J. CA19-9 in potentially resectable pancreatic cancer: Perspective to adjust surgical and perioperative therapy. *Ann. Surg. Oncol.* **2013**, *20*, 2188–2196. [CrossRef]
17. Combs, S.E.; Habermehl, D.; Kessel, K.A.; Bergmann, F.; Werner, J.; Naumann, P.; Jager, D.; Buchler, M.W.; Debus, J. Prognostic impact of CA 19-9 on outcome after neoadjuvant chemoradiation in patients with locally advanced pancreatic cancer. *Ann. Surg. Oncol.* **2014**, *21*, 2801–2807. [CrossRef]
18. Boone, B.A.; Steve, J.; Zenati, M.S.; Hogg, M.E.; Singhi, A.D.; Bartlett, D.L.; Zureikat, A.H.; Bahary, N.; Zeh, H.J., 3rd. Serum CA 19-9 response to neoadjuvant therapy is associated with outcome in pancreatic adenocarcinoma. *Ann. Surg. Oncol.* **2014**, *21*, 4351–4358. [CrossRef]
19. Humphris, J.L.; Chang, D.K.; Johns, A.L.; Scarlett, C.J.; Pajic, M.; Jones, M.D.; Colvin, E.K.; Nagrial, A.; Chin, V.T.; Chantrill, L.A.; et al. The prognostic and predictive value of serum CA19.9 in pancreatic cancer. *Ann. Oncol.* **2012**, *23*, 1713–1722. [CrossRef]
20. Ferrone, C.R.; Finkelstein, D.M.; Thayer, S.P.; Muzikansky, A.; Fernandez-delCastillo, C.; Warshaw, A.L. Perioperative CA19-9 levels can predict stage and survival in patients with resectable pancreatic adenocarcinoma. *J. Clin. Oncol.* **2006**, *24*, 2897–2902. [CrossRef]
21. Luo, G.; Liu, C.; Guo, M.; Cheng, H.; Lu, Y.; Jin, K.; Liu, L.; Long, J.; Xu, J.; Lu, R.; et al. Potential Biomarkers in Lewis Negative Patients With Pancreatic Cancer. *Ann. Surg.* **2017**, *265*, 800–805. [CrossRef] [PubMed]
22. Katz, M.H.; Varadhachary, G.R.; Fleming, J.B.; Wolff, R.A.; Lee, J.E.; Pisters, P.W.; Vauthey, J.N.; Abdalla, E.K.; Sun, C.C.; Wang, H.; et al. Serum CA 19-9 as a marker of resectability and survival in patients with potentially resectable pancreatic cancer treated with neoadjuvant chemoradiation. *Ann. Surg. Oncol.* **2010**, *17*, 1794–1801. [CrossRef] [PubMed]
23. Xia, B.T.; Fu, B.; Wang, J.; Kim, Y.; Ahmad, S.A.; Dhar, V.K.; Levinsky, N.C.; Hanseman, D.J.; Habib, D.A.; Wilson, G.C.; et al. Does radiologic response correlate to pathologic response in patients undergoing neoadjuvant therapy for borderline resectable pancreatic malignancy? *J. Surg. Oncol.* **2017**, *115*, 376–383. [CrossRef] [PubMed]
24. Mellon, E.A.; Jin, W.H.; Frakes, J.M.; Centeno, B.A.; Strom, T.J.; Springett, G.M.; Malafa, M.P.; Shridhar, R.; Hodul, P.J.; Hoffe, S.E. Predictors and survival for pathologic tumor response grade in borderline resectable and locally advanced pancreatic cancer treated with induction chemotherapy and neoadjuvant stereotactic body radiotherapy. *Acta Oncol.* **2017**, *56*, 391–397. [CrossRef]
25. Cassinotto, C.; Sa-Cunha, A.; Trillaud, H. Radiological evaluation of response to neoadjuvant treatment in pancreatic cancer. *Diagn. Interv. Imaging* **2016**, *97*, 1225–1232. [CrossRef]
26. Akita, H.; Takahashi, H.; Ohigashi, H.; Tomokuni, A.; Kobayashi, S.; Sugimura, K.; Miyoshi, N.; Moon, J.H.; Yasui, M.; Omori, T.; et al. FDG-PET predicts treatment efficacy and surgical outcome of pre-operative chemoradiation therapy for resectable and borderline resectable pancreatic cancer. *Eur. J. Surg. Oncol.* **2017**, *43*, 1061–1067. [CrossRef]
27. Kittaka, H.; Takahashi, H.; Ohigashi, H.; Gotoh, K.; Yamada, T.; Tomita, Y.; Hasegawa, Y.; Yano, M.; Ishikawa, O. Role of (18)F-fluorodeoxyglucose positron emission tomography/computed tomography in predicting the pathologic response to preoperative chemoradiation therapy in patients with resectable T3 pancreatic cancer. *World J. Surg.* **2013**, *37*, 169–178. [CrossRef]

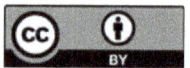

© 2020 by the authors. Licensee MDPI, Basel, Switzerland. This article is an open access article distributed under the terms and conditions of the Creative Commons Attribution (CC BY) license (http://creativecommons.org/licenses/by/4.0/).

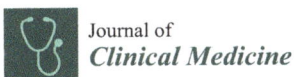

Article

Prognostic Implications of 18-FDG Positron Emission Tomography/Computed Tomography in Resectable Pancreatic Cancer

Cosimo Sperti [1,*], Alberto Friziero [1], Simone Serafini [1], Sergio Bissoli [2], Alberto Ponzoni [3], Andrea Grego [1], Emanuele Grego [4] and Lucia Moletta [1]

1. Department of Surgery, Oncology and Gastroenterology, 3rd Surgical Clinic, University of Padua, Via Giustiniani 2, 35128 Padua, Italy; alberto.friziero@unipd.it (A.F.); simone.serafini@ymail.com (S.S.); andrea.grego@studenti.unipd.it (A.G.); lucia.moletta@unipd.it (L.M.)
2. Nuclear Medicine, Belluno General Hospital, Viale Europa 22, 32100 Belluno, Italy; sergiocelico@gmail.com
3. Department of Radiology, Padua General Hospital, Via Giustiniani 2, 35128 Padua, Italy; alberto.ponzoni@aopd.veneto.it
4. University of Padua, Via Giustiniani 2, 35128 Padua, Italy; emanuele.grego@studenti.unipd.it
* Correspondence: cosimo.sperti@unipd.it; Tel.: +39-049-821-8845

Received: 5 June 2020; Accepted: 7 July 2020; Published: 9 July 2020

Abstract: There are currently no known preoperative factors for determining the prognosis in pancreatic cancer. The aim of this study was to examine the role of 18-fluorodeoxyglucose (18-FDG) positron emission tomography/computed tomography (18-FDG-PET/CT) as a prognostic factor for patients with resectable pancreatic cancer. Data were obtained from a retrospective analysis of patients who had a preoperative PET scan and then underwent pancreatic resection from January 2007 to December 2015. The maximum standardized uptake value (SUVmax) of 18-FDG-PET/CT was calculated. Patients were divided into high (>3.65) and low (≤3.65) SUVmax groups, and compared in terms of their TNM classification (Union for International Cancer Contro classification), pathological grade, surgical treatment, state of resection margins, lymph node involvement, age, sex, diabetes and serum Carbohydrate Antigen 19-9 (CA 19-9) levels. The study involved 144 patients, 82 with high SUVmax pancreatic cancer and 62 with low SUVmax disease. The two groups' disease-free and overall survival rates were significantly influenced by tumor stage, lymph node involvement, pathological grade, resection margins and SUVmax. Patients with an SUVmax ≤ 3.65 had a significantly better survival than those with SUVmax > 3.65 ($p < 0.001$). The same variables were independent predictors of survival on multivariate analysis. The SUVmax calculated with 18-FDG-PET/CT is an important prognostic factor for patients with pancreatic cancer, and may be useful in decisions concerning patients' therapeutic management.

Keywords: fluorodeoxyglucose; pancreatectomy; pancreatic cancer; positron emission tomography; prognosis; standardized uptake value

1. Introduction

Pancreatic cancer is only the 12th most common cancer worldwide, but it is the 7th most common cause of cancer-related death [1]. The number of new cases of pancreatic cancer will continue to rise in future, largely due to population aging and growth. In the United States, pancreatic cancer was the second most common gastrointestinal malignancy in 2018 [2]. In the European Union (EU), it was estimated that deaths from pancreatic cancer surpassed those due to breast cancer in 2017, making the disease the third most important cause of cancer-related death in the EU, after lung and colorectal cancer [3]. The prognosis for pancreatic cancer is generally poor, with five-year survival rates in the range of 6% to 10% [4,5]. Approximately 80% of patients have regional spread or metastatic disease at the time of their diagnosis. Hence the need for enhanced screening modalities, early detection, accurate preoperative staging, and improved treatment options. Surgery is the only potentially curative treatment for pancreatic cancer [6]. Unfortunately, only 15–20% of patients are candidates for pancreatectomy due to the above-mentioned high proportion of cases of advanced disease at presentation. Neoadjuvant therapy, defined as treatment (chemotherapy and/or radiation) administered prior to surgery, has been advocated for locally-advanced pancreatic cancer, and also for potentially resectable disease. The possible benefits lie in earlier treatment reducing the likelihood of distant disease, and tumor downsizing optimizing resection. The potential problems associated with neoadjuvant treatments for resectable tumors concern the risk of the cancer progressing to unresectable tumor during such therapy, the differences in the neoadjuvant therapy protocols adopted at different centers, and the current lack of strong evidence to support its efficacy [7].

Many circulating, molecular and clinicopathological factors have been thoroughly investigated in efforts to predict the survival of patients with pancreatic cancer [8]. Attention has focused especially on tumor stage and pathological grade [9,10], resection margins [11], preoperative serum CA 19-9 levels, postoperative normalization of tumor markers [12,13], and the demonstration of disseminated tumor cells [14]. There have been conflicting results, however, and a different survival for patients with the same stage of disease is not infrequent.

18-fluorodeoxyglucose positron emission tomography (18-FDG-PET) is a noninvasive imaging technique based on the principle of specific tissue metabolism, with a selective 18-FDG uptake and retention by malignant cells [15,16]. PET has been proposed for diagnosing and staging various malignancies, including pancreatic carcinoma [17,18]. There is evidence of 18-FDG uptake in malignant tumors being related to a tumor's aggressiveness. Some authors [19–21] have reported on prognostic information obtained with 18-FDG-PET in patients with pancreatic cancer, or outlined the role of PET in predicting early recurrences after surgery [22–24]. The numbers of patients included in these studies were too small to draw any final conclusions, however. This is particularly true for patients with localized pancreatic cancer (stage I–II) amenable to resection as part of a multimodality approach to pancreatic adenocarcinoma. We previously found PET an independent prognostic marker in a series of patients with pancreatic cancer, including a small subset of resectable tumors ($n = 16$) [25].

The aim of the present study on a series of patients with resectable pancreatic adenocarcinoma was to ascertain whether glucose metabolism, as assessed with 18-fluorodeoxyglucose positron emission tomography/computed tomography (PET/CT), provides additional prognostic information, over and above the established prognostic factors, in patients with pancreatic cancer.

2. Materials and Methods

2.1. Patients Population

Data were obtained from a retrospective analysis of a prospective database of patients who underwent pancreatic resection at our department between January 2007 and December 2015. Patients with intraductal papillary mucinous neoplasms, endocrine tumors, cystic neoplasms, pancreatic metastases, and duodenal, ampullary and bile duct cancers were excluded. This left 144 consecutive patients with pancreatic cancer who had a PET/CT scan (with semiquantitative analysis of the tracer uptake) as part of their preoperative work-up within 30 days before undergoing pancreatic resection, who were enrolled in the present study. Informed consent was obtained from each patient.

The sample was a mean 66.3 years old (range 48–82), and consisted of 70 males and 74 females. Pancreatic ductal adenocarcinoma was confirmed at histology on surgical specimens in all cases. All resection procedures were performed by the same surgical team. A limited involvement of the superior mesenteric-portal axis (less than 2 cm) in the absence of extrapancreatic disease, or involvement of the superior mesenteric artery and/or celiac trunk, were not considered as contraindications to surgery. None of the patients received neoadjuvant therapies. Resection of the pancreas entailed pylorus-preserving pancreaticoduodenectomy (PD) for tumors of the head of the pancreas, and distal pancreatectomy with splenectomy for tumors of the body and tail. Total pancreatectomy was reserved for cases where the resection margin of the pancreas was involved by the tumor or when a pancreatic anastomosis was judged at high risk of leakage. All patients underwent standard lymph node dissection—5, 6, 8a, 12b1, 12b2, 12c, 13a, 13b, 14a and 14b right lateral side, 17a, 17b, [26] and para-aortic node sampling for pancreatic head carcinoma, and 8a, 9,10,11, 18 for patients with pancreatic body and tail cancers. Para-aortic nodes were excised by harvesting the lymphocellular aortocaval tissue located below the left renal vein up to the origin of the inferior mesenteric artery (station 16b1). Resections were defined as curative (R0) when the pathology report confirmed negative resection margins, or R1 in the presence of tumor ≤ 1 mm from the resection margins, according to Leeds criteria [27]. Tumors were staged according to the Union for International Cancer Control (UICC)TNM classification [28]. Each patient's clinical and pathological records were reviewed, and the following characteristics were included in our analysis—age, sex, diabetes, type of surgery, preoperative serum CA 19-9 levels (RIA, Centocor Inc., Malvern, PA, reference: < 37 kU/L), tumor stage, lymph node status, pathological grade, R0 resection, disease-free survival and overall survival. Disease-free survival (DFS) was measured from the date of surgery to the date of radiologically detected recurrence or censoring. Overall survival (OS) was measured from the date of surgery to the date of death or censoring. All patients underwent regular follow-up, which included a physical examination, abdominal CT or US, and tumor marker assay every 3 months for the first 2 years, and every 6 months thereafter. Adjuvant gemcitabine-based chemotherapy was scheduled for all patients, whenever applicable.

Ethical approval: All procedures performed in studies involving human participants were in accordance with the ethical standards of the institutional and/or national research committee and with the 1964 Helsinki Declaration and its later amendments or comparable ethical standards.

2.2. 18-FDG-PET/CT Imaging

18-FDG-PET/CT images were obtained using two different dedicated tomographs—Biograph-16™, Siemens Healthcare GmbH, Erlangen-Germany from 2007 to 2012, and Discovery™, GE-Healthcare, Boston USA in the years 2013–2015.

Each scan was performed 50–70 min postinjection of 150–400 MBq of FDG in fasting patients (almost 6 hours), with serum levels of glucose < 110 mg/dL for nondiabetic patients and < 200 mg/dL in diabetic ones; in order to avoid interferences due to hyperglycaemia, blood glucose was checked just before the procedure.

The acquisitions were performed with standard modalities (scan length from base skull to 1/3 prox of legs, 6–7 beds, 2–3 min/bed); when necessary, a limited second scan of 2 beds with the same modalities was repeated on the hepato-pancreatic region at 90-100 min postinjection.

Images were reconstructed with standard algorithms, and the SUV value was calculated in the suspected neoplastic foci (SUV = tissue tracer concentration/injected dose/body weight); for the SUV analysis, a circular region of interest was placed over the area of maximal focal FDG uptake suspected to be a tumorous focus (SUVmax).

After acquisition, scan images were interpreted and referred by an experienced Nuclear Medicine physician, well-trained in PET/TC (almost five years).

2.3. Statistical Analyses

Statistical analyses were run using STATA, version 14.1 (4905 Lakeway Drive College Station, Texas, 77845, USA). Receiver operating characteristic (ROC) curve analysis was used to ascertain the optimal cut-off for predicting DFS and OS after pancreatectomy. The optimal cut-off was identified as the point of intersection nearest the top left-hand corner between the ROC curve and the diagonal line from the top right-hand corner to the bottom left-hand corner of the graph. For the univariate analysis, the patients were divided into two groups, with SUVmax (> vs. ≤ 3.65) as the cut-off. Differences between the characteristics of the patients in the two groups were tested for significance using the

Mann–Whitney U test, chi-square test, Fisher's exact test or t-student test. Univariate and multivariate analysis were used to investigate the effect of the following variables on survival—age, sex, tumor stage, pathological grade, lymph node involvement, resection margins, diabetes, and serum CA 19-9 levels. Survival data were estimated with the Kaplan–Meier method and examined using the log-rank test. Multivariate analysis of survival was performed using Cox's proportional hazards model. Significance was set at $p < 0.05$.

3. Results

Table 1 shows the clinical and pathological details of the 144 patients. Fifty-three patients had diabetes, and 93 had preoperative serum CA 19-9 levels above the normal limit. The surgical procedure involved pylorus-preserving PD in 106 patients, distal pancreatectomy with splenectomy in 34, and total pancreatectomy in four. A segmental portal-mesenteric vein resection was included in 21 cases. The resection margins were positive (R1) in 38 patients (26.4%). Lymph node metastases (stage II1) were identified in 103 patients, 114 had stage I-II tumor, and 95 tumors (66%) were well- or moderately-differentiated. A total of 132 patients (92%) received gemcitabine-based adjuvant chemotherapy.

Table 1. Standardized Uptake Values and Patients' Clinical and Pathological Details.

	All Patients	SUVmax ≤ 3.65	SUVmax > 3.65	p Value
Patients, n (%)	144	62 (43.1%)	82 (56.9%)	
Age, yrs (mean ± SD)	66.32 ± 11.40	66.48 ± 09.32	67.55 ± 10.31	
Sex M	70	32	38	
F	74	30	44	
UICC I–II, n (%)	114 (79.2%)	52 (45.6%)	62 (54.4%)	0.158
III–IV, n (%)	30 (20.8%)	10 (33.3%)	20 (66.7%)	
Grade, n (%) Well- or moderately differentiated (G1–G2)	95 (66%)	47 (49.5%)	48 (50.5%)	0.023
Poorly-differentiated (G3)	49 (34%)	15 (30.6%)	34 (69.4%)	
Resection margins R0, n (%)	106 (73.6%)	48 (45.3%)	58 (54.7%)	0.232
R1, n (%)	38 (26.4%)	14 (36.8%)	24 (63.2%)	
Lymph nodes Negative, n (%)	41 (28.5%)	23 (56.1%)	18 (43.9%)	0.036
Positive, n (%)	103 (71.5%)	39 (37.9%)	64 (62.1%)	
Diabetes No, n (%)	90 (62.5%)	42 (46.7%)	48 (53.3%)	0.170
Yes, n (%)	54 (37.5%)	20 (37%)	34 (63%)	
SUVmax, mean (±SD)	5 (±3.2)	2.6 (±1.2)	6.9 (±3.1)	
Serum CA 19-9, mean (±SD)	524.5 (±1123)	392.9 (±1051.9)	623.9 (±1172.1)	0.88
Serum CA 19-9, median (IQR), range	114 (IQR 23–382) range 1–6637	52.9 (IQR 18–256) range 1–6637	154.35 (IQR 27–470) range 1–5460	0.032
CA 19-9 < 114 kU/L	81 (56.3%)	41 (50.6%)	40 (49.4%)	0.028
CA 19-9 > 114 kU/L	63 (43.7%)	21 (33.3%)	42 (66.7%)	
OS, median (95%CI)	22 (19–27)	28 (24–37)	19 (16–22)	0.002
DFS, median (95%CI)	12 (10–14)	20 (14–23)	9 (8–11)	0.001

The median SUVmax of the 144 patients was 4.0 (range 1.0 to 12.0). From the ROC analysis, the best cut-off was identified at 3.65. The area under the ROC curve (AUC) was 0.66 (95%CI 0.542–0.77) (Figure 1). When patients were grouped by low SUVmax (≤ 3.65) versus high SUVmax (> 3.65), the two groups did not differ statistically in terms of age, sex, number of patients with of diabetes, tumor stage, type of treatment, or number of patients given adjuvant therapy. Median values of CA 19-9, numbers of patients with lymph node metastases and those with poorly-differentiated tumors were significantly higher in the high SUVmax group (Table 1). The 144 patients' median serum CA 19-9 level was 114 kU/L (range 1.0 to 6637 kU/L). Follow-up was available for all patients, and ranged from 6 to 152 months.

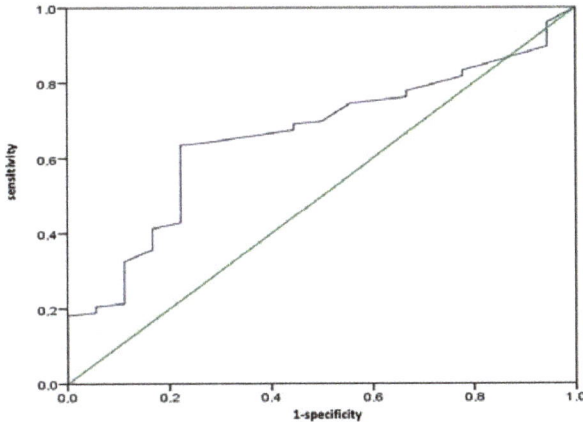

Figure 1. Receiver operator characteristic (ROC) curve for maximum standardized uptake value (SUVmax) cut-off, showing that the most effective cut-off was 3.65 (AUC 0.659, 95%CI 0.542–0.77).

3.1. Disease-Free Survival

With a median follow-up of 56.7 months (range 2–70), pancreatic cancer recurred in 126/144 patients (87.5%). The median DFS was 11.6 months.

On univariate Cox regression analysis (Table 2), lymph node metastases, pathological grade, resection margins, tumor stage, and SUVmax correlated significantly with DFS, while diabetes and serum CA 19-9 levels did not. Multivariate Cox regression analysis (Table 2) showed that the same parameters were independent predictors of DFS. Patients with a preoperative SUVmax > 3.65 had a significantly shorter DFS than patients with a SUVmax ≤ 3.65 ($p = 0.001$) (Figure 2). When the patients grouped by SUVmax were stratified by stage of disease, 18-FDG-PET/CT uptake correlated with survival even among patients in stage I-II, with a better survival for patients with SUVmax ≤3.65 ($p = 0.0004$) (Figure 3)

Table 2. Association Between Preoperative Variables and Disease-Free Survival on Univariate [a] and Multivariate [b] Cox Regression Model. HR = hazard ratio.

Variables	HR [a]	95%CI [a]	P Value [a]	HR [b]	95%CI [b]	P Value [b]
Lymph node metastases	2.33	1.511–3.596	<0.0001	1.779	1.130–2.800	0.013
Pathological grade	1.581	1.090–2.293	0.016	1.661	1.137–2.426	0.009
Radicality	2.047	1.377–3.044	<0.0001	1.840	1.223–2.769	0.003
Stage	2.181	1.429–3.330	<0.0001	1.787	1.144–2.794	0.011
Diabetes	1.352	0.942–1.941	0.102	-	-	-
SUVmax	1.106	1.051–1.165	<0.0001	1.085	1.025–1.148	0.004
CA 19-9	1.001	0.999–1.001	0.312	-	-	-

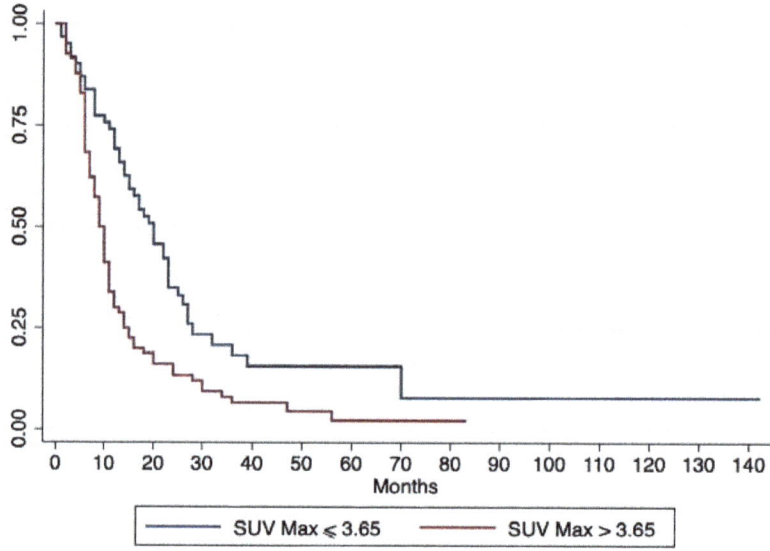

Figure 2. Kaplan–Meier curve for disease-free survival estimated for patients with preoperative SUVmax > 3.65 and those with SUVmax ≤ 3.65.

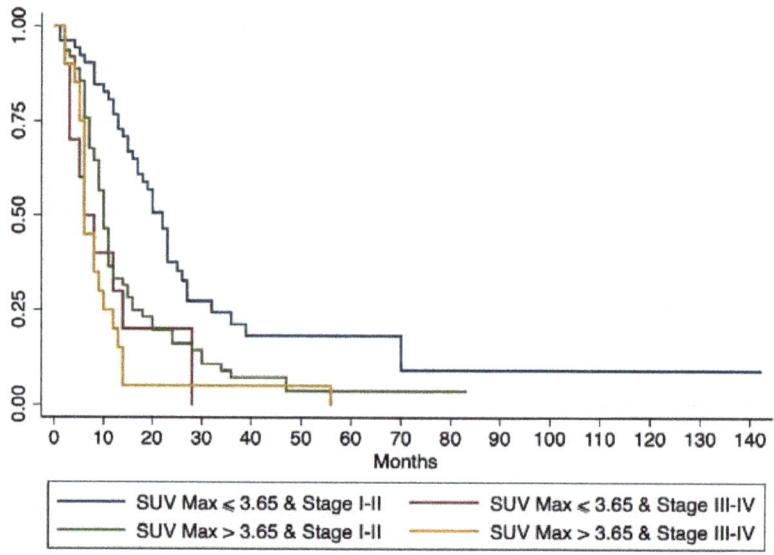

Figure 3. Kaplan–Meyer estimates for disease-free survival based on preoperative tumor stage and high or low SUVmax.

3.2. Overall Survival

With a median follow-up of 100.8 months (range 6–152), 125/144 patients (87%) died of pancreatic cancer, and another two patients died of causes unrelated to their pancreatic disease. The median OS for the whole cohort was 22.4 months (range 19–27). At univariate Cox regression analysis (Table 3) lymph node metastases, pathological grade, resection margins, tumor stage, and SUVmax correlated significantly with OS. Multivariate Cox regression analysis (Table 3) identified the same variables as being significantly associated with OS. As in the case of DFS, diabetes and CA 19-9 serum levels were not independent predictors of OS. Survival analysis with the Kaplan–Meier method showed a significantly lower OS for patients with a preoperative SUVmax > 3.65 than for those with a SUVmax ≤ 3.65 ($p < 0.001$) (Figure 4). When the patients grouped by SUVmax were stratified by tumor stage, 18-FDG uptake correlated with OS among patients with stage I-II (better survival for patients with SUVmax ≤ 3.65, $p = 0.0002$), but not for those with stage III–IV tumors ($p = 0.71$). The survival curves for patients with stage I–II and SUVmax > 3.65 did not differ statistically from those of patients with stage III–IV and SUVmax ≤ 3.65. (Figure 5). At latest follow-up, 17 patients were alive (16 disease-free): 13 in the group with SUVmax ≤ 3.65, and 4 in the group with SUVmax > 3.65 (one with recurrent cancer).

Table 3. Association Between Preoperative Variables and Overall Survival on Univariate [a] and Multivariate [b] Cox Regression Model.

Variables	HR [a]	95%CI [a]	P Value [a]	HR [b]	95%CI [b]	P Value [b]
Lymph node metastases	2.433	1.588–3.721	<0.0001	1.730	1.101–2.719	0.017
Pathological grade	1.493	1.030–2.165	0.034	1.484	1.017–2.163	0.040
Radicality	2.352	1.583–3.495	<0.0001	2.079	1.374–3.147	0.001
Tumor stage	2.489	1.637–3.784	<0.0001	2.127	1.369–3.305	0.001
Diabetes	1.222	0.851–1.756	0.278	-	-	-
SUVmax	1.074	1.025–1.124	0.002	1.055	1.001–1.111	0.044
CA 19-9	1.001	0.999–1.001	0.196	-	-	-

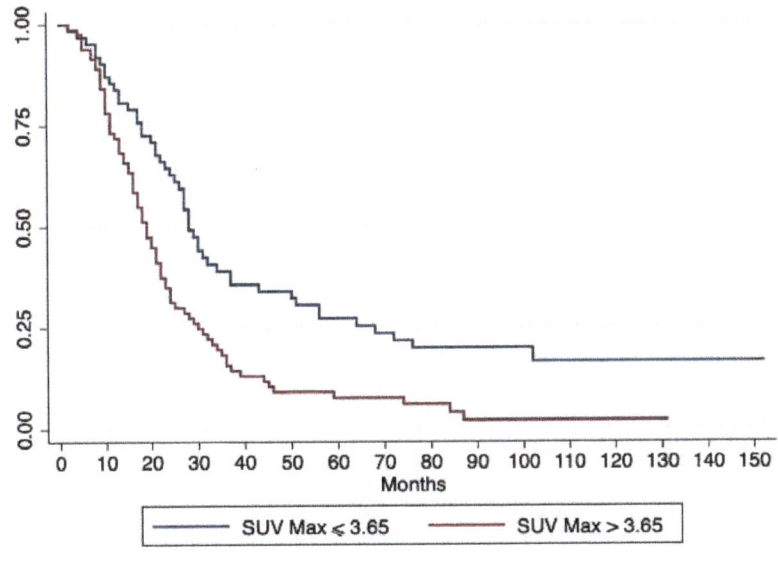

Figure 4. Kaplan–Meier curves for overall survival of patients with preoperative SUVmax > 3.65 and those with SUVmax ≤ 3.65.

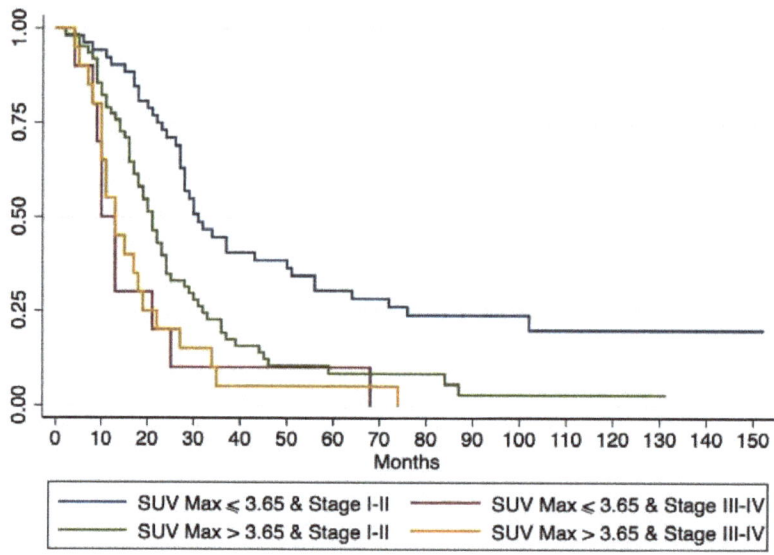

Figure 5. Kaplan-Meyer curves for overall patient survival by preoperative stage and SUVmax category.

4. Discussion

An accurate pretreatment prognosis for patients with pancreatic cancer would be very helpful for the purpose of tailoring their treatment (either surgery or multimodality clinical management). This is particularly true for apparently localized, resectable carcinoma of the pancreas because several authors have recommended neoadjuvant therapy for such patients rather than upfront surgery, the benefits of which have yet to be definitely established. The rationale for using PET/CT preoperatively for prognostic purposes in cases of pancreatic cancer stems from evidence of an accelerated glucose transport rate and increased rate of glycolysis being among the most characteristic biochemical markers of malignant transformation. Overexpression of glucose transporter 1 (Glut-1) [29] and glycolytic enzymes [30] has been demonstrated in human pancreatic adenocarcinoma. 18-FDG is a glucose analog actively taken up into the pancreatic cell by Glut-1 and phosphorylated by hexokinase in the first step of glycolysis. Its accumulation thus reflects the rate of carbohydrate metabolism and the malignant activity of a pancreatic cancer [22]. The standardized uptake value (SUV), a semiquantitative parameter of glucose consumption that enables a quantitative estimation of 18-FDG accumulation, can easily be obtained preoperatively on PET/CT. 18-FDG-PET/CT is therefore useful for distinguishing benign from malignant tumors, for diagnosing tumor recurrences, and for assessing the effects of neoadjuvant chemoradiation therapies [20,31,32]. Preliminary evidence of the correlation between 18-FDG uptake and prognosis for pancreatic adenocarcinoma has been reported in small series of patients [21,25,33]. Nakata et al. [33] introduced 18-FDG PET and SUV as metabolic prognostic factors in patients with pancreatic carcinoma. In a small series of 14 patients, they found survival significantly shorter in the high SUV group (>3.0) than in the low SUV group (<3.0) ($p < 0.05$). These results were only partially confirmed, however, by the same authors four years later [19] in 37 patients with histologically-confirmed pancreatic cancer. While SUV was unable to predict survival for patients with resectable tumor, among those with unresectable disease, patients with a low SUV survived significantly longer than those with a high SUV ($p = 0.03$); furthermore, multivariate analysis confirmed tumor SUV as an independent prognostic indicator for patients with unresectable tumors.

In the present study, we analyzed 18-FDG uptake in a cohort of patients ($n = 144$) with histologically-confirmed pancreatic cancer. When grouped by high (> 3.65) versus low (≤ 3.65)

SUVmax, patients did not differ statistically in terms of age, sex, tumor stage, pathological grade, serum CA 19-9 levels, diabetes, or type of treatment. DFS and OS were significantly influenced by SUVmax, however, being 20 and 28 months, respectively, for low-SUVmax patients as opposed to 9 and 19 months for high-SUVmax patients ($p = 0.001$). Among the clinicopathological variables considered, tumor stage, pathological grade, lymph node involvement, and resection margins correlated significantly with both DFS and OS after univariate analysis. Multivariate analysis confirmed SUVmax, tumor stage, grade, resection margins and lymph node status as independent predictors of DFS and OS.

Interestingly, when patients in the two SUVmax groups were stratified by tumor stage, 18-FDG uptake significantly influenced survival for cases in stage I–II, but not for those in stage III–IV. Serum CA 19-9 levels and diabetes had no influence on survival. The different biological aggressiveness of the tumor indicated by the SUVmax may explain the different survival rates after potentially curative resection with otherwise similar prognostic variables. 18-FDG-PET/CT is known to be a less accurate indicator in diabetic patients, and may be unable to predict their survival adequately. Some authors [34,35] recently reported that preoperative SUVmax and serum CA 19-9 independently predicted pathological stages and OS. However, it is hard to establish an optimal cut-off value of CA 19-9 as a reproducible preoperative prognostic factor, because 10–15% of the population does not express CA 19-9 and because the levels of such tumor markers are notoriously influenced by liver and renal insufficiency [36].

Our results confirm previous evidence [22,23,37–42] of SUVmax (measured in terms of the tumor's uptake of 18-FDG) being a simple and reliable pretreatment prognostic parameter, as in other malignancies. A summary of the results of other studies on SUVmax as a prognostic factor in cases of resectable pancreatic cancer is given in Table 4.

Table 4. The Literature Reporting Differences in Overall Survival and Disease-Free Survival by SUVmax.

Author	Year	Design	n	SUVmax	OS (mo)	p	DFS (mo)	p
Okamoto et al. [22]	2011	R	56	<5.5 >5.5	NA	-	NA	0.025
Choi et al. [38]	2013	R	64	≤3.5 >3.5	45.4 vs. 23.5	0.011	26.1 vs. 9.2	0.002
Lee et al. [40]	2014	R	87	≤4.7 >4.7	34.4 vs. 20.6	0.03	12.9 vs. 9.9	0.03
Kitasato et al. [39]	2014	R	41	≤3.4 >3.4	NR	-	610 vs. 354 days	0.04
Yamamoto et al. [23]	2015	R	128	<6.0 ≥6.0	37 vs. 18	<0.001	23 vs. 6	<0.001
Ariake et al. [41]	2018	R	138	<4.85 ≥4.85	50.4 vs. 21.5	<0.001	24.3 vs. 10.3	<0.001
Present series	2020	R	144	≤3.65 >3.65		<0.001		<0.001

R = retrospective; OS = overall survival; DFS = disease-free survival; NR = not reported; NA = not applicable; mo = months.

Including ours, seven studies have been published [22,23,38–41], all retrospective, concerning a total of 658 patients. SUVmax cut-offs vary greatly, but all the studies report a significantly longer DFS for patients with a low SUVmax, and 4 studies also describe a significantly better OS [23,38,40,41]. Since SUVmax only gives an indication of peak metabolic activity, not of tumor burden, some authors have explored the value of metabolic tumor volume (MTV) and total lesion glycolysis (TLG) as predictors of pancreatic cancer outcome [40,43,44]. Xu et al. [44] found that MTV and TLG independently predicted OS and DFS, and did so better than CA 19-9 levels, SUVmax, or tumor size. These findings were confirmed by Lee et al. [40] in 87 patients with resectable carcinoma of the pancreas (30 treated with neoadjuvant therapy)—MTV and TLG were independent prognostic factors irrespective of neoadjuvant therapy. On the other hand, SUVmax is less time-consuming and easier to calculate, and in our and others' experience, it provides the same important information.

Several previous studies found the tumor's histological characteristics important in establishing the prognosis for pancreatic cancer patients [8–14], but most of them are only available after surgery. The great advantage of the SUVmax calculated on 18-FDG-PET/CT is that it can be obtained before any treatment is undertaken. As the prognostic value of SUVmax is equivalent to that of tumor staging, stratifying patients by extent of disease on multidetector CT scans and SUVmax may improve our understanding of the actual effect of different treatments.

There is evidence to suggest that glycolytic activity as measured from 18-FDG uptake gives an indication of a tumor's growth and biological behavior, enabling a prediction of patients' DFS and OS. 18-FDG-PET/CT might therefore be used to identify patients with resectable pancreatic cancer at higher risk of early recurrence and shorter survival who could benefit from neoadjuvant therapy. The feasibility and clinical usefulness of this approach would need to be confirmed in prospective trials.

Another topic of interest could be the evaluation of SUVmax with 18-FDG PET/CT measured before and after chemotherapy in those patients scheduled for neoadjuvant therapy and its association with their survival.

There are some limitations of our study to mention. First, it was a retrospective study conducted at a single institution. Second, various drugs were used for adjuvant therapy during the study period, and this may have influenced the results. The significant number of patients and PET findings considered nonetheless sufficed to show statistically significant and clinically relevant differences.

5. Conclusions

The SUVmax calculated on 18-FDG-PET/CT provides useful prognostic informations in patients with pancreatic cancer before any surgical or medical treatment is administered, and may therefore help stratify patients for prospective studies comparing different treatment options (surgery versus chemotherapy).

Author Contributions: Study conception and design: C.S., S.S., L.M.; data acquisition: A.F, S.S., S.B., A.P., A.G.; data analysis and interpretation f: A.F., S.S., S.B., A.G., L.M., E.G.; drafting of manuscript: A.F., S.S, A.P., A.G., E.G.; critical revision: C.S., A.F., S.S., L.M. All authors have read and agreed to the published version of the manuscript.

Funding: This research received no external funding.

Conflicts of Interest: The authors have no conflict of interest to disclose. The institutional review boards of the hospitals involved approved this retrospective study, and the requirement to obtain informed consent was waived.

References

1. Arnold, M.; Abnet, C.C.; Neale, R.E.; Vignat, J.; Giovannucci, E.L.; McGlynn, K.A.; Bray, F. Global burden of 5 major types of gastrointestinal cancer. *Gastroenterology* **2020**. [CrossRef] [PubMed]
2. Vareedayah, A.A.; Alkaade, S.; Taylor, J.R. Pancreatic adenocarcinoma. *Mo. Med.* **2018**, *115*, 230–235.
3. Ferlay, J.; Partensky, C.; Bray, F. More deaths from pancreatic cancer than breast cancer in the EU by 2017. *Acta. Oncol.* **2016**, *55*, 1158–1160. [CrossRef] [PubMed]
4. Siegel, R.L.; Miller, K.D.; Jemal, A. Cancer statistics. *CA Cancer J. Clin.* **2020**, *70*, 7–30. [CrossRef] [PubMed]
5. Arnold, M.; Rutherford, M.J.; Bardot, A.; Ferlay, J.; Andersson, T.M.; Myklebust, T.Å.; Tervonen, H.; Thursfield, V.; Ransom, D.; Shack, L.; et al. Progress in cancer survival, mortality, and incidence in seven high-income countries 1995-2014 (ICBP SURVMARK-2): A population-based study. *Lancet Oncol.* **2019**, *20*, 1493–1505. [CrossRef]
6. Shaib, Y.; Davila, J.; Naumann, C.; El-Serag, H. The impact of curative intent surgery on the survival of pancreatic cancer patients: A US Population-based study. *Am. J. Gastroenterol.* **2007**, *102*, 1377–1382. [CrossRef]
7. Cloyd, J.M.; Heh, V.; Pawlik, T.M.; Ejaz, A.; Dillhoff, M.; Tsung, A.; Williams, T.; Abushahin, L.; Bridges, J.F.P.; Santry, H. Neoadjuvant therapy for resectable and borderline resectable pancreatic cancer: A meta-analysis of randomized controlled trials. *J. Clin. Med.* **2020**, *9*, 1129. [CrossRef] [PubMed]
8. Dell'Aquila, E.; Fulgenzi, C.A.M.; Minelli, A.; Citarella, F.; Stellato, M.; Pantano, F.; Russano, M.; Cursano, M.C.; Napolitano, A.; Zeppola, T.; et al. Prognostic and predictive factors in pancreatic cancer. *Oncotarget* **2020**, *11*, 924–941. [CrossRef]
9. Lim, J.E.; Chien, M.W.; Earle, C.C. Prognostic factors following curative resection for pancreatic adenocarcinoma. A population-based, linked database analysis of 396 patients. *Ann. Surg.* **2003**, *237*, 74–85. [CrossRef] [PubMed]

10. Bilici, A. Prognostic factors related with survival in patients with pancreatic adenocarcinoma. *World J. Gastroenterol.* **2014**, *20*, 10802–10812. [CrossRef]
11. Kim, K.S.; Kwon, J.; Kim, K.; Chie, E.K. Impact of resection margin distance on survival of pancreatic cancer: A systematic review and meta-analysis. *Cancer Res. Treat.* **2017**, *49*, 824–833. [CrossRef] [PubMed]
12. Sperti, C.; Pasquali, C.; Catalini, S.; Cappellazzo, F.; Bonadimani, B.; Behboo, R.; Pedrazzoli, S. CA 19-9 as a prognostic index after resection for pancreatic cancer. *J. Surg. Oncol.* **1993**, *52*, 137–141. [CrossRef] [PubMed]
13. Winter, J.M.; Yeo, C.J.; Brody, J.R. Diagnostic, prognostic, and predictive biomarkers in pancreatic cancer. *J. Surg. Oncol.* **2013**, *107*, 15–22. [CrossRef]
14. Vogel, I.; Kalthoff, H.; Henne-Bruns, D.; Kremer, B. Detection and prognostic impact of disseminated tumor cells in pancreatic carcinoma. *Pancreatology* **2002**, *2*, 79–88. [CrossRef]
15. Delbeke, D.; Martin, W.H. Positron emission tomography imaging in oncology. *Radiol. Clin. N. Am.* **2001**, *39*, 883–917. [CrossRef]
16. Hustinx, R.; Benard, F.; Alavi, A. Whole-body imaging in the management of patients with cancer. *Semin. Nucl. Med.* **2002**, *32*, 35–46. [CrossRef] [PubMed]
17. Rose, M.; Delbeke, D.; Beauchamp, D.; Chapman, W.C.; Sandler, M.P.; Sharp, K.W.; Richards, W.O.; Write, J.K.; Frexes, M.E.; Pinson, C.W.; et al. 18-Fluorodeoxyglucose positron emission tomography in the management of patients with suspected pancreatic cancer. *Ann. Surg.* **1998**, *229*, 729–738. [CrossRef]
18. Van Heertum, R.L.; Fawrwaz, R.A. The role of nuclear medicine in the evaluation of pancreatic disease. *Surg. Clin. N. Am.* **2001**, *82*, 345–348. [CrossRef]
19. Nakata, B.; Nishimura, S.; Ishikawa, T.; Ohira, M.; Nishino, H.; Kawabe, J.; Ochi, H.; Hirakawa, K. Prognostic predictive value of 18-fluorodeoxyglucose positron emission tomography for patients with pancreatic cancer. *Int. J. Oncol.* **2001**, *19*, 53–58.
20. Maisey, N.R.; Webb, A.; Flux, G.D.; Padhani, A.; Cunningham, D.C.; Ott, R.J.; Norman, A. FDG-PET in the prediction of survival of patients with cancer of the pancreas: A pilot study. *Br. J. Cancer* **2000**, *83*, 287–293. [CrossRef]
21. Zimny, M.; Fass, J.; Bares, R.; Cremerius, U.; Sabri, O.; Buechin, P.; Schumpelick, V.; Buell, U. Fluorodeoxyglucose positron emission tomography and the prognosis of pancreatic carcinoma. *Scand. J. Gastroenterol.* **2000**, *35*, 883–888. [PubMed]
22. Okamoto, K.; Koyama, I.; Miyazawa, M.; Toshimitsu, Y.; Aikawa, M.; Okada, K.; Imabayashi, E.; Matsuda, H. Preoperative 18[F]-fluorodeoxyglucose positron emission tomography/computed tomography predicts early recurrence after pancreatic cancer resection. *Int. J. Clin. Oncol.* **2011**, *16*, 39–44. [CrossRef] [PubMed]
23. Yamamoto, T.; Sugiura, T.; Mizuno, T.; Okamura, Y.; Aramaki, T.; Endo, M.; Uesaka, K. Preoperative FDG-PET predicts early recurrence and a poor prognosis after resection of pancreatic adenocarcinoma. *Ann. Surg. Oncol.* **2015**, *22*, 677–684. [CrossRef] [PubMed]
24. Wang, L.; Dong, P.; Wang, W.; Li, M.; Hu, W.; Liu, X.; Tian, B. Early recurrence detected by 18F-FDG PET/CT in patients with resected pancreatic ductal adenocarcinoma. *Medicine* **2020**, *99*, e19504. [CrossRef] [PubMed]
25. Sperti, C.; Pasquali, C.; Chierichetti, F.; Ferronato, A.; Decet, G.; Pedrazzoli, S. 18-Fluorodeoxyglucose positron emission tomography in predicting survival of patients with pancreatic carcinoma. *J. Gastrointest. Surg.* **2003**, *7*, 953–959. [CrossRef]
26. Japan Pancreas Society. *Classification of Pancreatic Carcinoma*, 2nd English ed.; Kanehara & Co.: Tokyo, Japan, 2003.
27. Menon, K.V.; Gomez, D.; Smith, A.M.; Anthoney, A.; Verbeke, C.S. Impact of margin status on survival following pancreatoduodenectomy for cancer: The Leeds Pathology Protocol (LEEPP). *HPB* **2009**, *11*, 18–24. [CrossRef] [PubMed]
28. Brierley, J.D.; Gospodarowicz, M.K.; Wittekind, C. *TNM Classification of Malignant Tumors*, 8th ed.; UICC: Geneva, Switzerland, 2017.
29. Pizzi, S.; Porzionato, A.; Pasquali, C.; Guidolin, D.; Sperti, C.; Fogar, P.; Macchi, V.; De Caro, R.; Pedrazzoli, S.; Parenti, A. Glucose transporter-1 expression and prognostic significance in pancreatic carcinogenesis. *Histol. Histopathol.* **2009**, *24*, 175–185.
30. Schek, N.; Hall, B.L.; Finn, O.J. Increased glyceraldehyde-3-phosphate dehydrogenase gene expression in human pancreatic adenocarcinoma. *Cancer Res.* **1988**, *48*, 6354–6359.

31. Choi, M.; Heilbrun, L.K.; Venkatramanamoorthy, R.; Lawhorn-Crews, J.M.; Zalupski, M.M.; Shields, A.F. Using 18F-fluorodeoxyglucose positron emission tomography to monitor clinical outcomes in patients treated with neoadjuvant chemo-radiotherapy for locally advanced pancreatic cancer. *Am. J. Clin. Oncol.* **2010**, *33*, 257–261. [CrossRef]
32. Chang, J.S.; Choi, S.H.; Lee, Y.; Kim, K.H.; Park, J.Y.; Song, S.Y.; Cho, A.; Yun, M.; Lee, J.D.; Seong, J. Clinical usefulness of 18F-fluorodeoxyglucose positron emission tomography in patients with locally advanced pancreatic cancer planned to undergo concurrent chemoradiation therapy. *Int. J. Radiat. Oncol. Biol. Phys.* **2014**, *90*, 126–133. [CrossRef]
33. Nakata, B.; Chung, Y.S.; Nishimura, S.; Nishihara, T.; Sakurai, Y.; Sawada, T.; Okamura, T.; Kawabe, J.; Ochi, H.; Sowa, M. 18F-fluorodeoxyglucose positron emission tomography and the prognosis of patients with pancreatic adenocarcinoma. *Cancer* **1997**, *79*, 695–699. [CrossRef]
34. Zhao, J.G.; Hu, Y.; Liao, Q.; Niu, Z.Y.; Zhao, Y.P. Prognostic significance of SUVmax and serum carbohydrate antigen 19-9 in pancreatic cancer. *World J. Gastroenterol.* **2014**, *20*, 5875–5880. [CrossRef] [PubMed]
35. Gu, X.; Zhou, R.; Li, C.; Liu, R.; Zhao, Z.; Gao, Y.; Xu, Y. Preoperative maximum standardized uptake value and carbohydrate antigen 19-9 were independent predictors of pathological stages and overall survival in Chinese patients with pancreatic duct adenocarcinoma. *BMC Cancer* **2019**, *19*, 456. [CrossRef] [PubMed]
36. Goonetilleke, K.S.; Siriwardena, A.K. Systematic review of carbohydrate antigen (CA 19-9) as a biochemical marker in the diagnosis of pancreatic cancer. *Eur. J. Surg. Oncol.* **2007**, *33*, 266–270. [CrossRef]
37. Hwang, J.P.; Lim, I.; Chang, K.J.; Kim, B.I.; Choi, C.W.; Lim, S.M. Prognostic value of SUVmax measured by fluorine-18 fluorodeoxyglucose positron emission tomography with computed tomography in patients with pancreatic cancer. *Nucl. Med. Mol. Imaging* **2012**, *46*, 207–214. [CrossRef] [PubMed]
38. Choi, H.J.; Kang, C.M.; Lee, W.J.; Song, S.Y.; Cho, A.; Yun, M.; Lee, J.D.; Kim, J.H.; Lee, J.H. Prognostic value of 18-fluorodeoxyglucose positron emission tomography in patients with resectable pancreatic cancer. *Yonsei Med. J.* **2013**, *54*, 1377–1383. [CrossRef] [PubMed]
39. Kitasato, Y.; Yasunaga, M.; Okuda, K.; Kinoshita, H.; Tanaka, H.; Okabe, Y.; Kawahara, A.; Kage, M.; Kaida, H.; Ishibashi, M. Maximum standardized uptake value on 18F-fluoro-2-deoxy-glucose positron emission tomography/computed tomography and glucose transporter-1 expression correlates with survival in invasive ductal carcinoma of the pancreas. *Pancreas* **2014**, *43*, 1060–1065. [CrossRef] [PubMed]
40. Lee, J.W.; Kang, C.M.; Choi, W.J.; Lee, W.J.; Song, S.Y.; Lee, J.H. Prognostic value of metabolic tumor volume and total lesion glycolysis on preoperative 18FDG PET/CT in patients with pancreatic cancer. *J. Nucl. Med.* **2014**, *55*, 896–904. [CrossRef]
41. Ariake, K.; Motoi, F.; Shimomura, H.; Mizuma, M.; Maeda, S.; Terao, C.; Tatewaki, Y.; Ohtsuka, H.; Fukase, K.; Masuda, K.; et al. 18-Fuorodeoxyglucose positron emission tomography predicts recurrence in resected pancreatic ductal adenocarcinoma. *J. Gastrointest. Surg.* **2018**, *22*, 279–287. [CrossRef]
42. Nunna, P.; Sheikhbahaei, S.; Ahn, S.; Young, B.; Subramaniam, R.M. The role of positron emission tomography/computed tomography in management and prediction of survival in pancreatic cancer. *J. Comput. Assist. Tomogr.* **2016**, *40*, 142–151. [CrossRef]
43. Parlak, C.; Topkan, E.; Onal, C.; Reyhan, M.; Selek, U. Prognostic value of gross tumor volume delineated by FDG-PET-CT based radiotherapy treatment planning in patients with locally advanced pancreatic cancer treated with chemoradiotherapy. *Radiat. Oncol.* **2012**, *7*, 37. [CrossRef] [PubMed]
44. Xu, H.X.; Chen, T.; Wang, W.Q.; Wu, C.T.; Liu, C.; Long, J.; Xu, J.; Zhang, Y.J.; Chen, R.H.; Liu, L.; et al. Metabolic tumor burden assessed by 18F-FDG PET/CT associated with serum CA 19-9 predicts pancreatic cancer outcome. *Eur. J. Nucl. Med. Mol. Imaging* **2014**, *41*, 1093–1102. [CrossRef] [PubMed]

© 2020 by the authors. Licensee MDPI, Basel, Switzerland. This article is an open access article distributed under the terms and conditions of the Creative Commons Attribution (CC BY) license (http://creativecommons.org/licenses/by/4.0/).

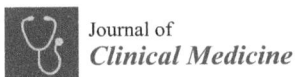

Article

Identification and Validation of Circulating Micrornas as Prognostic Biomarkers in Pancreatic Ductal Adenocarcinoma Patients Undergoing Surgical Resection

Natalia Gablo [1], Karolina Trachtova [1], Vladimir Prochazka [2], Jan Hlavsa [2], Tomas Grolich [2], Igor Kiss [3], Josef Srovnal [4], Alona Rehulkova [4], Martin Lovecek [5], Pavel Skalicky [5], Ioana Berindan-Neagoe [6], Zdenek Kala [2,*] and Ondrej Slaby [1,7,8,*]

1. Central European Institute of Technology, Masaryk University, 625 00 Brno, Czech Republic; gablon@wp.pl (N.G.); trachtova@mail.muni.cz (K.T.)
2. Department of Surgery, Faculty Hospital Brno and Faculty of Medicine, Masaryk University, 601 77 Brno, Czech Republic; Prochazka.Vladimir@fnbrno.cz (V.P.); Hlavsa.Jan@fnbrno.cz (J.H.); Grolich.Tomas@fnbrno.cz (T.G.)
3. Masaryk Memorial Cancer Institute, Department of Comprehensive Cancer Care, 602 00 Brno, Czech Republic; kiss@mou.cz
4. Laboratory of Experimental Medicine, Institute of Molecular and Translational Medicine, Faculty of Medicine and Dentistry, Palacky University and University Hospital Olomouc, 771 47 Olomouc, Czech Republic; josef.srovnal@fnol.cz (J.S.); alona.rehulkova@upol.cz (A.R.)
5. 1st Department of Surgery, Faculty of Medicine and Dentistry, Palacky University and University Hospital 771 47 Olomouc, Czech Republic; Martin.Lovecek@fnol.cz (M.L.); pavel.skalicky@upol.cz (P.S.)
6. MEDFUTURE-Research Center for Advanced Medicine, University of Medicine, and Pharmacy Iuliu-Hatieganu, 400000 Cluj-Napoca, Romania; ioana.neagoe@umfcluj.ro
7. Department of Pathology, Faculty Hospital Brno and Faculty of Medicine, Masaryk University, 625 00 Brno, Czech Republic
8. Department of Biology, Faculty of Medicine, Masaryk University, 625 00 Brno, Czech Republic
* Correspondence: Kala.Zdenek@fnbrno.cz (Z.K.); oslaby@med.muni.cz (O.S.); Tel.: +42-0532232966 (Z.K.)

Received: 31 May 2020; Accepted: 27 July 2020; Published: 30 July 2020

Abstract: Pancreatic ductal adenocarcinoma (PDAC) is one of the most lethal and aggressive cancers with a less than 6% five-year survival rate. Circulating microRNAs (miRNAs) are emerging as a useful tool for non-invasive diagnosis and prognosis estimation in the various cancer types, including PDAC. Our study aimed to evaluate whether miRNAs in the pre-operative blood plasma specimen have the potential to predict the prognosis of PDAC patients. In total, 112 PDAC patients planned for surgical resection were enrolled in our prospective study. To identify prognostic miRNAs, we used small RNA sequencing in 24 plasma samples of PDAC patients with poor prognosis (overall survival (OS) < 16 months) and 24 plasma samples of PDAC patients with a good prognosis (OS > 20 months). qPCR validation of selected miRNA candidates was performed in the independent cohort of PDAC patients ($n = 64$). In the discovery phase of the study, we identified 44 miRNAs with significantly different levels in the plasma samples of the group of good and poor prognosis patients. Among these miRNAs, 23 showed lower levels, and 21 showed higher levels in plasma specimens from PDAC patients with poor prognosis. Eleven miRNAs were selected for the validation, but only miR-99a-5p and miR-365a-3p were confirmed to have significantly lower levels and miR-200c-3p higher levels in plasma samples of poor prognosis cases. Using the combination of these 3-miRNA levels, we were able to identify the patients with poor prognosis with sensitivity 85% and specificity 80% (Area Under the Curve = 0.890). Overall, 3-miRNA prognostic score associated with OS was identified in the pre-operative blood plasma samples of PDAC patients undergoing surgical resection. Following further independent validations, the detection of these miRNA may enable identification of PDAC patients who have no survival benefit from the surgical treatment, which is associated with the high morbidity rates.

Keywords: Pancreatic ductal adenocarcinoma; prognosis; microRNAs

1. Introduction

Pancreatic ductal adenocarcinoma (PDAC) constitutes 90% of all pancreatic cancers and is associated with the worst survival, with only 5–7% of patients living longer than five years from diagnosis [1,2]. In comparison to other types of pancreatic cancer [3], PDAC, due to its aggressive biological behavior, has a high incidence/mortality ratio reaching 94%, which makes this disease the 4th most common cause of cancer-associated mortality in developed countries [2]. Among the available treatment strategies, including radical pancreatectomy, chemotherapy, radiotherapy, or integrated multimodal treatment, radical surgical resection of the tumor in its early stages (IA–IIB) remains the only option that may increase the five-year survival rate to 16–21% [4–6]. Nevertheless, most of the patients are diagnosed at an advanced inoperable stage of the disease, and only 15–20% of PDAC patients can be considered candidates for radical surgical resection. Clinical studies revealed that there is a subset of PDAC patients, who develop disease recurrence shortly after resection without any improvement in survival [7–9]. Compared to PDAC patients with inoperable disease receiving only chemotherapy, this subset of poor prognosis patients has no clinical benefit from the surgical resection, which is associated with a high morbidity rate. Therefore, pre-operative estimation of the prognosis is essential to avoid treatment-related risks for those patients who would unlikely benefit from this treatment approach [10,11]. One of the reasons behind poor outcomes is the presence of micro-metastatic disease, which cannot be detected during pre-operative staging examination and even during intraoperative assessment [10]. Unfortunately, there is still a lack of powerful biomarkers, that would contribute to better individualization of PDAC patients' treatment strategies. Currently, all PDAC patients with localized disease and operable tumors evaluated through imaging methods are candidates for surgical treatment [12]. Carbohydrate antigen 19-9 (CA19-9) is the only approved blood-based biomarker used in PDAC patients, but it is mainly useful for monitoring of PDAC patients following the surgical resection rather than for pre-operative survival prognostication [13]. In the last few years, there has been increasing evidence suggesting circulating cell-free microRNAs (miRNAs) present promising non-invasive biomarkers in cancer.

MiRNAs are highly conserved, small, non-coding RNAs, 18–25 nucleotides in length. miRNAs are involved in post-transcriptional regulation of gene expression. miRNAs act as powerful regulators of gene expression, mostly via interacting with the 3' UTR of target mRNAs, which inhibit translation or induces mRNA degradation [14]. Additionally, they can also bind to 5'UTR of target mRNAs or bind to coding sequence regions [15]. A number of studies have revealed that miRNAs are involved in the regulation of cell homeostasis by controlling important cellular processes including the development, differentiation, proliferation, apoptosis and stress reaction. Furthermore, aberrant expression of miRNAs can promote carcinogenesis through direct or indirect regulation of oncogenes or tumor suppressor genes [16].

In PDAC, many investigators have detected changes in miRNA expression patterns, which influenced multiple genetic aberrations that contribute to initiation of tumorigenesis progression, invasion, and metastatic processes. Subsequently, miRNAs correlate with disease-free, overall survival of PDAC patients, and their response to treatment [17].

Interest in the minimally invasive biomarkers is growing because they would significantly contribute to improving the outcome of PDAC patients by individualization of the therapeutic approach. The presence of tumor-derived miRNAs in body fluids offers an opportunity to obtain such biomarker and became the subject of intense investigation. miRNAs are selectively and specifically released into circulation under various pathological conditions including cancer. Moreover, circulating miRNAs present many favorable advantages for application as liquid biopsy-based biomarkers, such as high stability, high abundance, and their presence in nearly all body fluids including blood plasma [18–20].

The aim of our study was to enable identification of the PDAC patients who will not benefit from the surgical resection (patients with the same or shorter overall survival (OS) as PDAC patients without surgical resection) and therefore give the rationale for the clinical decision, whether to perform surgical resection or give preference to non-surgical therapeutic modalities and quality of life.

To this end, we performed global profiling of blood plasma miRNAs using small RNA sequencing followed by the validation of miRNA candidates in the independent cohort of PDAC patients to assess the potential of plasma miRNAs for pre-operative prognostic stratification of PDAC patients planned for radical surgical resection.

2. Material and Methods

2.1. Study Population Characteristic

Treatment-naive patients with histologically confirmed pancreatic ductal adenocarcinoma were recruited from the University Hospital Brno (UHB; Brno, Czech Republic), University Hospital Olomouc (UHO; Olomouc, Czech Republic), and Masaryk Memorial Cancer Institute (MMCI; Brno, Czech Republic). Only patients undergoing radical surgical resection were enrolled in our study. Subjects were of the same ethnicity (Caucasian). Patient characteristics are summarized in Table 1. The study was approved by multi-centric Ethical Board (UHB) and written informed consent was provided by each study participant. Approximately 10 mL of peripheral venous blood was collected in an ethylenediaminetetraacetic acid (EDTA)-treated Vacutainer before surgical resection and any other treatment. Within one hour after collection, plasma fraction was separated by centrifugation at 1200× g for 10 min at 4 °C and stored at −80 °C till further processed.

Table 1. Clinical and histopathological characteristics of pancreatic ductal adenocarcinoma patients.

	Discovery Cohort	Validation Cohort
n (Patients)	48	64
Age		
65 years	15	24
>65 years	33	40
Sex		
Male	24	24
Female	24	40
Tumor location		
pancreatic head	38	50
pancreatic body/tail	10	14
pT stage		
T2	0	9
T3	48	55
pN stage		
N0	5	20
N1-2	43	44
pM stage		
M0	48	64
CA19-9		
High	22	30
Low	18	20
NA	8	14
Adjuvant chemotherapy		
Yes	42	44
No	6	20
Poor survival group (median 9, range 4–14 months)	24	14
Good survival group (median 27, range 20–47 months)	24	16

2.1.1. RNA Isolation from Blood Plasma Specimens

Cell-free miRNAs were isolated from 250 μL of blood plasma using Qiagen miRNeasy Serum/Plasma Kit (Qiagen, GmbH, Hilden, Germany) according to manufacturers' protocol. We used glycogen during isolation step as an RNA carrier, since exogenous RNA can interfere—via non-specific hybridization or amplification—with the results of small RNA sequencing [21]. Concentration and purity of RNA was measuring by both UV spectrophotometry (NanoDrop ND-2000, Thermo Fisher Scientific, Walthman, MA, USA) and fluorometry (Qubit, Thermofisher Scientific, Walthamn, MA, USA). The purified RNA was stored at −80 °C until further analysis or processed immediately.

2.1.2. Small RNA Libraries Preparation and Next Generation Sequencing

In the discovery phase of the study, we used a blood plasma samples collected pre-operatively from PDAC patients, which have been already available in the biobank of Masaryk Memorial Cancer Institute (Brno, Czech Republic). For small RNA sequencing, libraries were prepared from 2 μL of total RNA using the QIAseq™ miRNA Library Kit and QIAseq miRNA NGS 48 Index IL (Qiagen, Hilden, Germany). Following 3' and 5' adapter ligation, small RNAs were reverse transcribed, using unique molecular identifier (UMI) primers of random 12-nucleotide sequences. This way, precise linear quantification of miRNAs is achieved, overcoming potential PCR-induced biases. cDNA libraries were amplified by PCR for 24 cycles, with a 3' primer that includes a 6-nucleotide unique index. Following size selection and cleaning of the sequencing libraries with magnetic beads, quality control was performed by measuring library concentration with a Qubit fluorometer using a dsDNA High Sensitivity (HS) assay kit (Thermo Fisher Scientific, Walthamn, MA, USA) and confirming library size with TapeStation D1000 (Agilent). Further, libraries were multiplexed and sequenced on a single NextSeq 500/550 v2 flow cell (Illumina, San Diego, CA, USA) with 75bp single read and 6bp index read (80 cycles).

2.1.3. Quantitative Real-Time PCR (qRT-PCR)

In the validation phase of the study, we used a prospectively collected plasma samples withdrawn pre-operatively from PDAC patients at University Hospital Brno (Brno, Czech Republic) and University Hospital Olomouc (Olomouc, Czech Republic). For miRNA qRT-PCR, plasma RNA was reverse-transcribed to complementary DNA (cDNA) using a miRCURY LNA Universal RT cDNA Synthesis Kit (Qiagen, Hilden, Germany). Initial RNA input used in reverse transcription reaction was optimized by running a few individual assays with different volumes of RNA samples according to manufacture requirements. We used 2 μL of RNA template in 10 μL of final reaction volume for all samples, which correspond to 16 μL of original blood plasma specimens. Reverse Transcription was performed using T100™ Thermal Cycler (Bio-Rad, Hercules, CA, USA) at 42 °C for 60 min and 90 °C for 5 min. The final product of reaction was diluted in ratio 1:30 with nuclease free water. Three microliters of diluted cDNA were added to qPCR mixture (miRCURY SYBR Green PCR Kit) containing LNA-enhanced primers specific for each miRNA (miRCURY LNA miRNA PCR primers; hsa-miR-9-5p; hsa-miR-30e-5p; hsa-miR-365a-3p; hsa-miR-22-3p; hsa-miR-885-5p; hsa-miR-99b-5p; hsa-miR-99a-5p; hsa-miR-200c-3p; hsa-miR-122-5p; hsa-miR-100-5p; hsa-let-7e-5p; hsa-miR-93-5p). All samples were run using Quant Studio 12K Flex Sstem (Applied Biosystems, Foster City, CA, USA).

2.1.4. Data Normalization and Statistical Analysis

The raw sequencing images from Illumina NextSeq 550 (change for the right machine used) were demultiplexed and converted to fastq format using bcl2fastq (version 2.20.0). Adapter sequences in raw sequencing data were identified by Kraken package (15-065) and trimmed using Cutadapt (version 1.18). Collapsing was performed utilizing unique molecular identifiers (UMIs) with FASTX-Toolkit (version 0.0.14). Subsequently, reads were quality trimmed and these shorter than 15bp were discarded. Reads originating from snoRNAs, snRNAs, rRNAs, tRNAs, piRNAs, and YRNAs (downloaded from Ensembl and RefSeq) were identified using Bowtie (version 1.2.2) and removed from the data. Remaining reads were mapped against the miRBase (version 21) using the miraligner tool (version 1.2.4). Statistical analysis, including normalization for library depth, was carried out in R (version 3.4.3) with DESeq2 package (version 1.18.1).

The threshold cycle data were calculated by QuantStudio 12K Flex software. All real-time PCR reactions were run in duplicates. All PCR reactions where the difference between Ct values in duplicate were higher than 0.25 were repeated. The average expression levels of all measured miRNAs were normalized using miR-93-5p which was found to be suitable reference gene based on consensus of two algorithm, namely NormFinder and geNorm. Quantification of target miRNA relative to reference endogenous control was determined by the $2^{-\Delta Ct}$ method [22]. Statistical differences between the levels of analyzed miRNAs in plasma samples of poor and good prognosis cases were evaluated by two-tailed non-parametric Mann–Whitney U-test. Further, receiver operating curve (ROC) analyses were performed to assess the diagnostic performance of analyzed miRNAs. Survival analyses were carried out using the log-rank test and Kaplan–Meier analysis. All calculations were performed using GraphPad Prism version 7.01 (GraphPad Software) p-values of less than 0.05 were considered statistically significant.

3. Results

In total, 112 patients with PDAC were enrolled in the study. These patients were divided into two cohorts: discovery (n = 48) and validation (n = 64) cohort. In terms of prognosis, patients with overall survival (OS) shorter than 16 months were classified as poor prognosis cases, conversely patients with OS longer than 20 months (without event) were classified as good prognosis cases. According to this definition of prognostic groups, there was 24 good prognosis and 24 poor prognosis cases in the discovery cohort and 16 good prognosis and 14 poor prognosis cases in the validation cohort. Remaining 34 cases in the validation cohort were included in the survival analysis but were not used for the group analysis due to the short follow-up or intermediate OS between the good and poor prognosis survival ranges.

In this discovery phase of the study, we performed small RNA sequencing of the pre-operative blood plasma specimens, and we identified 44 miRNAs to have significantly different levels in the plasma samples of the 24 patients with good prognosis cases and 24 with poor prognosis ($p < 0.05$). Among these miRNAs, 21 showed higher expression and 23 showed lower expression in blood plasma from PDAC patients with poor prognosis (Table 2). Out of these 44 miRNAs identified in discovery phase, 11 miRNAs (miR-99a-5p, miR-9-5p, miR-365a-3p, miR-22-3p, miR-885-5p, miR-200c-3p, let-7e-5p, miR-100-5p, miR-122-5p, miR-99b-5p, miR-30e-5p) were selected for the validation phase of the study to evaluate their ability to distinguish PDAC patients with poor and good prognosis. These miRNAs were selected based on the p-value ($p < 0.02$), log2(fold-change) ≥ 0.45 or ≤ -0.45, and the average number of reads across all sequenced samples (at least 10). Lower threshold for the fold-change was selected based on the pleiotropic regulatory effects of miRNAs and related biological relevance of even subtle expression changes compared to the mRNAs.

The blood plasma levels of miRNA candidates from the discovery cohort were determined by use of individual qPCR assays and statistically evaluated between the groups of patients with good and poor prognosis. Using two-tailed non-parametric Mann–Whitney U test and ROC analysis, only miR-99a-5p and miR-365a-3p were confirmed to have significantly lower levels and miR-200c-3p significantly higher levels in the blood plasma of the patients with poor prognosis (p-values and AUC values are summarized in Table 3 and Figure 1A–F). Other tested miRNAs were not confirmed to have different levels in blood plasma samples of PDAC patients with different prognosis. These results were also confirmed using the Kaplan–Meier analysis. Patients with lower levels of miR-99a-5p and miR-365a-3p and higher levels of miR-200c-3p in blood plasma had significantly shorter overall survival (Figure 1D–I).

Table 2. List of the miRNAs with significantly different levels in blood plasma of patients with good (overall survival (OS) > 20 months) and poor prognosis (OS < 16 months) identified in the discovery phase of the study.

microRNA	BaseMean	log2FC	p-Value
miR-99a-5p	200.59	−1.19	**0.001**
miR-9-5p	12.70	1.48	**0.002**
miR-365a-3p	16.54	−1.75	**0.002**
miR-362-5p	3.39	1.07	0.005
miR-627-5p	4.33	−1.26	0.006
miR-22-3p	566.82	−0.61	**0.006**
miR-885-5p	27.65	−1.50	**0.008**
miR-1273h-5p	7.55	0.90	0.009
miR-940	0.89	1.49	0.011
miR-499a-5p	2.38	−1.50	0.011
miR-34c-3p	2.09	2.11	0.012
miR-200c-3p	79.59	0.49	**0.012**
miR-101-5p	1.28	−2.17	0.012
miR-18b-3p	0.66	−2.01	0.014
let-7e-5p	843.66	0.54	**0.014**
miR-30e-5p	3565.64	−0.35	**0.015**
miR-100-5p	99.16	−0.97	**0.015**
miR-122-5p	196,465.98	−1.14	**0.016**
miR-99b-5p	298.30	0.45	**0.019**
let-7b-3p	9.59	−1.02	0.020
let-7f-5p	24,401.75	0.33	0.024
miR-6770-3p	0.64	1.65	0.025
miR-181c-5p	6.71	0.81	0.026
miR-5010-5p	9.20	0.74	0.028
miR-30a-5p	954.09	−0.66	0.030
miR-4676-3p	2.38	1.11	0.030
miR-885-3p	109.35	−1.16	0.030
miR-193b-3p	1.43	−1.69	0.034
miR-12135	3.27	0.95	0.035
miR-1275	5.86	−0.69	0.037
miR-202-3p	2.46	−1.30	0.037
miR-552-5p	2.50	−1.03	0.037
miR-99b-3p	29.24	0.74	0.038
miR-210-3p	14.32	−0.69	0.041
miR-3146	2.11	1.31	0.043
miR-148a-3p	12,136.24	−0.66	0.043
miR-1249-3p	0.83	2.18	0.043
miR-6875-5p	1.63	1.25	0.044
miR-6796-5p	0.68	1.51	0.045
miR-548bc	2.49	1.47	0.046
miR-191-5p	8975.04	0.45	0.047
miR-378a-3p	677.18	−0.63	0.047
miR-224-5p	485.23	−0.66	0.049
miR-96-5p	63.60	−0.78	0.050

Log2FC: Logarithm to the base 2 of fold-change; baseMean: Average of the normalized read numbers; bolded miRNAs were selected for validation in the independent cohort of PDAC patients based on the pre-defined selection criteria. Bold: miRNAs selected for independent validation.

Table 3. Results of the validation of miRNA candidates by qPCR in the independent cohort of PDAC patients.

microRNA	NGS Discovery Cohort		qPCR Group Comparison Validation Cohort		qPCR Survival Analysis Validation Cohort
	Log2FC	p-Value	Log2FC	p-Value	p-Value
miR-99a-5p	−1.188	0.001	−1.324	0.03	0.006
miR-365a-3p	−1.752	0.002	−1.39	0.003	0.013
miR-200c-3p	0.493	0.012	0.766	0.04	0.012

Log2FC: Logarithm to the base 2 of fold-change; NGS: Next-generation sequencing; qPCR: Quantitative polymerase chain reaction.

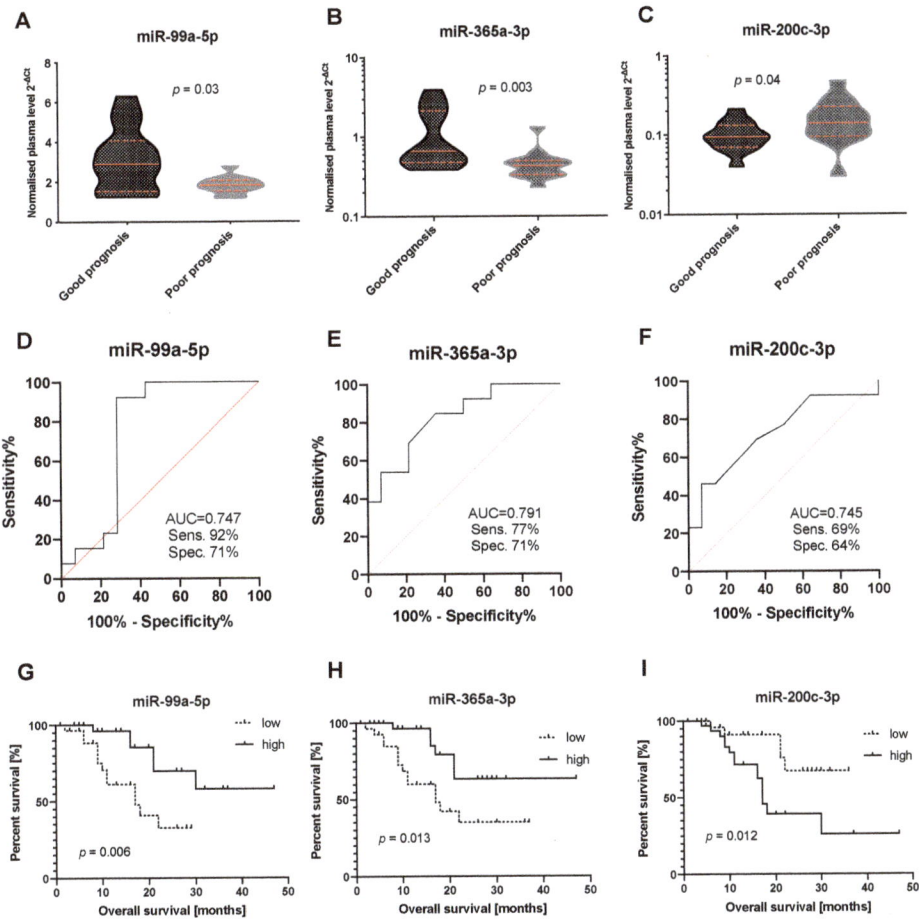

Figure 1. miRNAs with significantly different levels in blood plasma of pancreatic ductal adenocarcinoma (PDAC) patients with good and poor prognosis after surgical resection. Results of Mann–Whitney U-test for miR-99a-5p (**A**), miR-365a-3p (**B**), and miR-200c-3p (**C**); ROC analysis for miR-99a-5p (**D**), miR-365a-3p (**E**) and miR-200c-3p (**F**); and Kaplan-Meier survival analysis for miR-99a-5p (**G**), miR-365a-3p (**H**) and miR-200c-3p (**I**). AUC: Area under the curve; Sens.: Sensitivity; Spec.: Specificity.

Subsequent ROC analysis revealed that the usage of 3-miRNA-combined prognostic score (PScore = −0.6430 + 0.8689 *miR-99a-5p + 0.9261 *miR-365a-3p-17.5256 *miR-200c-3p), as established by a bidirectional stepwise logistic regression, enabled the identification of the patients with poor prognosis after surgical resection (OS < 16 months) with sensitivity of 85% and specificity of 80% (area under the curve (AUC) = 0.890; cut-off value = 0.5522; Figure 2). Prognostic score based on the combination of three miRNAs enabled us to increase the AUC from 0.791, which was the highest in reached by individual miRNA, to 0.890.

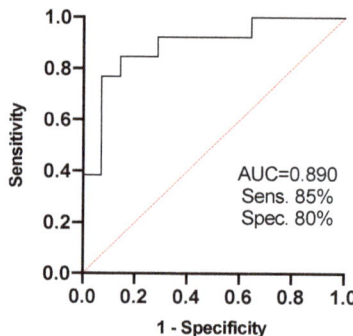

Figure 2. Receiver operating characteristic analysis of the use of miR-99a-5p, miR-365a-3p, and miR-200c-3p combination (Pscore) in the discriminating between the PDAC patients with good and poor prognosis. AUC: area under the curve.

4. Discussion

Complete removal of the tumor at its early stage is considered only as an curative option for PDAC patients. However, a significant percentage of PDAC patients that undergo primary tumor resection rapidly develop a disease recurrence, whereas other patients benefit from surgery and have long disease-free survival. Identifying the patients at risk of early disease recurrence could enable adjustments in rational treatment selection to perform surgical resection or give preference to non-surgical treatment modalities and quality of life. There is increasing evidence that cell-free miRNAs are suitable candidates for the prediction of PDAC progression due to their altered expression during tumorigenesis and their stability in the body fluids [19,23].

Herein, we present results of a multicenter study where we sought to identify circulating cell-free miRNAs with the potential of pre-operative prognostic stratification of PDAC patients in a minimally invasive way. For this purpose, we implemented a small RNA sequencing technique for global miRNA in pre-operative plasma samples from treatment-naive patients with PDAC at the operable stage of the disease. Patient populations in both the discovery and validation cohorts were divided into two prognostic groups according to their survival after curative-intend surgery. The cut-off for prognostic stratification was established according to the median overall survival of inoperable, advanced PDAC patients. Small RNA sequencing revealed 44 miRNAs significantly associated with the PDAC patients' survival after surgery. Out of these, the most promising miRNAs that met the established selection criteria were subjected to further evaluation as prognostic biomarkers in the independent patients' cohort. Finally, a comparison of miRNA expression level in the validation phase confirmed ability of three miRNAs (miR-99a-5p, miR-200c-3p, and miR-365a-3p) to discriminate PDAC patients with poor outcomes after resection from those with longer survival. Validation confirmed that a high level of miR-99a-5p in pre-operative plasma is associated with better survival of PDAC patients who underwent curative surgery. This finding is indicating its dual role during tumorigenesis and cancer progression. MiR-99a-5p belongs to the twenty most abundant miRNAs in human plasma exosomes, indicating that its appearance in bloodstream is a result of coordinated release from cell in response to different stimuli and could reflect disease status [24]. The role of miR-99a-5p in various cancer types has been described; aberrant expression of this miRNA has been linked with both oncogenic and tumor suppressive function. While results provided by Dhayata et al. imply pro-oncogenic regulatory activity of miR-99a-5p, our observation indicates its protective functioning in the progression of PDAC [25,26]. However, a number of other reports support our observation, indicating miR-99a roles in a suppression of various cancer types. Decreased expression of miR-99a-5p was found to predict worse survival in lung adenocarcinoma [27], cervical cancer [28], and breast cancer [29]. MiR-99a-5p was found to play important tumor-suppressive roles, including inhibition of cell proliferation and tumorigenesis by suppressing mTOR signaling pathway and downregulation of insulin-like growth factor 1 receptor [30], and also inhibition of migration and invasion of cancer cells by decreasing MTMR3 protein (Myotubularin-related protein 3) in oral cancer [31].

The second successfully validated miRNA was miR-200c-3p. However, log2(FC) in both discovery and validation cohort was below 1, which could limit its application as a potential biomarker. This miRNA belongs to the miR-200 family and is well described as an epithelial marker in solid tumors, including PDAC. It plays an important role in regulating of epithelial phenotype of tumor cells during both epithelial mesenchymal transition (EMT) and mesenchymal epithelial transition (MET) processes. Results of the metanalysis of Wang et al. demonstrated that low expression of miR-200c in tumor tissue and high expression in serum is correlated with poorer survival in solid tumors [32]. The main targets of or miR-200c are transcriptional repressors, namely E-cadherin and ZEB1 and ZEB2. Insufficient expression of this miRNA led to the loss of epithelial features of cancer cells, thereby, cells acquire the ability to escape from primary localization and further enter to circulation. During reverse process, miR-200c-3p is upregulated, and tumor cells with mesenchymal phenotype acquire epithelial phenotype necessary to final metastatic colonization and formation of macroscopic metastases in the distant organs. The reason for poor prognosis in PDAC patients is rapid disease progression and early dissemination [10]. Therefore, we speculate that higher levels of miR-200c in the blood plasma of PDAC patients with shorter survival results from the presence a non-detectable metastatic disease in the time of tumor resection suggesting diverse roles of miR-200c-3p in different stages of PDAC development.

Finally, we found that a higher level of miR-365a-3p in pre-operative plasma might predict the longer survival of PDAC patients following curative radical resection. To support our observation, reports of Yin et al. note an association between low expression of miR-356a-3p and PDAC progression by in vitro, in vivo, and patient tissue studies [33]. Increased expression of miR-365a-3p inhibits NF-κB activity by downregulating c-Rel and thus reduced the viability of PDAC cells and induced apoptosis.

A combination of circulating miRNAs may considerably improve cancer diagnosis and prognosis, and some miRNAs panels have already been described as non-invasive biomarkers for PDAC disease. For example, Cao et al. established two plasma miRNAs-based panels with high diagnostic accuracy. The first panel comprising three miRNAs, namely, miR-486-5p, miR-126-3p, and miR-106b-3p, had high accuracy for distinguishing pancreatic cancer (PC) from chronic pancreatitis (CHP) with AUC values of 0.891. Furthermore, panel including 6 microRNAs; miR-486-5p, miR-126-3p, miR-106b-3p, miR-938, miR-26b-3p, miR-1285 accurately discriminate between PC patients and CHP with AUC 0.889. Moreover, both miRNA panels showed higher diagnostic accuracy than CA19-9 (AUC = 0.775) [34]. Most recently, Zou et al. identified a panel of six serum miRNAs (let-7b-5p, miR-192-5p, miR-19a-3p, miR-19b-3p, miR-223-3p, and miR-25-3p) with potential to distinguish PC patients and healthy donors with AUC = 0.910. Besides, the analysis provided in their study revealed that the combination of miRNAs showed higher diagnostic value than the individual miRNA [35].

Herein, we showed that three miRNAs-based biomarkers can significantly predict PDAC patients' survival time after curative surgery. Multiple miRNAs combined are considered as a more superior diagnostic tool than a single miRNA-based test. This thesis can be verified based on the mechanisms of miRNAs in cancer development and progression, whereas a series of miRNAs, rather than a single one, are involved in the pathological process. Moreover, the same miRNAs are deregulated in different types of malignancies suggesting that single miRNAs could not be specific to a cancer type. In this sense, it is reasonable that a combination of miRNAs guarantee that the biomarker is specific to a cancer type. miRNA panels are based on the combination of two miRNAs up to several miRNAs. Nevertheless, an optimal clinical model must have a high sensitivity and specificity and a suitable cost and time-effectiveness.

5. Conclusions

In conclusion, we identified miRNAs associated with OS in the pre-operative blood plasma samples of PDAC patients undergoing surgical resection. Following further independent validations, the detection of these miRNA may enable identification of PDAC patients who have no survival benefit from the surgical treatment, which is associated with the high morbidity rates. However, our study suffers from some limitations. As the main limitation, we recognize that the validation part of the study is based on a small prospective sample cohort and further validation with larger sample size is required to validate the efficacy of candidate miRNAs. Although several challenges remain to be addressed, plasma miRNAs can potentially be useful for the prognostic stratification of PDAC patients undergoing curative resection.

Author Contributions: Conceptualization, I.K., Z.K. and O.S.; Data curation, N.G., K.T., V.P., J.H., T.G., J.S., A.R., M.L., P.S. and I.B.-N.; Formal analysis, K.T., I.K., I.B.-N., Z.K. and O.S.; Funding acquisition, Z.K. and O.S.; Investigation, N.G., V.P., J.H., T.G., J.S., A.R., M.L. and P.S.; Methodology, N.G. and I.B.-N.; Resources, V.P.; Software, K.T.; Supervision, I.K., Z.K. and O.S.; Validation, N.G., J.H., T.G., J.S., A.R., M.L. and P.S.; Writing—original draft, N.G. and O.S.; Writing—review & editing, I.K., Z.K. and O.S. All authors have read and agreed to the published version of the manuscript.

Funding: This study was supported by the Ministry of Health of the Czech Republic by the Czech Health Research Council project No. 16-31314A.

Conflicts of Interest: The authors declare no conflict of interest. The funders had no role in the design of the study; in the collection, analyses, or interpretation of data; in the writing of the manuscript, or in the decision to publish the results.

References

1. Kleeff, J.; Korc, M.; Apte, M.; La Vecchia, C.; Johnson, C.D.; Biankin, A.V.; Neale, R.E.; Tempero, M.; Tuveson, D.A.; Hruban, R.H.; et al. Pancreatic cancer. *Nat. Rev. Dis. Primers* **2016**, *2*, 16022. [CrossRef]
2. Rawla, P.; Sunkara, T.; Gaduputi, V. Epidemiology of Pancreatic Cancer: Global Trends, Etiology and Risk Factors. *World J. Oncol.* **2019**, *10*, 10–27. [CrossRef] [PubMed]
3. Poredska, K.; Kunovsky, L.; Prochazka, V.; Dolina, J.; Chovancova, M.; Vlazny, J.; Andrasina, T.; Eid, M.; Jabandziev, P.; Kysela, P. Triple malignancy (NET, GIST and pheochromocytoma) as a first manifestation of neurofibromatosis type-1 in an adult patient. *Diag. Pathol.* **2019**, *14*, 77. [CrossRef] [PubMed]
4. Neoptolemos, J.P.; Stocken, D.D.; Friess, H.; Bassi, C.; Dunn, J.A.; Hickey, H.; Beger, H.; Fernandez-Cruz, L.; Dervenis, C.; Lacaine, F.; et al. A Randomized Trial of Chemoradiotherapy and Chemotherapy after Resection of Pancreatic Cancer. *N. Engl. J. Med.* **2004**, *350*, 1200–1210. [CrossRef] [PubMed]
5. Neoptolemos, J.P.; Stocken, D.D.; Smith, C.T.; Bassi, C.; Ghaneh, P.; Owen, E.; Moore, M.; Padbury, R.; Doi, R.; Smith, D.; et al. Adjuvant 5-fluorouracil and folinic acid vs observation for pancreatic cancer: Composite data from the ESPAC-1 and -3(v1) trials. *Br. J. Cancer* **2009**, *100*, 246–250. [CrossRef] [PubMed]
6. Neoptolemos, J.P.; Palmer, D.H.; Ghaneh, P.; E Psarelli, E.; Valle, J.W.; Halloran, C.M.; Faluyi, O.; A O'Reilly, D.; Cunningham, D.; Wadsley, J.; et al. Comparison of adjuvant gemcitabine and capecitabine with gemcitabine monotherapy in patients with resected pancreatic cancer (ESPAC-4): A multicentre, open-label, randomised, phase 3 trial. *Lancet* **2017**, *389*, 1011–1024. [CrossRef]

7. Jang, J.-Y.; Kang, M.; Heo, J.S.; Choi, S.H.; Choi, D.W.; Park, S.-J.; Han, S.-S.; Yoon, D.S.; Yu, H.C.; Kang, K.J.; et al. A Prospective Randomized Controlled Study Comparing Outcomes of Standard Resection and Extended Resection, Including Dissection of the Nerve Plexus and Various Lymph Nodes, in Patients with Pancreatic Head Cancer. *Ann. Surg.* **2014**, *259*, 656–664. [CrossRef]
8. Farnell, M.B.; Pearson, R.K.; Sarr, M.G.; DiMagno, E.P.; Burgart, L.J.; Dahl, T.R.; Foster, N.; Sargent, D.; the Pancreas Cancer Working Group. A prospective randomized trial comparing standard pancreatoduodenectomy with pancreatoduodenectomy with extended lymphadenectomy in resectable pancreatic head adenocarcinoma. *Surgery* **2005**, *138*, 618–630. [CrossRef]
9. Zheng, L.; Wolfgang, C.L. Which patients with resectable pancreatic cancer truly benefit from oncological resection: Is it destiny or biology? *Cancer Boil.* **2015**, *16*, 360–362. [CrossRef]
10. Rhim, A.D.; Mirek, E.T.; Aiello, N.M.; Maitra, A.; Bailey, J.M.; McAllister, F.; Reichert, M.; Beatty, G.L.; Rustgi, A.K.; Vonderheide, R.H.; et al. EMT and Dissemination Precede Pancreatic Tumor Formation. *Cell* **2012**, *148*, 349–361. [CrossRef]
11. Strobel, O.; Neoptolemos, J.P.; Jäger, D.; Büchler, M.W. Optimizing the outcomes of pancreatic cancer surgery. *Nat. Rev. Clin. Oncol.* **2018**, *16*, 11–26. [CrossRef] [PubMed]
12. Hong, S.B.; Lee, S.S.; Kim, J.H.; Kim, H.J.; Byun, J.H.; Hong, S.-M.; Song, K.-B.; Kim, S. Pancreatic Cancer CT: Prediction of Resectability according to NCCN Criteria. *Radiology* **2018**, *289*, 710–718. [CrossRef]
13. Pandiaraja, J.; Viswanathan, S.; Antomy, T.B.; Thirumuruganand, S.; Kumaresan, D.S. The Role of CA19-9 in Predicting Tumour Resectability in Carcinoma Head of Pancreas. *J. Clin. Diagn. Res.* **2016**, *10*, PC06–PC09. [CrossRef]
14. Schanen, B.C.; Li, X. Transcriptional regulation of mammalian miRNA genes. *Genomics* **2011**, *97*, 1–6. [CrossRef] [PubMed]
15. Jabandziev, P.; Bohosova, J.; Pinkasova, T.; Kunovsky, L.; Slaby, O.; Goel, A. The Emerging Role of Noncoding RNAs in Pediatric Inflammatory Bowel Disease. *Inflamm. Bowel. Dis.* **2020**, *26*, 985–993. [CrossRef] [PubMed]
16. Galatenko, V.V.; Galatenko, A.V.; Samatov, T.R.; Turchinovich, A.A.; Shkurnikov, M.Y.; Makarova, J.A.; Tonevitsky, A.G. Comprehensive network of miRNA-induced intergenic interactions and a biological role of its core in cancer. *Sci. Rep.* **2018**, *8*, 2418. [CrossRef]
17. Vorvis, C.; Koutsioumpa, M.; Iliopoulos, D. Developments in miRNA gene signaling pathways in pancreatic cancer. *Futur. Oncol.* **2016**, *12*, 1135–1150. [CrossRef]
18. Chen, X.; Ba, Y.; Ma, L.; Cai, X.; Yin, Y.; Wang, K.; Guo, J.; Zhang, Y.; Chen, J.; Guo, X.; et al. Characterization of microRNAs in serum: A novel class of biomarkers for diagnosis of cancer and other diseases. *Cell Res.* **2008**, *18*, 997–1006. [CrossRef]
19. Mitchell, P.S.; Parkin, R.K.; Kroh, E.M.; Fritz, B.R.; Wyman, S.K.; Pogosova-Agadjanyan, E.L.; Peterson, A.; Noteboom, J.; O'Briant, K.C.; Allen, A.; et al. Circulating microRNAs as stable blood-based markers for cancer detection. *Proc. Natl. Acad. Sci. USA* **2008**, *105*, 10513–10518. [CrossRef]
20. Weber, J.A.; Baxter, D.H.; Zhang, S.; Huang, D.Y.; Huang, K.H.; Lee, M.-J.; Galas, D.J.; Wang, K. The MicroRNA Spectrum in 12 Body Fluids. *Clin. Chem.* **2010**, *56*, 1733–1741. [CrossRef]
21. McAlexander, M.A.; Phillips, M.J.; Witwer, K.W. Comparison of Methods for miRNA Extraction from Plasma and Quantitative Recovery of RNA from Cerebrospinal Fluid. *Front. Genet.* **2013**, *4*, 83. [CrossRef] [PubMed]
22. Marabita, F.; De Candia, P.; Torri, A.; Tegnér, J.; Abrignani, S.; Rossi, R.L. Normalization of circulating microRNA expression data obtained by quantitative real-time RT-PCR. *Brief. Bioinform.* **2015**, *17*, 204–212. [CrossRef] [PubMed]
23. Karasek, P.; Gablo, N.; Hlavsa, J.; Kiss, I.; Vychytilova-Faltejskova, P.; Hermanová, M.; Kala, Z.; Slaby, O.; Prochazka, V. Pre-operative Plasma miR-21-5p Is a Sensitive Biomarker and Independent Prognostic Factor in Patients with Pancreatic Ductal Adenocarcinoma Undergoing Surgical Resection. *Cancer Genom. Proteom.* **2018**, *15*, 321–327. [CrossRef] [PubMed]
24. Huang, X.; Yuan, T.; Tschannen, M.; Sun, Z.; Jacob, H.J.; Du, M.; Liang, M.; Dittmar, R.L.; Liu, Y.; Liang, M.; et al. Characterization of human plasma-derived exosomal RNAs by deep sequencing. *BMC Genom.* **2013**, *14*, 1–14. [CrossRef]
25. Stroese, A.J.; Ullerich, H.; Koehler, G.; Raetzel, V.; Senninger, N.; Dhayat, S.A. Circulating microRNA-99 family as liquid biopsy marker in pancreatic adenocarcinoma. *J. Cancer Res. Clin. Oncol.* **2018**, *144*, 2377–2390. [CrossRef]

26. Dhayat, S.A.; Mardin, W.A.; Seggewiß, J.; Ströse, A.J.; Matuszcak, C.; Hummel, R.; Senninger, N.; Mees, S.T.; Haier, J. MicroRNA Profiling Implies New Markers of Gemcitabine Chemoresistance in Mutant p53 Pancreatic Ductal Adenocarcinoma. *PLoS ONE* **2015**, *10*, e0143755. [CrossRef]
27. Song, Y.; Dou, H.; Wang, P.; Zhao, S.; Wang, T.; Gong, W.; Zhao, J.; Li, E.; Tan, R.; Hou, Y.; et al. A novel small-molecule compound diaporine A inhibits non-small cell lung cancer growth by regulating miR-99a/mTOR signaling. *Cancer Biol. Ther.* **2014**, *15*, 1423–1430. [CrossRef]
28. Wang, L.; Chang, L.; Li, Z.; Gao, Q.; Cai, D.; Tian, Y.; Zeng, L.; Li, M. MiR-99a and -99b inhibit cervical cancer cell proliferation and invasion by targeting mTOR signaling pathway. *Med. Oncol.* **2014**, *31*, 934. [CrossRef]
29. Hu, Y.; Zhu, Q.; Tang, L. MiR-99a Antitumor Activity in Human Breast Cancer Cells through Targeting of mTOR Expression. *PLoS ONE* **2014**, *9*, e92099. [CrossRef]
30. Cheng, H.; Xue, J.; Yang, S.; Chen, Y.; Wang, Y.; Zhu, Y.; Wang, X.; Kuang, D.; Ruan, Q.; Duan, Y.; et al. Co-targeting of IGF1R/mTOR pathway by miR-497 and miR-99a impairs hepatocellular carcinoma development. *Oncotarget* **2017**, *8*, 47984–47997. [CrossRef]
31. Kuo, Y.-Z.; Tai, Y.-H.; Lo, H.-I.; Chen, Y.-L.; Cheng, H.-C.; Fang, W.-Y.; Lin, S.-H.; Yang, C.-L.; Tsai, S.-T.; Wu, L.-W. MiR-99a exerts anti-metastasis through inhibiting myotubularin-related protein 3 expression in oral cancer. *Oral Dis.* **2013**, *20*, e65–e74. [CrossRef] [PubMed]
32. Wang, H.; Shen, J.; Jiang, C.-P.; Liu, B. How to Explain the Contradiction of microRNA 200c Expression and Survival in Solid Tumors?: A Meta-analysis. *Asian Pac. J. Cancer Prev.* **2014**, *15*, 3687–3690. [CrossRef] [PubMed]
33. Yin, L.; Xiao, X.; Georgikou, C.; Yin, Y.; Liu, L.; Karakhanova, S.; Luo, Y.; Gladkich, J.; Fellenberg, J.; Sticht, C.; et al. MicroRNA-365a-3p inhibits c-Rel-mediated NF-kappaB signaling and the progression of pancreatic cancer. *Cancer Lett.* **2019**, *452*, 203–212. [CrossRef]
34. Cao, Z.; Liu, C.; Xu, J.; You, L.; Wang, C.; Lou, W.; Sun, B.; Miao, Y.; Liu, X.; Wang, X.; et al. Plasma microRNA panels to diagnose pancreatic cancer: Results from a multicenter study. *Oncotarget* **2016**, *7*, 41575–41583. [CrossRef] [PubMed]
35. Zou, X.; Wei, J.; Huang, Z.; Zhou, X.; Lu, Z.; Zhu, W.; Miao, Y. Identification of a six-miRNA panel in serum benefiting pancreatic cancer diagnosis. *Cancer Med.* **2019**, *8*, 2810–2822. [CrossRef] [PubMed]

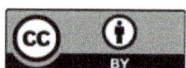

© 2020 by the authors. Licensee MDPI, Basel, Switzerland. This article is an open access article distributed under the terms and conditions of the Creative Commons Attribution (CC BY) license (http://creativecommons.org/licenses/by/4.0/).

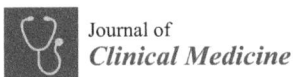

Article

Effect of Flowable Thrombin-Containing Collagen-Based Hemostatic Matrix for Preventing Pancreatic Fistula after Pancreatectomy: A Randomized Clinical Trial

Yejong Park [1,†], Jae Hyung Ko [2,†], Dae Ryong Kang [3,4], Jun Hyeok Lee [3], Dae Wook Hwang [1], Jae Hoon Lee [1], Woohyung Lee [1], Jaewoo Kwon [1], Si-Nae Park [2,*], Ki-Byung Song [1,*] and Song Cheol Kim [1,5,*]

[1] Division of Hepato-Biliary Pancreatic Surgery, Department of Surgery, University of Ulsan College of Medicine & Asan Medical Center, 88, Olympic-ro 43-gil, Songpa-gu, Seoul 05505, Korea; blackpig856@gmail.com (Y.P.); dwhwang@amc.seoul.kr (D.W.H.); gooddr23@naver.com (J.H.L.); ywhnet@gmail.com (W.L.); skunlvup@naver.com (J.K.)
[2] Regenerative Medicine Research Center, Dalim Tissen Co., Ltd., 31, Yeonhui-ro, Mapo-gu, Seoul 05505, Korea; rnd10@dalimtissen.com
[3] Department of Precision Medicine, Wonju College of Medicine, Yonsei University, 1 Yonseidae-gil, Wonju, Gangwon-do 26493, Korea; dr.kang@yonsei.ac.kr (D.R.K.); ljh0101@yonsei.ac.kr (J.H.L.)
[4] Department of Biostatistics, Wonju College of Medicine, Yonsei University, 1 Yonseidae-gil, Wonju, Gangwon-do 26493, Korea
[5] Asan Medical Institute of Convergence Science and Technology (AMIST), 88, Olympic-ro 43-gil, Songpa-gu, Seoul 05505, Korea
* Correspondence: snpark@dalimtissen.com (S.-N.P.); mtsong21c@naver.com (K.-B.S.); drksc@amc.seoul.kr (S.C.K.)
† These two authors contributed equally to this study as co-first authors.

Received: 30 August 2020; Accepted: 21 September 2020; Published: 24 September 2020

Abstract: Background: The aim of this study was to evaluate the safety and efficacy of a flowable hemostatic matrix, and their effects for postoperative pancreatic fistula (POPF) after pancreatectomy. Methods: This was a randomized, clinical, single-center, single-blind (participant), non-inferiority, phase IV, and parallel-group trial. The primary endpoint was the incidence of POPF. The secondary endpoints were risk factors for POPF, drain removal days, incidence of complication, 90-day mortality, and length of hospital stay. Results: This study evaluated a total of 53 patients, of whom 26 patients were in the intervention group (flowable hemostatic matrix) and 27 patients were in the control group (thrombin-coated collagen patch). POPF was more common in the control group than in the intervention group (59.3% vs. 30.8%, $p = 0.037$). Among participants who underwent distal pancreatectomy, POPF (33.3% vs. 92.3%, $p = 0.004$), and clinically relevant POPF (8.3% vs. 46.2%, $p = 0.027$) was more common in the control group. A multivariate logistic regression model identified flowable hemostatic matrix use as an independent negative risk factor for POPF, especially in cases of distal pancreatectomy (DP) (odds ratio 17.379, 95% confidential interval 1.453–207.870, $p = 0.024$). Conclusion: Flowable hemostatic matrix application is a simple, feasible, and effective method of preventing POPF after pancreatectomy, especially for patients with DP. Non-inferiority was demonstrated in the efficacy of preventing POPF in the intervention group compared to the control group.

Keywords: pancreatic fistula; pancreatectomy; pancreatic neoplasm

1. Introduction

Pancreatectomy including pancreaticoduodenectomy (PD) and distal pancreatectomy (DP) are standard surgical procedures in cases of pancreatic neoplasms, respectively [1–3]. However, the morbidity of this procedure is still high, ranging from 30% to 40% for PD [1,4]. The complication rate of PD is higher than that of other operations, and the high morbidity is mainly attributed to the occurrence of postoperative pancreatic fistula (POPF). In addition, POPF remains the leading cause of morbidity after DP, with a frequency ranging from 13% to 64% [3,5,6]. The clinically significant complication after pancreatectomy is POPF, which can lead to secondary complications such as intra-abdominal abscess, sepsis, and bleeding.

Despite attempts at reducing the incidence of POPF, which include pancreaticoenteric anastomosis, use of fibrin sealants, pancreatic stent insertion, and administration of octreotide, the incidence of POPF after PD has not considerably decreased. In addition, there are no validated recommendations or guidelines for the closure of the pancreatic remnant after DP, and no consensus exists on an optimal method for closure of the pancreatic stump [7,8]. The use of several different methods to secure the pancreatic remnant, including duct ligation, ultrasonic dissection, fibrin glue, patches and meshes, pancreaticoenteric anastomosis, and handsewn and stapler closure, possibly with bovine pericardial buttress, demonstrates the ongoing controversy [9–11].

Collagen has low antigenicity, hemostatic effects, and cell adhesion ability, and it is commonly used as a major component of hemostatic agents and artificial tissue substitutes [7,12–19]. In addition, collagen provides an environment in which fibroblasts can proliferate and induces wound healing by inactivating elastase and matrix metalloproteinases (MMPs) [20–22]. The prevention of POPF by applying collagen-based fibrin sealant patches to the anastomosis site or pancreatic stump has been reported previously. However, the usefulness of using fibrin sealant patches at the pancreatectomy site is still unclear [7,12–17,23].

CollaStat® (Dalim Tissen Co. Ltd., Seoul, Korea) is a novel flowable hemostatic agent that combines a collagen matrix with thrombin, a paste-like matrix that exhibits both passive and active mechanisms of actions, which are similar to FloSeal® (Baxter Healthcare, Deerfield, IL, USA) [18,19]. To the best of our knowledge, no studies have evaluated the efficacy of a flowable hemostatic matrix for the prevention of POPF. The aim of this study was to evaluate the safety and efficacy of a flowable hemostatic agent compared with a thrombin-coated collagen patch (CollaSeal®, Dalim Tissen Co. Ltd., Seoul, Korea) and their effect on clinical outcomes including POPF in a randomized controlled clinical trial.

2. Methods

2.1. Trial Design

We enrolled patients who underwent pancreatectomy in the Division of Hepato-Biliary and Pancreatic Surgery of the Department of Surgery at Asan Medical Center between February 2018 and September 2018. This was a randomized, clinical, single-center, single-blind (participant), non-inferiority, phase IV, and parallel-group trial. The study complied with the Declaration of Helsinki and was approved and overseen by the institutional review board (Number: 2017-1062) of Asan Medical Center. This study was registered at clinicaltrials.gov (NCT04357483) and performed according to CONSORT guidelines [24].

2.2. Inclusion and Exclusion Criteria

Patients were included if they (1) were 20–80 years on the day of enrollment; (2) had Eastern Cooperative Oncology Group (ECOG) performance scores of 0–2; (3) had potentially curable benign, premalignant, or malignant pancreatic disease, as shown by preoperative imaging (computed tomography, magnetic resonance imaging, and/or positron emission tomography); (4) had appropriate bone marrow function (WBC count of at least 3000/mm^3, platelet count of at least 100,000/mm^3); (5) had appropriate liver function (AST/ALT less than 3 times the upper limit of normal); (6) had appropriate renal function (creatinine level greater than 1.5 times the upper limit of normal); (7) provided written informed consent. Patients were excluded if they (1) had active or uncontrolled infections; (2) had severe psychiatric or neurological disorders; (3) had alcohol or other drug addictions; (4) were included in other clinical studies that may affect this study; (5) had uncontrolled heart disease; (6) had moderate or severe comorbidities that are thought to have affected the quality of life or nutritional status; (7) had pelvic tumors, benign tumors, or malignant tumors in other organs; (8) were pregnant or planning on becoming pregnant during the follow-up period; (9) had lymphatic or coagulation disease; or (10) had known sensitivity or allergy to bovine and/or porcine substance(s).

2.3. Surgical Technique and Study Protocol

The procedures for PD and DP in our institution have been reported previously [4,6,17,25,26]. Furthermore, the detailed description of pancreaticojejunostomy (PJ) during PD is in detail in our previous study [17]. PJ was carried out using the double-layered, end-to-side duct-to-mucosa method. In addition, when left-sided pancreatectomy was performed, to transect the pancreas safely in both the open and laparoscopic procedures, straight or rotated endoscopic linear staplers of various sizes (staple height, 3.5 to 4.2 mm) were used depending on the thickness or hardness of the pancreas. After transecting the pancreas, 4 or 5 small titanium clips were applied along the stapling line to prevent pancreatic fistula and bleeding from the resected stump.

Before closure, a 1–3 closed suction drain was inserted into the bed of the removed portion of the pancreas and maintained for at least 3 days postoperatively to prevent intra-abdominal fluid collection and identify POPF. Each patient was allowed sips of water on postoperative day (POD) 1 and a soft blended diet on POD 2. Postoperative assessment included repeated measurements of amylase concentrations in the serum and drainage fluid while the drain was in place. POPF was defined as a drain fluid amylase concentration greater than 3 times the upper normal serum concentration after POD 3 as defined by the International Study Group on Pancreatic Surgery (ISGPS) criteria [27].

2.4. Application of Thrombin-Containing Collagen Hemostatic Matrix (T-C Matrix) in the Intervention Group

The T-C matrix (CollaStat®; Dalim Tissen Co. Ltd., Seoul, Korea) is a flowable collagen-based hemostatic matrix [18,19]. The T-C matrix is comprised of two connectable syringes, syringe A and syringe B. Syringe A contains porcine skin-derived atelocollagen, thrombin. Syringe B contains calcium chloride solution (Figure 1). The collagen granules of T-C matrix are made from highly purified type I atelocollagen derived from the porcine dermis, which shows biocompatibility due to the minimally immunogenic, biocompatible, and biodegradable properties of atelocollagen. The matrix can be prepared after mixing the materials in the syringes. In the intervention group, T-C matrix was applied to the anastomosis site and pancreatic stump after PJ or DP. The matrix was approved for use by the Korean Food and Drug Administration.

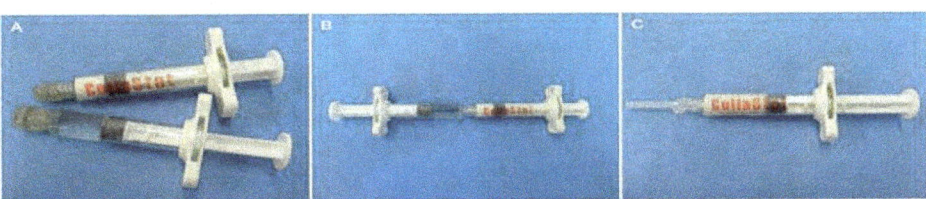

Figure 1. Preparation of CollaStat®. (**A**) CollaStat consists of two syringes: one for collagen granules and thrombin and the other for CaCl$_2$ solution. (**B**) CollaStat® can be easily prepared by connecting the two syringes and mixing them. (**C**) After mixing and detaching the CaCl$_2$ syringe, CollaStat is ready for use by connecting the enclosed application tip.

2.5. Application of Thrombin-Coated L-Dopa-Containing Collagen Patch (T-CD Patch) in the Control Group

For patients in the active control group, a 5.0 cm × 5.0 cm T-CD patch (CollaSeal®; Dalim Tissen Co. Ltd., Seoul, Korea) was applied to the front and back of the anastomosis site. The T-CD patch, which has been clinically used for the prevention of POPF and postpancreatectomy hemorrhage (PPH), is a sponge-like wound dressing incorporated with thrombin and L-DOPA. Owing to thrombin and L-DOPA, a T-CD patch can effectively accomplish hemostasis and adhere to the wound site. In addition, a T-CD patch has a honeycomb-like porous structure, which contributes to a good absorption capacity for blood or exudates.

2.6. Outcome Measures

The primary endpoint of this study was the incidence of POPF. The evaluation of pancreatic fistula was based on the ISGPS criteria [27]. According to the criteria, POPF was defined as a drain fluid amylase concentration greater than 3 times the upper normal serum concentration after POD 3. The secondary endpoints were risk factors for POPF, drain removal days, incidence of complication according to the Clavien–Dindo classification [28], 90-day mortality, and length of hospital stay.

2.7. Sample Size

The POPF prevention rate of fibrin sealants has been reported as 88% previously [7]. The non-inferiority limit was calculated to be 0.22 based on the case where more than 75% of 88% of existing treatments were confirmed. When the lower limit of the 95% CI for the difference between the two groups was greater than −0.22, it was judged that TC-matrix was not inferior to T-CD patch. Based on this hypothesis, a sample size of 54 patients (27 in each group) was estimated based on type 1 error $\alpha = 0.05$ and power $(1 - \beta) = 0.8$ using a two-sided χ^2 test. Factoring in a 10% dropout rate, we recruited 60 patients (30 per group).

2.8. Randomization

A total of 58 patients were randomized with block randomization before surgery. We performed block randomization to correct the imbalance between the intervention and control groups. We assigned A to the intervention group and the groups were determined as follows: (1) ABBA, (2) BBAA, (3) ABAB, (4) BABA, (5) AABB, and (6) BAAB. We selected blocks and allocated surgical procedures based on the number of a die rolled once. Independent researchers randomized patients for this study.

2.9. Statistical Analysis

The results are presented as the mean with standard deviation (SD) or median with interquartile range (IQR). Patient demographics and clinical characteristics were compared using the χ^2 test or Fisher's exact test for categorical variables and the Student's t-test and Mann–Whitney test for continuous variables. In assessing the risk factors associated with overall POPF and clinically relevant POPF, only variables statistically significant in univariate analysis were included in multivariate analysis, which was performed using logistic regression. All statistical analyses were performed using SPSS version 21.0 (IBM Corp., Armonk, NY, USA) with p values less than 0.05 considered statistically significant.

3. Results

Participants were recruited from February 2018 to September 2018 and followed up until February 2019. A total of 60 patients were enrolled; however, 2 patients declined to participate. Of the 58 randomized patients, 4 patients had to withdraw consent to undergo surgery, and the remaining 54 patients were allocated to two groups (intervention group: $n = 26$, active control group: $n = 28$). One patient in the control group did not undergo pancreatectomy due to the progression of pancreatic cancer; thus, this participant was excluded from further analysis. Therefore, this study evaluated a total of 53 patients, with 26 patients in the intervention group and 27 patients in the control group (Figure 2).

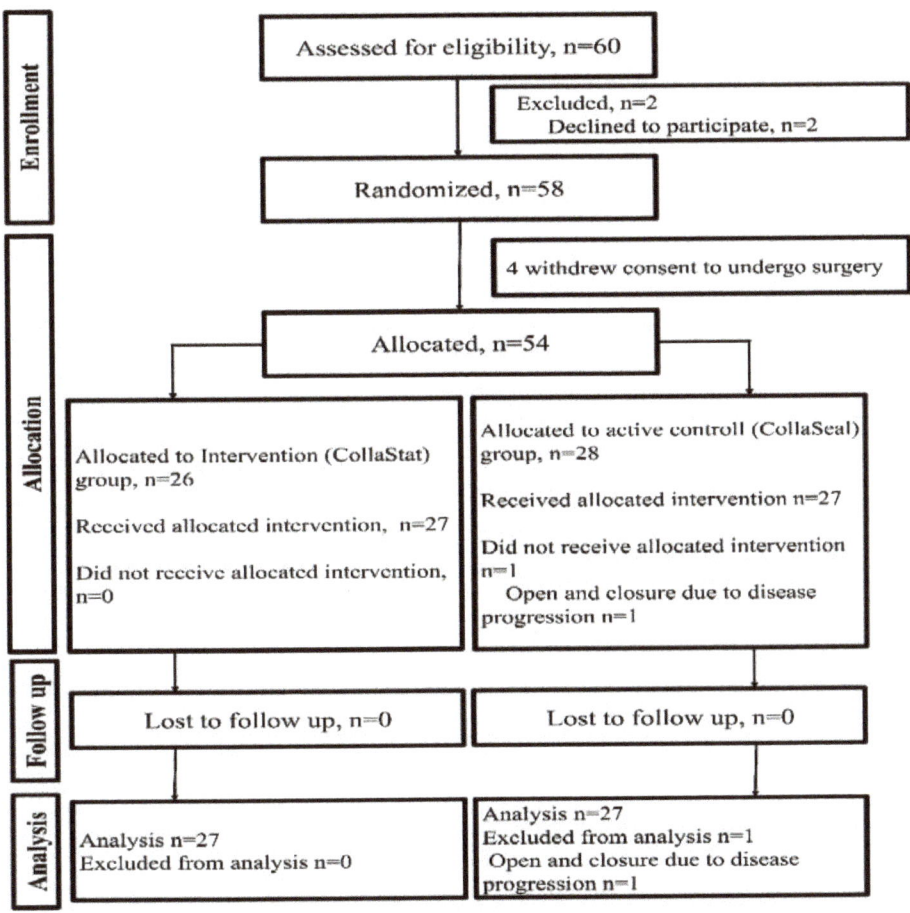

Figure 2. CONSORT flow diagram of the trial.

Age, sex, Charlson comorbidity score, operative type, operative name, additional organ resection, operative time, estimated blood loss, pathological diagnosis, pancreatic texture, mass size, pancreatic duct size, alternative fistula risk score, and neoadjuvant chemotherapy were not statistically different between the two groups (Table 1).

Table 1. Clinicopathological features of patients who underwent pancreatectomy.

Variable		Intervention (n = 26)	Control (n = 27)	p Value [1]
Age (years)	Median, IQR	59 (56~63)	63 (52~70)	0.849
Sex, n (%)	Female	14 (53.8%)	12 (44.4%)	0.494
	Male	12 (46.2%)	15 (55.6%)	
Diabetes Mellitus	Yes	2 (7.7%)	7 (25.9%)	0.077
Preoperative Fasting glucose (mg/dL)	Yes	9 (34.6%)	13 (48.1%)	0.406
BMI (kg/m^2)	Mean, SD	24.2 ± 3.2	22.4 ± 2.4	0.026
ASA classification, n (%)	<3	26 (100.0%)	26 (96.3%)	>0.999
	≥3	0 (0.0%)	1 (3.7%)	
Charlson comorbidity score, n (%)	<4	13 (50.0%)	9 (33.3%)	0.218
	≥4	13 (50.0%)	18 (66.7%)	
Operative type, n (%)	Laparotomy	13 (50.0%)	12 (44.4%)	0.685
	Minimal invasive	13 (50.0%)	15 (55.6%)	
Operative name, n (%)	Whipple's operation	14 (53.8%)	14 (51.9%)	>0.999
	Distal pancreatectomy	12 (46.2%)	13 (48.1%)	
Additional resection, n (%)	Yes	6 (22.2%)	3 (11.1%)	0.467
	Gallbladder	0	1	
	SMV or PV	3	2	
	Total gastrectomy/celiac axis	1	0	
	Right hemicolectomy	1	0	
	Liver	1	0	
Operative time, min	Mean, SD	293.5 ± 108.3	280.0 ± 110.9	0.656
Estimated blood loss, n (%)	≤400 mL	24 (92.4%)	25 (92.6%)	>0.999
	401~700 mL	1 (3.8%)	1 (3.7%)	
	≥701 mL	1 (3.8%)	1 (3.7%)	
Pathological diagnosis, n (%)	Malignancy	15 (57.7%)	11 (40.7%)	0.217
	PDAC	14 (53.8%)	9 (33.3%)	
	Benign	11 (42.3%)	16 (59.3%)	
Pancreas texture, n (%)	Soft	12 (46.2%)	15 (55.6%)	0.494
	Firm or hard	14 (53.8%)	12 (44.4%)	
Mass size, cm	Mean, SD	3.4 ± 2.1	3.3 ± 1.7	0.793
Pancreatic duct size, mm	Mean, SD	3.1 ± 1.9	3.0 ± 1.7	0.816
Neoadjuvant therapy, n (%)	Yes	4 (15.4%)	1 (3.7%)	0.192
Alternative fistula risk score, n (%) [2]	Low	4 (14.8%)	8 (29.6%)	0.264
	Intermediate	15 (55.6%)	15 (55.6%)	
	High	8 (29.6%)	4 (14.8%)	

[1] The p value was calculated using Student's t-test or Mann–Whitney U test for continuous variables and χ^2 test or Fisher's exact test for binary variables; [2] The alternative fistula risk score was determined according to the definition of the Dutch Pancreatic Cancer Group; IQR, interquartile range; ASA classification, American Society of Anesthesiologists physical status classification; SD, standard deviation; BMI, body mass index; PDAC, pancreatic ductal adenocarcinoma; SMV, superior mesenteric vein; PV, portal vein.

3.1. Primary Outcomes

POPF was more common in the active control group than in the intervention group (59.3% vs. 30.8%, p = 0.037; Table 2). However, there was no statistical difference in clinically relevant POPF between the two groups (15.4% vs. 29.6%, p = 0.409).

As a result of evaluating the POPF prevention rate in this study, it was 60.2% (18/26 patients) for the intervention group and 40.7% (11/27 patients) for the control group. The upper limit of the 95% confidence interval for the difference in the POPF prevention rate between the two groups was −2.83%, which was less than the non-inferiority margin of 22%.

Table 2. Outcomes of postoperative pancreatic fistula and morbidities for all patients.

Variable		Intervention ($n = 26$)	Control ($n = 27$)	p Value [1]
Drain removal, days	Median, IQR	4 (3~5)	5 (3~6)	0.241
POPF, n (%) [2]	Yes	8 (30.8%)	16 (59.3%)	0.037
POPF grade, n (%) [2]	BL	4 (15.4%)	8 (29.6%)	0.438
	B	4 (15.4%)	7 (25.9%)	
	C	0 (0.0%)	1 (3.7%)	
Clinically relevant POPF, n (%) [2]	Yes	4 (15.4%)	8 (29.6%)	0.409
Postoperative complication, n (%) [2]	Yes	9 (34.6%)	17 (63.0%)	0.039
Complication grade, n (%) [2]	≥Grade III	5 (19.2%)	3 (11.1%)	0.444
Length of hospital stay, days	Median, IQR	8 (7~11)	9 (7~14)	0.284
90-day mortality, n (%)	Yes	0 (0.0%)	0 (0.0%)	>0.999
Readmission, n (%)	Yes	5 (19.2%)	3 (11.1%)	0.409

[1] The p value was calculated using Student's t-test or Mann–Whitney U test for continuous variables and χ^2 test or Fisher's exact test for binary variables; [2] Postoperative pancreatic fistula (POPF) and overall complications were assessed and graded based on the criteria of the International Study Group on Pancreatic Surgery (ISGPS) and the Clavien–Dindo complication classification, respectively; IQR, interquartile range; BL, biochemical leakage.

3.2. Secondary Outcomes

The postoperative outcomes of all patients are shown in Table 2. There were no significant differences in postoperative outcomes except for the occurrence of POPF (Table 2). The median length of hospital stay (8 days vs. 9 days, $p = 0.284$) and median drain removal days (4 days vs. 5 days, $p = 0.241$) were not significantly different between the two groups. In addition, the complication rate was significantly different (34.6% vs. 63.0%, $p = 0.039$). By limiting the Clavien–Dindo classification to ≥grade 3, there was no significant difference in the complication grade between the intervention and control groups (19.2% vs. 11.1%, $p = 0.444$). There was no difference in the 90-day mortality between the two groups.

There were 4 patients with clinically relevant POPF in the intervention group, and all of them had grade B POPF. Among these patients, 1 patient underwent antibiotic therapy, and 2 patients underwent endoscopic ultrasound-guided gastrocystostomy for intra-abdominal complicated fluid collection. The other patient underwent embolization for pseudoaneurysm of the gastroduodenal artery stump. In the control group, there were 8 patients with clinically relevant POPF, and 1 of them had grade C POPF (this patient underwent reoperation for surgical site infection). A total of 6 patients underwent antibiotic therapy, and 1 patient underwent anticoagulation therapy for portal vein thrombosis. Red blood cell (RBC) transfusions were made only to 2 patients in each group. The amount of RBC was the same as 720 ± 113.14 mL in both groups. The readmission rate (19.2% vs. 11.1%, $p = 0.409$) was not different between the two groups.

3.3. Sub-Analysis of Patients Who Underwent Distal Pancreatectomy

Among patients who underwent DP, POPF (33.3% vs. 92.3%, $p = 0.004$) and clinically relevant POPF (8.3% vs. 46.2%, $p = 0.027$) were more common in the control group than in the intervention group. There were no statistically significant differences in drain removal days, length of hospital stay, 90-day mortality, readmission rate, and complication rate. Furthermore, the complication rate was significantly different (33.3% vs. 92.3%, $p = 0.004$). By limiting the Clavien–Dindo classification to ≥ grade 3, there was no significant difference in the complication grade between the intervention and control groups (8.3% vs. 23.1%, $p = 0.593$) (Table 3).

Table 3. Sub-analysis of postoperative pancreatic fistula and morbidities for patients who underwent distal pancreatectomy.

Variable		Intervention (n = 12)	Control (n = 13)	p Value [1]
Drain removal, days	Median, IQR	4 (3~5)	4 (3~6)	0.167
POPF, n (%) [2]	Yes	4 (33.3%)	12 (92.3%)	0.004
POPF grade, n (%) [2]	BL	3 (25.0%)	6 (46.2%)	0.018
	B	1 (8.3%)	5 (38.5%)	
	C	0 (0.0%)	1 (7.7%)	
Clinically relevant POPF, n (%) [2]	Yes	1 (8.3%)	6 (46.2%)	0.027
Postoperative complication, n (%) [2]	Yes	4 (33.3%)	12 (92.3%)	0.004
Complication grade, n (%) [2]	≥Grade III	1 (8.3%)	3 (23.1%)	0.593
Length of hospital stay, days	Median, IQR	7 (6–9)	7 (6–14)	0.274
90-day mortality, n (%)	Yes	0 (0.0%)	0 (0.0%)	>0.999
Readmission, n (%)	Yes	1 (8.3%)	1 (7.7%)	>0.999

[1] The p value was calculated using Student's t-test or Mann–Whitney U test for continuous variables and χ^2 test or Fisher's exact test for binary variables; [2], Postoperative pancreatic fistula (POPF) and overall complications were assessed and graded based on the criteria of the International Study Group on Pancreatic Surgery and the Clavien–Dindo complication classification, respectively; IQR, interquartile range; BL, biochemical leakage.

The POPF rate was 28.6% (p > 0.999) in both the intervention and control groups, showing no statistically significant difference. In addition, CR-POPF (21.4% vs. 14.3%, p > 0.999), postoperative complication (35.7% vs. 35.7%, p > 0.999), complication ≥ Grade III (21.4% vs. 0.0%, p = 0.119), median length of hospital stay (10 days vs. 9 days, p > 0.999), and readmission rate (28.6% vs. 14.3%, p = 0.648) showed no difference between the two groups.

3.4. Risk Factors for POPF and Clinically Relevant POPF

A multivariate logistic regression model identified T-C matrix use (OR 4.744, 95% CI 1.172–19.210, p = 0.029), pancreatic duct ≥ 3 mm (OR 7.120, 95% CI 1.399–36.241, p = 0.018), and form or hard pancreatic texture (OR 6.525, 95% CI 1.668–25.529, p = 0.007) as independent negative risk factors for POPF in the current study (Table 4). In addition, multivariate logistic regression analysis of clinically relevant POPF identified soft pancreatic as an independent risk factor (OR: 7.353, 95% CI: 1.429~37.847, p = 0.017).

Table 4. Univariate and multivariate logistic regression analyses of risk factors for postoperative pancreatic fistula.

Variable	Univariate			Multivariate		
	OR [1]	95% CI	p Value [2]	OR [1]	95% CI	p Value [2]
All patients (n = 53)						
Intervention			0.031			0.029
Control	3.455	1.119~10.669		4.744	1.172~19.210	
Pancreatic duct size, mm			0.012			0.018
≥3						
<3	6.125	1.501~24.997		7.120	1.399~36.241	
Pancreatic texture			0.002			0.007
Firm or hard						
Soft	7.000	2.088~23.468		6.525	1.668~25.529	
Patients who underwent distal pancreatectomy (n = 25)						
Intervention			0.006			0.024
Control	27.000	2.561~284.696		17.379	1.453~207.870	
Pancreatic texture			0.011			0.096
Firm or hard						
Soft	12.000	1.762~81.745		6.666	0.712~62.374	

[1] The odds ratio (OR) was estimated using a logistic regression model excluding possible confounding variables; [2] The p value was calculated using a logistic regression model; 95% CI, 95% confidence interval; DP, distal pancreatectomy.

T-C matrix application was a negative risk factor for POPF (Table 4) and clinically relevant POPF (OR: 10.286, 95% CI: 1.018~103.948, p = 0.048) among patients who underwent left-sided pancreatectomy.

4. Discussion

This prospective study showed that applying a T-C matrix to the PJ or pancreatic stump after pancreatectomy significantly reduced the incidence of POPF compared with that in the active control group (T-CD patch). POPF was more common in the control group than in the intervention group (59.3% vs. 30.8%, p = 0.037; Table 2). In a multivariate logistic regression model, T-C matrix application was a negative risk factor for POPF (Table 4), especially among patients who underwent DP.

To the best of our knowledge, no studies have evaluated the efficacy of a flowable hemostatic matrix for the prevention of POPF. Two retrospective studies reported that fibrin sealant patches are feasible and safe with 7.4%–20% POPF rates after PD with pancreaticojejunostomy [13,29]. Schindl et al. [30] conducted a multicenter, randomized clinical trial to investigate the effect of using thrombin-coated collagen patches after PD. In the study, the rates of POPF were 63% in the intervention group and 56% in the control group, and clinically relevant POPF rates were 23% in the intervention group and 14% in the control group. The study reported that there was no POPF reduction with the use of thrombin-coated collagen patches after PD. Similarly, there was no POPF reduction in a prospective study of patients who underwent PD in our center [17]. The POPF rate was 25.8% in the intervention group and 37.1 in the control group (p = 0.246). In the current study, we attempted to evaluate the safety and efficacy of a flowable hemostatic agent compared with a thrombin-coated collagen patch and their effect on clinical outcomes including POPF. The POPF rate was 28.6% among patients who underwent PD in the control group (thrombin-coated collagen patch) and was 28.6% among patients who underwent PD in the intervention group (flowable hemostatic matrix); thus, there was no POPF reduction effect. Clinically relevant POPF rates were 21.4% in the intervention group and 14.3% in the control group (p > 0.999) among the patients who underwent PD.

Several studies have been conducted on the use of thrombin-coated collagen patches for preventing POPF after DP. Silvestri et al. [14] reported that the use of fibrin sealant patches appeared to be associated with a lower incidence of grade C POPF. However, the POPF rate was not different in both groups (intervention: 36.1% vs. control: 41.6%, p = n.s). Two previous multicenter, randomized controlled trials reported that there was no significant effect on the rate of POPF after DP. Montorsi et al. [7] reported POPF rates of 62% and 68% in the intervention and control groups, respectively ($p = 0.267$), and Sa Cunha et al. [31] reported rates of 54.5% and 56.6%, respectively ($p = 0.807$). There was no statistically significant difference in clinically relevant POPF. In another randomized trial, the POPF rate was reported as 70.8% in the intervention group and 54.7% in the control group [10]. The study indicated there are no clinically relevant benefits in applying a patch in terms of reducing the incidence and severity of POPF after DP. In the current study, the POPF rate was reduced among patients who underwent DP, and a low incidence of clinically relevant POPF was observed when a flowable hemostatic matrix was applied (Table 3). Moreover, in a multivariate logistic regression model, T-C matrix application was a negative risk factor for POPF, especially among patients who underwent DP (Table 4).

In this study, the overall incidence of POPF, especially after DP, was 64.0%, and the rate of clinically relevant POPF was 28.0%, which was greater than that reported in previous studies [7,14,31]. As mentioned previously [10], this may be explained by the rigid application of the ISGPS criteria by an independent research coordinator and not the doctors who were involved in this study. In addition, several studies omitted grade A (or BL) fistula from the analyses because intra-abdominal drains were not routinely used during surgery [32,33]. Similar to previous studies [7,31], most of the POPF cases were biochemical leakage ($n = 12$, 50%) in this study.

A T-C matrix is a novel flowable collagen-based hemostatic agent. The matrix can be prepared via the following simple steps: (1) connecting two syringes, (2) mixing the contents, and (3) application of the mixed matrix on the defect site. This simple procedure allows the preparation of a hemostatic matrix without a time-consuming thrombin re-constitution process. In addition, flowable hemostatic agents may be more advantageous than non-flowable ones as they can cover irregular wound surfaces, fill deep lesions, and easily remove excess material with irrigation [18,19]. In fact, like T-CD patch, T-C matrix achieved successful hemostasis as intended in all cases.

This study may be underpowered as it was designed to be conducted at a single institution in a short period, and considering the recruitment capacity, it was designed to have 80% statistical power. Risk factor interpretation was limited because the number of cases was not high. A multicenter randomized clinical trial with a large number of patients is needed to clarify the effects of a T-C matrix. Furthermore, there is heterogeneity among the enrolled patients. PD and DP, which have been reported to have differences in POPF rates, were included in this study. Consequently, the sample size in sub-analysis is reduced, and the conclusions may be limited.

Nevertheless, this is the first prospective study to report the efficacy of a flowable hemostatic matrix for the prevention of POPF after pancreatectomy. When the T-C matrix was applied after pancreatectomy, POPF rates were effectively reduced, especially in cases of DP. In addition, the T-C matrix application was a negative risk factor for POPF in this study. In addition, the upper limit of the 95% confidence interval for the difference in the POPF prevention rate between the two groups was −2.83%, which was less than the non-inferiority margin of 22%, thus demonstrating non-inferiority in the efficacy of preventing POPF in the intervention group compared to the control group.

5. Conclusions

In conclusion, our findings indicated that flowable thrombin-containing collagen hemostatic matrix (T-C matrix) application is a simple, feasible, and effective method of preventing POPF after pancreatectomy, especially in cases of DP. A larger, randomized controlled trial may be required to confirm the effectiveness of this method.

Author Contributions: Substantial contributions to the conception or design of the work: Y.P., J.H.K., D.R.K., J.H.L. (Jun Hyeok Lee), S.-N.P., K.-B.S., S.C.K.; Acquisition of data: Y.P., J.H.K., D.R.K., J.H.L. (Jun Hyeok Lee), S.-N.P.; Analysis and interpretation of data: Y.P., J.H.K., D.W.H., J.H.L. (Jae Hoon Lee), W.L., J.K., S.C.K.; Statistical Analysis: Y.P., J.H.K., D.R.K., J.H.L. (Jun Hyeok Lee), D.W.H.; Drafting of manuscript: Y.P., J.H.K.; Critical revision; Y.P., J.H.K., D.R.K., J.H.L. (Jun Hyeok Lee), D.W.H., J.H.L. (Jae Hoon Lee), W.L., J.K., S.-N.P., K.-B.S., S.C.K. All authors have read and agree to the published version of the manuscript.

Funding: This research received no external funding.

Acknowledgments: This study was supported by a grant from Asan Institute for Life Science (2017-7004).

Conflicts of Interest: The authors declare no conflict of interest.

References

1. Kimura, W.; Miyata, H.; Gotoh, M.; Hirai, I.; Kenjo, A.; Kitagawa, Y.; Shimada, M.; Baba, H.; Tomita, N.; Nakagoe, T.; et al. A Pancreaticoduodenectomy Risk Model Derived From 8575 Cases From a National Single-Race Population (Japanese) Using a Web-Based Data Entry System The 30-Day and In-hospital Mortality Rates for Pancreaticoduodenectomy. *Ann. Surg.* **2014**, *259*, 773–780. [CrossRef]
2. Sakaguchi, T.; Nakamura, S.; Suzuki, S.; Kojima, Y.; Tsuchiya, Y.; Konno, H.; Nakaoka, J.; Nishiyama, R. Marginal ulceration after pylorus-preserving pancreaticoduodenectomy. *J. Hepatobiliary Pancreat. Surg.* **2000**, *7*, 193–197. [CrossRef] [PubMed]
3. Lillemoe, K.D.; Kaushal, S.; Cameron, J.L.; Sohn, T.A.; Pitt, H.A.; Yeo, C.J. Distal pancreatectomy: Indications and outcomes in 235 patients. *Ann. Surg.* **1999**, *229*, 693–698; discussion 698–700. [CrossRef] [PubMed]
4. Song, K.B.; Kim, S.C.; Hwang, D.W.; Lee, J.H.; Lee, D.J.; Lee, J.W.; Park, K.M.; Lee, Y.J. Matched Case-Control Analysis Comparing Laparoscopic and Open Pylorus-preserving Pancreaticoduodenectomy in Patients With Periampullary Tumors. *Ann. Surg.* **2015**, *262*, 146–155. [CrossRef] [PubMed]
5. Knaebel, H.P.; Diener, M.K.; Wente, M.N.; Buchler, M.W.; Seiler, C.M. Systematic review and meta-analysis of technique for closure of the pancreatic remnant after distal pancreatectomy. *Br. J. Surg.* **2005**, *92*, 539–546. [CrossRef] [PubMed]
6. Song, K.B.; Kim, S.C.; Park, J.B.; Kim, Y.H.; Jung, Y.S.; Kim, M.H.; Lee, S.K.; Seo, D.W.; Lee, S.S.; Park, D.H.; et al. Single-center experience of laparoscopic left pancreatic resection in 359 consecutive patients: Changing the surgical paradigm of left pancreatic resection. *Surg. Endosc.* **2011**, *25*, 3364–3372. [CrossRef]
7. Montorsi, M.; Zerbi, A.; Bassi, C.; Capussotti, L.; Coppola, R.; Sacchi, M.; Italian Tachosil Study, G. Efficacy of an absorbable fibrin sealant patch (TachoSil) after distal pancreatectomy: A multicenter, randomized, controlled trial. *Ann. Surg.* **2012**, *256*, 853–859. [CrossRef] [PubMed]
8. Reeh, M.; Nentwich, M.F.; Bogoevski, D.; Koenig, A.M.; Gebauer, F.; Tachezy, M.; Izbicki, J.R.; Bockhorn, M. High surgical morbidity following distal pancreatectomy: Still an unsolved problem. *World J. Surg.* **2011**, *35*, 1110–1117. [CrossRef]
9. Ecker, B.L.; McMillan, M.T.; Allegrini, V.; Bassi, C.; Beane, J.D.; Beckman, R.M.; Behrman, S.W.; Dickson, E.J.; Callery, M.P.; Christein, J.D.; et al. Risk Factors and Mitigation Strategies for Pancreatic Fistula After Distal Pancreatectomy: Analysis of 2026 Resections From the International, Multi-institutional Distal Pancreatectomy Study Group. *Ann. Surg.* **2019**, *269*, 143–149. [CrossRef]
10. Park, J.S.; Lee, D.-H.; Jang, J.-Y.; Han, Y.; Yoon, D.-S.; Kim, J.K.; Han, H.-S.; Yoon, Y.; Hwang, D.W.; Kim, K.S.; et al. Use of TachoSil® patches to prevent pancreatic leaks after distal pancreatectomy: A prospective, multicenter, randomized controlled study. *J. Hepatobiliary Pancreat. Sci.* **2016**, *23*, 110–117. [CrossRef]
11. Menahem, B.; Guittet, L.; Mulliri, A.; Alves, A.; Lubrano, J. Pancreaticogastrostomy Is Superior to Pancreaticojejunostomy for Prevention of Pancreatic Fistula after Pancreaticoduodenectomy: An updated meta-analysis of randomized controlled trials. *Ann. Surg.* **2015**, *261*, 882–887. [CrossRef] [PubMed]
12. Mita, K.; Ito, H.; Fukumoto, M.; Murabayashi, R.; Koizumi, K.; Hayashi, T.; Kikuchi, H. Pancreaticojejunostomy using a Fibrin Adhesive Sealant (TachoComb (R)) for the Prevention of Pancreatic Fistula after Pancreaticoduodenectomy. *Hepato-Gastroenterology* **2011**, *58*, 187–191. [PubMed]
13. Mita, K.; Ito, H.; Fukumoto, M.; Murabayashi, R.; Koizumi, K.; Hayashi, T.; Kikuchi, H.; Kagaya, T. A fibrin adhesive sealing method for the prevention of pancreatic fistula following distal pancreatectomy. *Hepato-Gastroenterology* **2011**, *58*, 604–608.
14. Silvestri, S.; Franchello, A.; Gonella, F.; Deiro, G.; Campra, D.; Cassine, D.; Fiore, A.; Ostuni, E.; Garino, M.; Resegotti, A.; et al. Role of TachoSil® in distal pancreatectomy: A single center experience. *Minerva Chir.* **2015**, *70*, 175–180. [PubMed]
15. Marangos, I.P.; Rosok, B.I.; Kazaryan, A.M.; Rosseland, A.R.; Edwin, B. Effect of TachoSil Patch in Prevention of Postoperative Pancreatic Fistula. *J. Gastrointest. Surg.* **2011**, *15*, 1625–1629. [CrossRef]
16. Kwon, H.E.; Seo, H.I.; Yun, S.P. Use of Neoveil or TachoSil to prevent pancreatic fistula following pancreaticoduodenectomy: A retrospective study. *Medicine* **2019**, *98*, e15293. [CrossRef]

17. Kwon, J.; Shin, S.H.; Lee, S.; Park, G.; Park, Y.; Lee, S.J.; Lee, W.; Song, K.B.; Hwang, D.W.; Kim, S.C.; et al. The Effect of Fibrinogen/Thrombin-Coated Collagen Patch (TachoSil®) Application in Pancreaticojejunostomy for Prevention of Pancreatic Fistula after Pancreaticoduodenectomy: A Randomized Clinical Trial. *World J. Surg.* **2019**, *43*, 3128–3137. [CrossRef]
18. Lee, H.; Lee, J.H.; Jeon, C.S.; Ko, J.H.; Park, S.N.; Lee, Y.T. Evaluation of a novel collagen hemostatic matrix in a porcine heart and cardiac vessel injury model. *J. Thorac. Dis.* **2019**, *11*, 2722–2729. [CrossRef]
19. Kim, M.J.; Kim, J.H.; Kim, J.S.; Choe, J.H. Evaluation of a Novel Collagen Hemostatic Matrix: Comparison of Two Hemostatic Matrices in a Rabbits Jejunal Artery Injury Model. *J. Surg. Res.* **2019**, *243*, 553–559. [CrossRef]
20. Stein, C.; Kuchler, S. Targeting inflammation and wound healing by opioids. *Trends Pharm. Sci.* **2013**, *34*, 303–312. [CrossRef]
21. Ruszczak, Z. Effect of collagen matrices on dermal wound healing. *Adv. Drug Deliv. Rev.* **2003**, *55*, 1595–1611. [CrossRef] [PubMed]
22. Chattopadhyay, S.; Raines, R.T. Review collagen-based biomaterials for wound healing. *Biopolymers* **2014**, *101*, 821–833. [CrossRef] [PubMed]
23. Hüttner, F.J.; Mihaljevic, A.L.; Hackert, T.; Ulrich, A.; Büchler, M.W.; Diener, M.K. Effectiveness of Tachosil®in the prevention of postoperative pancreatic fistula after distal pancreatectomy: A systematic review and meta-analysis. *Langenbecks Arch. Surg.* **2016**, *401*, 151–159. [CrossRef] [PubMed]
24. Moher, D.; Hopewell, S.; Schulz, K.F.; Montori, V.; Gotzsche, P.C.; Devereaux, P.J.; Elbourne, D.; Egger, M.; Altman, D.G. CONSORT 2010 explanation and elaboration: Updated guidelines for reporting parallel group randomised trials. *Int. J. Surg.* **2012**, *10*, 28–55. [CrossRef] [PubMed]
25. Shin, S.H.; Kim, S.C.; Song, K.B.; Hwang, D.W.; Lee, J.H.; Lee, D.; Lee, J.W.; Jun, E.; Park, K.M.; Lee, Y.J. A comparative study of laparoscopic vs. open distal pancreatectomy for left-sided ductal adenocarcinoma: A propensity score-matched analysis. *J. Am. Coll. Surg.* **2015**, *220*, 177–185. [CrossRef]
26. Park, Y.; Hwang, D.W.; Lee, J.H.; Song, K.B.; Jun, E.; Lee, W.; Kwon, J.; Kim, S.C. Analysis of Symptomatic Marginal Ulcers in Patients Who Underwent Pancreaticoduodenectomy for Periampullary Tumors. *Pancreas* **2020**, *49*, 208–215. [CrossRef]
27. Bassi, C.; Marchegiani, G.; Dervenis, C.; Sarr, M.; Abu Hilal, M.; Adham, M.; Allen, P.; Andersson, R.; Asbun, H.J.; Besselink, M.G.; et al. The 2016 update of the International Study Group (ISGPS) definition and grading of postoperative pancreatic fistula: 11 Years After. *Surgery* **2017**, *161*, 584–591. [CrossRef]
28. Dindo, D.; Demartines, N.; Clavien, P.A. Classification of surgical complications: A new proposal with evaluation in a cohort of 6336 patients and results of a survey. *Ann. Surg.* **2004**, *240*, 205–213. [CrossRef]
29. Chirletti, P.; Caronna, R.; Fanello, G.; Schiratti, M.; Stagnitti, F.; Peparini, N.; Benedetti, M.; Martino, G. Pancreaticojejunostomy with Applicationof Fibrinogen/Thrombin-Coated Collagen Patch (TachoSil®) in Roux-en-Y Reconstruction after Pancreaticoduodenectomy. *J. Gastrointest. Surg.* **2009**, *13*, 1396–1398. [CrossRef]
30. Schindl, M.; Fugger, R.; Gotzinger, P.; Langle, F.; Zitt, M.; Stattner, S.; Kornprat, P.; Sahora, K.; Hlauschek, D.; Gnant, M. Randomized clinical trial of the effect of a fibrin sealant patch on pancreatic fistula formation after pancreatoduodenectomy. *Br. J. Surg.* **2018**, *105*, 811–819. [CrossRef]
31. Cunha, A.S.; Carrere, N.; Meunier, B.; Fabre, J.-M.; Sauvanet, A.; Pessaux, P.; Ortega-Deballon, P.; Fingerhut, A.; Lacaine, F. Stump closure reinforcement with absorbable fibrin collagen sealant sponge (TachoSil) does not prevent pancreatic fistula after distal pancreatectomy: The FIABLE multicenter controlled randomized study. *Am. J. Surg.* **2015**, *210*, 739–748. [CrossRef] [PubMed]
32. Diener, M.K.; Seiler, C.M.; Rossion, I.; Kleeff, J.; Glanemann, M.; Butturini, G.; Tomazic, A.; Bruns, C.J.; Busch, O.R.; Farkas, S.; et al. Efficacy of stapler versus hand-sewn closure after distal pancreatectomy (DISPACT): A randomised, controlled multicentre trial. *Lancet* **2011**, *377*, 1514–1522. [CrossRef]
33. Nathan, H.; Cameron, J.L.; Goodwin, C.R.; Seth, A.K.; Edil, B.H.; Wolfgang, C.L.; Pawlik, T.M.; Schulick, R.D.; Choti, M.A. Risk factors for pancreatic leak after distal pancreatectomy. *Ann. Surg.* **2009**, *250*, 277–281. [CrossRef] [PubMed]

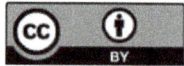

© 2020 by the authors. Licensee MDPI, Basel, Switzerland. This article is an open access article distributed under the terms and conditions of the Creative Commons Attribution (CC BY) license (http://creativecommons.org/licenses/by/4.0/).

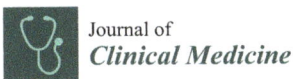

Article

A Plea for Surgery in Pancreatic Metastases from Renal Cell Carcinoma: Indications and Outcome from a Multicenter Surgical Experience

Anna Caterina Milanetto [1,*], Luca Morelli [2], Gregorio Di Franco [2], Alina David [1], Donata Campra [3], Paolo De Paolis [3] and Claudio Pasquali [1]

1. Clinica Chirurgica 1 - Pancreatic and Endocrine Digestive Surgical Unit. Department of Surgery, Oncology and Gastroenterology – University of Padua, via Giustiniani, 2 – 35128 Padova, Italy; davidalinagp@gmail.com (A.D.); claudio.pasquali@unipd.it (C.P.)
2. General Surgery Unit, Department of Translational Research and New Technologies in Medicine and Surgery, University of Pisa, via Paradisa, 2 – 56125 Pisa, Italy; luca.morelli@unipi.it (L.M.); gregorio.difranco@med.unipi.it (G.D.F.)
3. Chirurgia Generale e d'Urgenza 3, AOU Città della Salute e della Scienza di Torino, Corso Bramante, 88 – 10126 Torino, Italy; dcampra@cittadellasalute.to.it (D.C.); pdepaolis@cittadellasalute.to.it (P.D.P)
* Correspondence: acmilanetto@unipd.it; Tel.: +39-049-821-8831

Received: 22 August 2020; Accepted: 7 October 2020; Published: 13 October 2020

Abstract: Background: Pancreatic metastases from renal-cell carcinoma (RCC-PMs) are rare. Surgery may play a role in improving overall (OS) and disease-free survival (DFS). Methods: Clinical-pathological features, surgery and follow-up data of patients with RCC-PMs operated on in three pancreatic surgical centers (2000–2019) were retrospectively evaluated. Results: Thirty-nine patients (21 male/18 female, averaging 65 years) were enrolled. RCC-PMs were metachronous in 36 patients (mean 94 months, up to 24 years after nephrectomy), multiple in 21 patients, and with a median size of 2.5 (range, 0.7–7.5) cm. All the patients underwent pancreatic surgery (33 standard resections, 6 limited resections). Fifteen patients had post-operative complications (morbidity 38.5%). The median DFS was 63 months, and 19 out of 36 patients showed a disease recurrence. The median OS was 134 months, and 13 out of 36 patients were alive with no evidence of disease. At univariate analysis, lymph node positivity (HR 5.1, 95% CI 1.5–18), multi-visceral resection (HR 3.4, 95% CI 1.1–10) and synchronous RCC-PMs (HR 13, 95% CI 3–55) were significantly associated with a short OS. Conclusion: Surgery may allow a DFS up to 17 years in more than one third of patients, even after limited resections. Splenectomy and lymph node dissection are not mandatory.

Keywords: renal cell carcinoma; pancreatic neoplasms; pancreatectomy; PET-CT scan

1. Introduction

Renal cell carcinoma (RCC) incidence rate has increased, and it accounts for 2%–3% of all new adult malignancies [1]. More than 50% of RCCs are currently detected incidentally [2], and about 20%–30% of patients have metastatic disease at presentation [3]. In localised RCC, 20%–30% of patients will have a recurrence after nephrectomy [4]; distant metastases from RCC occur mostly to the liver, lung and bone, and in 2.8% of patients may present in the pancreas [5]. Pancreatic metastases from RCC (RCC-PMs) are characterized by a slow growing behavior and a long interval of about 10 years before recurrence after nephrectomy [6].

Follow-up after nephrectomy which may include chest and abdominal imaging is rarely performed beyond five years, unless clinically indicated [7]. Therefore, RCC-PMs are often detected incidentally by abdominal ultrasound, computed tomography scan (CT) scan and/or magnetic resonance imaging (MRI) performed for other reasons in asymptomatic patients. Currently, a total body functional imaging is not part of the routine follow-up of these patients, although the systemic spread of RCC is well known. Both on CT scan and MRI, RCC-PMs show an early enhancement after contrast medium injection; MRI can detect RCC-PMs even without contrast-enhancement, as hyper intense lesions at T2- and diffusion-weighted images [8]. These imaging features are common to both RCC-PMs and pancreatic neuroendocrine neoplasms (pNENs), and the differential diagnosis with a non-functioning pNEN may be challenging [9]. So far, a previous nephrectomy was strongly suggestive of RCC-PM, but nowadays the endoscopic ultrasound-guided biopsy may help in differential diagnosis.

Pancreatic surgery for RCC-PMs appears to confer a survival benefit to the patients [10], and a significantly longer overall survival (OS) when compared to PMs from other primary neoplasms may be achieved (median 109 vs. 36 months, respectively) [11]. A surgical treatment may have a role in improving OS and disease-free survival (DFS) in patients with RCC-PMs, even in the era of anti-vascular endothelial growth factor agents. Since the treatment with tyrosine kinase inhibitors (TKIs) failed to show a complete objective response in patients with metastatic setting [6], the question is whether surgery may be extended to a larger number of patients to give them OS and/or DFS benefits. This retrospective study collects the experience of three Italian high-volume pancreatic surgical centers on RCC-PM in the last 20 years. Clinical-pathological features, surgical management and DFS/OS were evaluated, and indications to pancreatic surgery and follow-up timing and imaging were discussed.

2. Patients and Methods

Clinical records of patients with RCC-PMs observed from November 2000–December 2019 in three Italian high-volume pancreatic surgical centers (Surgery Unit 1, Padua; General Surgery Unit, Pisa; and General and Emergency Surgery, Turin) were retrieved retrospectively. Patients who underwent surgery for a RCC-PM in the study period were enrolled. The following data were analyzed: age (years), gender, date and type of surgery for RCC; RCC staging (according to AJCC classification 8th ed.) [12]; date of diagnosis of PM (with "synchronous RCC-PM" defined as a PM diagnosed at the same time, or within six months of the RCC diagnosis); disease-free interval (DFI, defined as the time from resection of the primary RCC to the onset of PM); cross-sectional imaging studies (CT scan, MRI); functional imaging studies, such as ^{18}F- fluorodeoxyglucose positron emission tomography-CT (^{18}F-FDG PET-CT), ^{68}Gallium-DOTA-peptide PET-CT (^{68}Ga PET-CT), and ^{111}In-Octreotide scintigraphy; number and pancreatic location of PM; extra-pancreatic sites of RCC metastases.

We considered type of pancreatic surgery (standard resections: pancreatico-duodenectomy, distal pancreatectomy, total pancreatectomy; and limited resections: spleen-preserving distal pancreatectomy, duodenum-preserving pancreatic head resection, central pancreatectomy, enucleation); associated abdominal surgery (including splenectomy, and multi-visceral resections); operative time (min), blood loss (mL), and hospital stay (days). Surgical outcome included overall morbidity, early post-operative mortality (within 30 days from surgery), post-pancreatectomy haemorrhage, delayed gastric emptying, and post-operative pancreatic fistula (according to the International Study Group on Pancreatic Fistula definition) [13]. The following histological data were evaluated: tumor size (cm), lymph node metastases and lymph node ratio (defined as the number of positive lymph nodes on the total number of lymph nodes analyzed).

Follow-up closed at 31st December 2019. In all the patients with at least six months of follow-up we evaluated OS and DFS, defined by using a personal telephone interview or at the last follow-up visit, that included clinical evaluation and imaging studies (CT scan, MRI and/or ^{68}Ga PET-CT) to detect any tumor recurrences.

Kaplan-Meier survival curves for OS and DFS were plotted and compared using the log-rank test. The Chi-square test or Fisher's exact test were used for comparison of categorical variables, when appropriate. Cox proportional-hazard models were used to identify risk factors associated with OS and DFS at univariate analysis. The results were reported as hazard ratios (HRs) and 95% confidence intervals (95% CI). A p value less than 0.05 was considered statistically significant. Statistical analysis was performed using the R program version 3.6.3 [14].

Statement of Ethics

The research was conducted ethically in accordance with the World Medical Association Declaration of Helsinki. Subjects gave their written informed consent to data processing anonymously for research purposes. The ethics committee of the Azienda Ospedaliera di Padova approved the present study (project code: 2872p).

3. Results

Thirty-nine patients with RCC-PMs underwent open pancreatic resection and were enrolled in the study. Clinical features, surgery, and post-operative outcome are described in Table 1.

There were 21 men and 18 women, averaging 65 years (range, 45–81 years). All primary RCC were treated by R0 radical nephrectomy; all the patients had a clear cell RCC, and only one patient had histologically confirmed lymph node metastases. In 36 patients RCC-PMs were metachronous lesions, occurring after a median time of 84 (range, 7–291) months, and in one third of patients after a DFI longer than 10 years. In 21 patients RCC-PMs were multiple lesions, located in the body-tail of the pancreas in 28 cases (despite a left-sided nephrectomy in 23 patients), and with a median size of 2.5 (range, 0.7–7.5) cm. Only seven patients showed concomitant extra-pancreatic metastases. Concerning functional imaging studies, ^{18}F-FDG PET-CT showed a moderate tracer uptake in 9 out of 14 patients; ^{68}Ga PET-CT demonstrated a strong tracer uptake in all three patients in which it was performed (Figure 1), and when considered together, ^{68}Ga PET-CT and ^{111}In-Scintigraphy were strongly positive in five out of seven patients.

All the patients underwent open pancreatic surgery with curative intent, and in five patients a multi-visceral resection was needed due to other abdominal metastases. A pre-operative diagnosis was correctly assessed in 30 patients by imaging studies and medical history. Surgery consisted in 33 standard pancreatic resections (13 distal pancreatectomy, 12 total pancreatectomy, and eight pancreatico-duodenectomy), and six limited resections (three spleen-preserving distal pancreatectomy, one duodenum-preserving pancreatic head resection, and two central pancreatectomy). Ten patients underwent multi-visceral resections, which included: nephrectomy/ipsilateral adrenalectomy ($n = 2$) and hemicolectomy/ureteral resection ($n = 1$) for a synchronous RCC, partial/total gastrectomy ($n = 3$), hemicolectomy right/left ($n = 2$), adrenalectomy ipsilateral/contralateral ($n = 3$), and partial vena cava resection ($n = 1$). Histology showed an average of 18 lymph nodes counted, with an involvement of peri-pancreatic lymph nodes in five patients. Additional splenectomy was performed in 22 patients, and no splenic secondary lesions were detected. Fifteen patients had post-operative complications (morbidity 38.5%). Notably, there were four post-operative pancreatic fistulas grade B, and two post-pancreatectomy haemorrhages (in the standard resection group). Other post-operative complications included: pneumonia/pulmonary atelectasis ($n = 6$), respiratory failure ($n = 1$), splenic infarction after Warshaw operation ($n = 1$), and renal failure ($n = 1$). One patient with a liver hematoma required a reoperation, and one patient died from pulmonary embolism (mortality 2.6%).

Table 1. Clinical features, surgery, and post-operative outcome ($n = 39$).

Parameter	
Age (years), median (range)	65 (45–81)
Sex, n	
Male	21
Female	18
Nephrectomy, n	
Left	23
Right	16
Stage RCC [12], n	
I	2
II	14
III	20
IV	3
Timing of RCC-PM, n	
Synchronous	3
Metachronous	36
Disease free interval (months), median (range)	84 (7–291)
Number of RCC-PM, n	
Single	18
Multiple	21
Other sites of metastases, n	
No	32
Abdominal	3 local relapse, 1 contralateral kidney, 1 adrenal
Extra-abdominal	1 lung, 1 thyroid
Pancreatic metastases size (cm), median (range)	2.5 (0.7–7.5)
Type of pancreatic surgery, n	
Distal pancreatectomy	13
Total pancreatectomy	12
Pancreatico-duodenectomy	8 (1 associated enucleation)
Limited resections	3 spleen-preserving DP, 1 DPPHR, 2 CP (1 associated enucleation)
Associated surgery, n	
Splenectomy	22
Multi-visceral resections	12
Operation time (min), median (range)	350 (150–720)
Intra-operative blood loss (mL), median (range)	400 (100–1300)
Post-operative morbidity, n	
Post-operative pancreatic fistula	9 (5 biochemical leak, 4 post-operative pancreatic fistula grade B)
Post-pancreatectomy hemorrhage	2
Delayed gastric emptying	1
Other cause	9
Post-operative mortality, n	1
Reoperation rate, n	1
Hospital stay (days), median (range)	12 (6–133)

CP–central pancreatectomy, DP–distal pancreatectomy, DPPHR–duodenum-preserving pancreatic head resection, n.a.–not available, RCC renal cell carcinoma, RCC-PM–pancreatic metastasis from renal cell carcinoma.

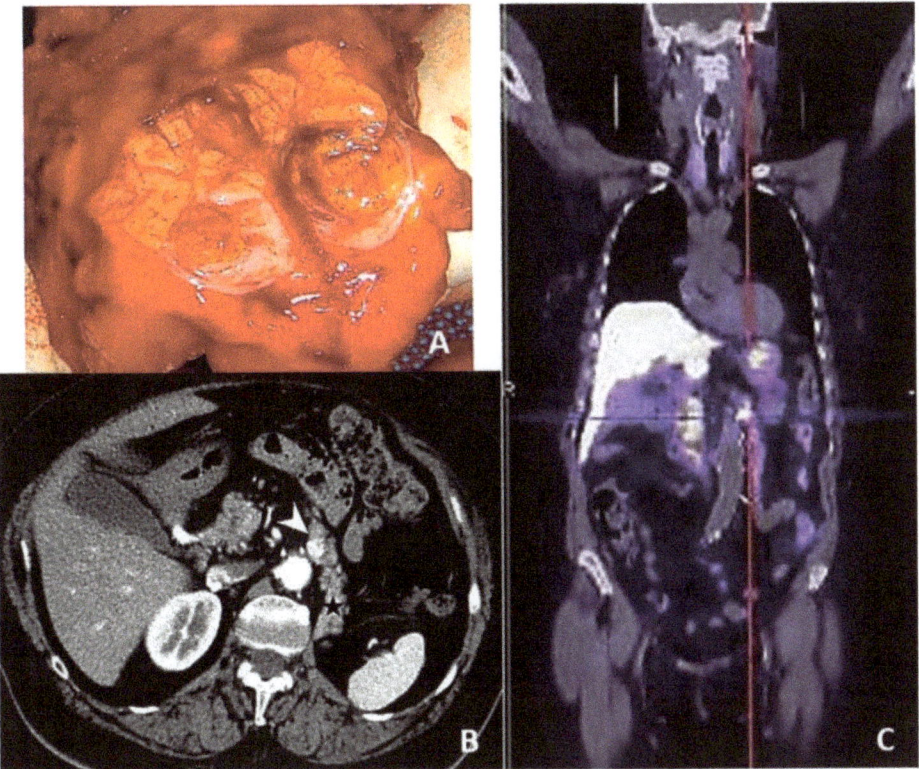

Figure 1. (**A**) Macroscopic appearance of a RCC-PM after cutting the specimen; (**B**) preoperative CT scan (white arrow for the lesion, black star for the pancreatic tail); (**C**) ^{68}Ga PET-CT of a single 1.2 cm-in size RCC metastasis in the pancreatic body.

Thirty-six patients were considered for the analysis of long-term outcome and survival as DFS and OS. Long-term follow-up is described in Table 2.

After a median follow-up of 68 (range, 4–201) months, post-operative diabetes and exocrine insufficiency were observed in 17 out of 36 and in 15 out of 35 patients, respectively. In the limited resection group, all the patients had normal endocrine and exocrine pancreatic functions. After a median DFS of 63 (range, 3–201) months, 19 patients experienced a disease recurrence, located in the pancreas in five cases. Notably, 4 out of 19 patients in follow-up after standard resection (excluding total pancreatectomy) showed a pancreatic recurrence after a median DFS of 20 months. When considering the 31 patients in follow-up with PMs only, 16 of them showed a recurrence after a median DFS of 25 (range, 3–130) months, and their median residual survival after recurrence was 50 (range, 4–121) months. The 1-, 3-, 5-, and 10-year DFS rates were 83%, 60%, 52%, and 38%, respectively (Figure 2). Finally, 11 patients in follow-up (median 68 months) died of disease; 20 patients were still alive, and 13 of them without evidence of disease. The median OS was 134 months; the 1-, 3-, 5-, and 10-year OS rates were 94%, 88%, 79%, and 55%, respectively (Figure 2).

Table 2. Long-term follow-up ($n = 36$).

Parameters	
Post-operative diabetes, n	17
Post-operative exocrine insufficiency, n	15
Disease recurrence, n	19
Site of recurrence, n	
Liver	7
Lung	7
Pancreas	5
Bone	2
Thyroid	1
Adrenal	1
Follow-up (months), median (range)	68 (4–201)
Status, n	
Died of disease	11
Died of other cause	5
Alive with disease	7
Alive and no evidence of disease	13

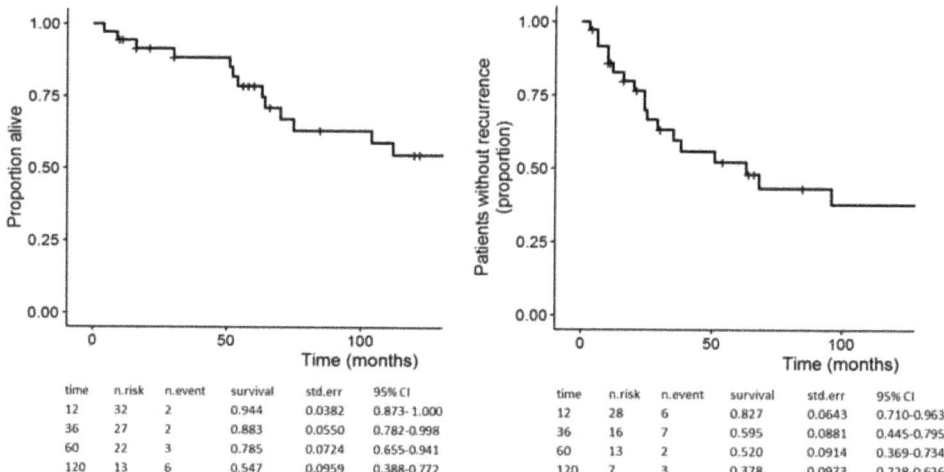

Figure 2. Kaplan-Meier estimates for overall survival (OS) (left) and disease-free survival (DFS) (right) of 36 patients after pancreatic surgery for RCC-PM.

At Cox-regression univariate analysis (Table 3), lymph node positivity (HR 5.1, 95% CI 1.5–18), multi-visceral resection (HR 3.4, 95% CI 1.1–10) and synchronous RCC-PMs (HR 13, 95% CI 3–55) were significantly associated with a short OS.

Table 3. Univariate Cox regression analysis for OS and DFS ($n = 36$).

	OS				DFS			
	Event	HR	95% CI	p Value	Event	HR	95% CI	p Value
Age (years)	16				19			
<65 ($n = 17$)	9	1			11	1		
≥65 ($n = 19$)	7	0.97	0.36–2.6	0.95	8	0.84	0.34–2.1	0.70
Stage RCC	16				19			
I-II ($n = 13$)	5	1			8	1		
III-IV ($n = 23$)	11	2.9	0.89–9.4	0.077	11	0.93	0.37–2.3	0.88
Timing RCC-PM	16				19			
Metachronous ($n = 33$)	13	1			17	1		
Synchronous ($n = 3$)	3	13	3–55	<0.001	2	4.2	0.91–19	0.065
Number RCC-PM	16				19			
Single ($n = 16$)	6	1			9	1		
Multiple ($n = 20$)	10	1.1	0.38–3	0.9	10	0.79	0.32–1.9	0.61
Extra-pancreatic metastases	16				19			
No ($n = 30$)	14	1			16	1		
Yes ($n = 6$)	2	2.8	0.54–15	0.22	3	2.0	0.57–7.4	0.27
Pancreatic resection	16				19			
Limited ($n = 5$)	2	1			4	1		
Standard ($n = 31$)	14	1.8	0.41–8.3	0.43	15	0.58	0.19–1.8	0.34
Multi-visceral resection	16				19			
No ($n = 26$)	10	1			13	1		
Yes ($n = 10$)	6	3.4	1.1–10	0.029	6	1.8	0.66–4.7	0.25
Splenectomy	16				19			
No ($n = 15$)	8	1			10	1		
Yes ($n = 21$)	8	0.94	0.35–2.5	0.89	9	0.74	0.3–1.8	0.52
Postoperative complications	16				19			
No ($n = 23$)	10	1			9	1		
Yes ($n = 13$)	6	0.84	0.3–2.3	0.74	10	1.9	0.77–4.7	0.17
Size RCC-PM (cm)	16				19			
<2.5 ($n = 14$)	10	1			6	1		
≥2.5 ($n = 22$)	6	1.1	0.4–3.2	0.80	13	1.7	0.63–4.5	0.31
Lymph-node positivity	16				19			
No ($n = 31$)	12	1			16	1		
Yes ($n = 5$)	4	5.1	1.5–18	0.011	3	1.4	0.4–5.1	0.59
Recurrence	16							
No ($n = 17$)	4	1			-	-	-	-
Yes ($n = 19$)	12	2.6	0.81–8.1	0.11	-	-	-	-
DFI (months)	13				17			
≥60 ($n = 22$)	9	1			12	1		
<60 ($n = 11$)	4	1	0.31–3.4	0.96	5	0.96	0.34–2.7	0.94

DFI–disease-free interval; DFS–disease-free survival; OS–overall survival; RCC–renal cell carcinoma; RCC-PM–pancreatic metastasis from renal cell carcinoma.

4. Discussion

Nephron-sparing or radical nephrectomy is the standard of care for localized RCC, with a 20-30% of recurrence rate [15], and RCC-PMs are reported to occur in 2.8% of patients [5]. In our experience, RCC-PMs were located in the body-tail of the pancreas in 28 cases (irrespective of the side of nephrectomy), multiple in 21 patients, and only seven patients had extra-pancreatic metastases. Confirming previous reports [6,16], 92% of RCC-PMs arose as metachronous, occurring after a median DFI of seven years (up to 24 years) after nephrectomy. Occasionally, metastases may have occurred earlier and been overlooked by the cross-sectional imaging studies [9]. The gold standard to detect hyper vascular RCC-PMs in the follow-up of RCC patients should be the CT scan, and MRI could be an acceptable alternative option [8]. One third of our patients developed RCC-PMs after a DFI of more than 10 years; a long follow-up over 10 years should be considered, even in asymptomatic patients. Due to the systemic spread of RCC, functional total-body imaging studies may have some relevance in the follow-up after nephrectomy for RCC. In our series, ^{18}F-FDG PET-CT had a sensitivity of 64% in detecting RCC metastases, as previously reported [17]. However, RCC-PMs showed a low/moderate FDG uptake, whereas ^{68}Ga PET-CT and ^{111}In-Scintigraphy together (both binding to somatostatin receptors) showed a strong positivity in five out of seven patients. The positivity of ^{111}In-Scintigraphy is a common finding in metastatic RCC [18]. Hence, ^{68}Ga PET-CT (which replaced ^{111}In-Scintigraphy) could be a promising tool for the RCC staging, and it may be advisable once RCC recurrence or metastases are suspected at CT scan.

In metastatic setting of RCC, the resection of RCC metastases is recommended as local treatment for most sites, except brain and bone metastases [19], since the surgical treatment can lead to a long DFS, even without a systemic therapy [20]. Concerning RCC-PMs, five-year survival was significantly longer in patients who underwent surgery (72–73%) when compared to patients without surgery (0–14%) [10,16]. In a recent multicenter study [6], surgery and TKIs showed comparable results, although evaluated as PFS and DFS, respectively, but patients treated with TKIs had no complete responses [6]. Moreover, TKI-related toxicity has been observed in most patients, with a decline in quality of life [21]. In our surgical series, we obtained a complete objective response in 13 patients, in terms of patients living without disease after a median follow-up of 148 months. In our study, in RCC-PMs without extra-pancreatic metastases, 19 showed a recurrence after a median DFS of 25 months, and their median residual survival after recurrence was 50 months. Even in a subset of patients older than 65 years, and those with a stage III-IV RCC at diagnosis, the five-year OS was found to be 80% and 71%, respectively, after pancreatic surgery. In our study, mortality rate was 2.6%, clinically relevant post-operative pancreatic fistula (excluding total pancreatectomy) occurred only in 15% of cases, and 62% of patients had an uneventful post-operative course. These results are in line with a recent study on "high-risk complication" patients who underwent pancreatic surgery [22], with morbidity and mortality rates of 42.5% and 3.5%, respectively. Particularly, morbidity and mortality rates of patients who underwent major pancreatic surgery (total pancreatectomy and pancreatico-duodenectomy) was 40% and nil, respectively. Thus, when performed in centers specialized in pancreatic surgery, a correct management of expected complications will minimize the risk of severe outcomes, and an aggressive approach for the treatment of RCC-PMs can be adopted to pursue the goal of an R0 resection, even if this could require a major pancreatic resection.

In the univariate analysis we analyzed the possible impact of the presence of single/multiple RCC-PMs, of the presence of extra-pancreatic disease, and of the DFI on the DFS and OS. High-volume analyses during the last 10 years on RCC-PMs showed that results of RCC-PMs surgical resection are not conditioned by the presence of single or multiple metastases, or the presence of synchronous or metachronous metastases [23–26]. In our study we also reported no difference in DFS or OS at Cox-regression univariate analysis between single or multiple metastases. On the contrary, at univariate analysis a significantly ($p < 0.001$) shorter OS was associated with synchronous RCC-PMs when compared to metachronous lesions with a HR of 13 (95% CI 3–55). However, this may be the result of low statistical power due to the small sample size of the patients with synchronous RCC-PMs. Furthermore, RCC-PMs without extra-pancreatic disease carry a favorable prognosis with a cumulative five-year survival after surgery of up to 88% [27], even if this finding was not confirmed in our study. A prolonged DFI is a characteristic feature of patients with RCC pancreatic metastases, and in our series, we reported 13 patients with a DFI of more than 10 years, nine of which were still alive without evidence of disease. Nevertheless, no associations between DFI and survival were observed, even when raising the DFI cut-off from 5 to 10 years, in accordance with data published recently in the literature [24,26,28]. Therefore, when a radical resection of RCC-PMs is obtainable, this should be taken in consideration both in the case of single or multiple RCC-PMs, or extra-pancreatic disease, and independently by the DFI. Moreover, we observed a disease recurrence in about half of patients either with single or multiple PMs, confirming a previous study [16]. However, as reported by Di Franco at al., an aggressive treatment could be taken into consideration also in case of recurrent disease after RCC pancreatic metastases resection and multiple surgical treatment of recurrent RCC metastases, diagnosed during the follow-up [11].

The usefulness of lymphadenectomy in pancreatic surgery performed for RCC-PMs is still debated. Several previous reports found that a peri-pancreatic lymph node involvement with PMs is uncommon [29], or even absent [30], especially with the pancreas as the only metastatic site [16]. In our study, only five patients had a RCC involvement of peri-pancreatic lymph nodes, but they showed a worse five-year OS than patients with negative lymph nodes (53 vs. 82%, respectively), confirmed at univariate analysis ($p = 0.011$). From our experience, lymph-node dissection should be performed only in case of suspected lymph node involvement detected intra- or pre-operatively. Similarly, splenectomy could be performed only for a pancreatic tail lesion close to the hilum, or if a lymph node involvement at the splenic hilum is suspected, since splenectomy was not related to any survival advantages. Some authors reported a high local recurrence rate after limited resections for RCC-PMs [31], but in our study no significant differences were shown between standard and limited resections in terms of DFS/OS. Considering long-life expectancy of these patients, limited pancreatic resections may be an alternative to standard procedures. Pancreatic recurrence occurred in five out of 24 patients in follow-up after pancreatic surgery (excluding total pancreatectomy), and all but one patient had undergone a standard pancreatic resection. Thus, a pancreatic "recurrence" may be related to undetected multiple PMs [32], rather than to the surgical procedure. Moreover, disease relapse after pancreatic surgery occurred mostly in distant extra-pancreatic sites. From our experience, a standard pancreatic resection with lymph node dissection (and splenectomy) may not prevent pancreatic (and systemic) recurrence of disease, since DFS depends mostly on extra-pancreatic metastases. Multi-visceral resections, performed with curative intent and mostly associated with total pancreatectomy, showed a significantly short OS ($p = 0.029$), confirming the bad prognosis when infiltration includes surrounding organs. Moreover, total pancreatectomy results in exocrine insufficiency and insulin-dependent diabetes mellitus, which may affect the global quality of life, especially for relatively young patients who had undergone nephrectomy.

Our study has some limitations due to the relatively small number of patients included and the retrospective design and data collection. Moreover, similarly to other published studies, the lack of a control group represents another limitation. In fact, the multicenter nature and the long period of the study made it difficult to obtain a really comparable control group of patients that did not undergo surgical resection in the last 20 years. However, patients with pancreatic metastases treated with sole systemic therapies were either patients not fit for surgery because of severe comorbidities with a high operative risk for pancreatic surgery, or patients not susceptible to undergo a R0 resection because of plurimetastatic disease with diffuse extra-pancreatic localizations. Therefore, any comparison with such group could have introduced a selection bias, because patients who were not operated on were more likely to have shorter survival rates. Nevertheless, this study reported the experience of three tertiary referral centers for pancreatic surgery, with a long time of follow-up.

In conclusion, the assessment of RCC-PMs may be improved using functional total body imaging, particularly ^{68}Ga PET-CT as a second-line imaging technique, and follow-up after nephrectomy for RCC should be extended after 10 years. Indications to surgery should be taken in consideration for RCC-PMs in which a radical resection could be obtained, both for single and multiple PMs; we have insufficient data to extend indications to patients with extra-pancreatic disease. Limited pancreatic resections are equivalent in terms of recurrence to standard pancreatic procedures, and splenectomy and lymph node dissection are not mandatory, since lymph node involvement is uncommon. In pancreatic units, resective surgery may obtain a complete objective response, with more than one third of patients living without disease after a median follow-up longer than 12 years. Moreover, in our opinion, with the introduction of new possible locally directed therapy, such as surgical, ablative or radiation-based approaches, and of new chemotherapy drugs, today each case of RCC-PM should be treated thorough multidisciplinary evaluation performed by general surgeons, radiation therapists, interventional radiologists, and medical oncologists. Probably, combination therapy with the newly available target therapies will be crucial for the management of these patients in the future.

Author Contributions: Conceptualization, A.C.M., L.M., P.D.P. and C.P.; Data curation, A.C.M., A.D., G.D.F. and D.C.; Writing—original draft, A.C.M.; Writing—review and editing, A.C.M., L.M., P.D.P. and C.P. All authors have read and agreed to the published version of the manuscript.

Funding: This research received no external funding.

Conflicts of Interest: The authors declare no conflict of interest.

References

1. Siegel, R.; Naishadham, D.; Jemal, A. Cancer statistics 2013. *CA Cancer J. Clin.* **2013**, *63*, 11–30. [CrossRef] [PubMed]
2. Novara, G.; Ficarra, V.; Antonelli, A.; Artibani, W.; Bertini, R.; Carini, M.; Cosciani Cunico, S.; Imbimbo, C.; Longo, N.; Martignoni, G.; et al. Validation of the 2009 TNM version in a large multi-institutional cohort of patients treated for renal cell carcinoma: Are further improvements needed? *Eur. Urol.* **2010**, *58*, 588–595. [CrossRef] [PubMed]
3. Lam, J.S.; Shvarts, O.; Leppert, J.T.; Figlin, R.A.; Belldegrun, A.S. Renal cell carcinoma 2005: New frontiers in staging, prognostication and targeted molecular therapy. *J. Urol.* **2005**, *1l73*, 1853–1862. [CrossRef]
4. Sandock, D.S.; Seftel, A.D.; Resnick, M.I. A new protocol for the followup of renal cell carcinoma based on pathological stage. *J. Urol.* **1995**, *154*, 28–31. [CrossRef]
5. Klugo, R.C.; Detmers, M.; Stiles, R.E.; Talley, R.W.; Cerny, J.C. Aggressive versus conservative management of stage IV renal cell carcinoma. *J. Urol.* **1977**, *118*, 244–246. [CrossRef]
6. Santoni, M.; Conti, A.; Partelli, S.; Porta, C.; Sternberg, C.N.; Procopio, G.; Bracarda, S.; Basso, U.; De Giorgi, U.; Derosa, L.; et al. Surgical resection does not improve survival in patients with renal metastases to the pancreas in the era of tyrosine kinase inhibitors. *Ann. Surg. Oncol.* **2015**, *22*, 2094–2100. [CrossRef]
7. Motzer, R.J.; Jonasch, E.; Agarwal, N.; Bhayani, S.; Bro, W.P.; Chang, S.S.; Choueiri, T.K.; Costello, B.A.; Derweesh, I.H.; Fishman, M.; et al. Kidney cancer, version 2.2017, NCCN clinical practice guidelines in oncology. *J. Natl. Compr. Canc. Netw. JNCCN* **2017**, *15*, 804–834. [CrossRef]
8. Vincenzi, M.; Pasquotti, G.; Polverosi, R.; Pasquali, C.; Pomerri, F. Imaging of pancreatic metastases from renal cell carcinoma. *Cancer Imaging* **2014**, *14*, 5. [CrossRef]
9. Moletta, L.; Milanetto, A.C.; Vincenzi, V.; Alaggio, R.; Pedrazzoli, S.; Pasquali, C. Pancreatic secondary lesions from renal cell carcinoma. *World J. Surg.* **2014**, *38*, 3002–3006. [CrossRef]
10. Tanis, P.J.; van der Gaag, N.A.; Busch, O.R.; van Gulik, T.M.; Gouma, D.J. Systematic review of pancreatic surgery for metastatic renal cell carcinoma. *Br. J. Surg.* **2009**, *96*, 579–592. [CrossRef]
11. Di Franco, G.; Gianardi, D.; Palmeri, M.; Furbetta, N.; Guadagni, S.; Bianchini, M.; Bonari, F.; Sbrana, A.; Vasile, E.; Pollina, L.E.; et al. Pancreatic resections for metastases: A twenty-year experience from a tertiary care center. *Eur. J. Surg. Oncol.* **2020**, *46*, 825–831. [CrossRef] [PubMed]
12. American Joint Committee on Cancer. Kidney. In *AJCC Cancer Staging Manual*, 8th ed.; Amin, M.B., Edge, S.B., Greene, F.L., Byrd, D.R., Brookland, R.K., Washington, M.K., Gershenwald, J.E., Compton, C.C., Hess, K.R., Sullivan, D.C., et al., Eds.; Springer: New York, NY, USA, 2017; pp. 739–748.
13. Bassi, C.; Marchegiani, G.; Dervenis, C.; Sarr, M.; Abu Hilal, M.; Adham, M.; Allen, P.; Andersson, R.; Asbun, H.J.; Besselink, M.G.; et al. The 2016 update of the international study group (ISGPS) definition and grading of postoperative pancreatic fistula: 11 years after. *Surgery* **2017**, *161*, 584–591. [CrossRef] [PubMed]
14. R Core Team. R: A language and environment for statistical computing. *R Foundation for Statistical Computing*, Vienna, Austria. 2020. Available online: https://www.R-project.org/ (accessed on 1st May 2020).
15. Janzen, N.K.; Kim, H.L.; Figlin, R.A.; Belldegrun, A.S. Surveillance after radical or partial nephrectomy for localized renal cell carcinoma and management of recurrent disease. *Urol. Clin. North. Am.* **2003**, *30*, 843–852. [CrossRef]

16. Sellner, F.; Tykalsky, N.; Se Santis, M.; Pont, J.; Klimpfinger, M. Solitary and multiple isolated metastases of clear cell renal carcinoma to the pancreas: An indication for pancreatic surgery. *Ann. Surg. Oncol.* **2006**, *13*, 75–85. [CrossRef] [PubMed]
17. Mueller-Lisse, U.G.; Mueller-Lisse, U.L. Imaging of advanced renal cell carcinoma. *World J. Urol.* **2010**, *28*, 253–261. [CrossRef]
18. Edgren, M.; Westlin, J.E.; Kälkner, K.M.; Sundin, A.; Nilsson, S. [^{111}In-DPTAD-Phe1]-octreotide scintigraphy in the management of patients with advanced renal cell carcinoma. *Cancer Biother. Radiopharm.* **1999**, *14*, 59–64. [CrossRef]
19. Bamias, A.; Escudier, B.; Sternberg, C.N.; Zagouri, F.; Dellis, A.; Djavan, B.; Tzannis, K.; Kontovinis, L.; Stravodimos, K.; Papatsoris, A.; et al. Current clinical practice guidelines for the treatment of renal cell carcinoma: A systematic review and critical evaluation. *Oncologist* **2017**, *22*, 667–679. [CrossRef]
20. Kwak, C.; Park, Y.H.; Jeong, C.W.; Lee, S.E.; Ku, J.H. Metastasectomy without systemic therapy in metastatic renal cell carcinoma: Comparison with conservative treatment. *Urol. Int.* **2007**, *79*, 145–151. [CrossRef]
21. Riaz, I.B.; Faridi, W.; Husnain, M.; Malik, S.U.; Sipra, Q.U.A.R.; Gondal, F.R.; Xie, H.; Yadav, S.; Kohli, M. Adjuvant therapy in high-risk renal cell cancer: A systematic review and meta-analysis. *Mayo Clin. Proc.* **2019**, *94*, 1524–1534. [CrossRef]
22. Primavesi, F.; Klieser, E.; Cardini, B.; Marsoner, K.; Fröschl, U.; Thalhammer, S.; Fischer, I.; Hauer, A.; Urbas, R.; Kiesslich, T.; et al. Exploring the surgical landscape of pancreatic neuroendocrine neoplasia in Austria: Results from the ASSO pNEN study group. *Eur. J. Surg. Oncol.* **2019**, *45*, 198–206. [CrossRef]
23. Schwarz, L.; Sauvanet, A.; Regenet, N.; Mabrut, J.Y.; Gigot, J.F.; Housseau, E.; Millat, B.; Ouaissi, M.; Gayet, B.; Fuks, D.; et al. Long-term survival after pancreatic resection for renal cell carcinoma metastasis. *Ann. Surg. Oncol.* **2014**, *21*, 4007–4013. [CrossRef] [PubMed]
24. Konstantinidis, I.T.; Dursun, A.; Zheng, H.; Wargo, J.A.; Thayer, S.P.; Fernandez-del Castillo, C.; Warshaw, A.L.; Ferrone, C.R. Metastatic tumors in the pancreas in the modern era. *J. Am. Coll. Surg.* **2010**, *211*, 749–753. [CrossRef]
25. Benhaim, R.; Oussoultzoglou, E.; Saeedi, Y.; Mouracade, P.; Bachellier, P.; Lang, H. Pancreatic metastasis from clear cell renal cell carcinoma: Outcome of an aggressive approach. *Urology* **2015**, *85*, 135–140. [CrossRef] [PubMed]
26. Tosoian, J.J.; Cameron, J.L.; Allaf, M.E.; Hruban, R.H.; Nahime, C.B.; Pawlik, T.M.; Pierorazio, P.M.; Reddy, S.; Wolfgang, C.L. Resection of isolated renal cell carcinoma metastases of the pancreas: Outcomes from the Johns Hopkins Hospital. *J. Gastrointest. Surg.* **2014**, *18*, 542–548. [CrossRef] [PubMed]
27. Sellner, F. Isolated pancreatic metastases from renal cell carcinoma: An outcome of a special metastatic pathway or of specific tumor cell selection? *Clin. Exp. Metastasis* **2018**, *35*, 91–102. [CrossRef] [PubMed]
28. Jakubowski, C.D.; Vertosick, E.A.; Untch, B.R.; Sjoberg, D.; Wei, E.; Palmer, F.L.; Patel, S.G.; Downey, R.J.; Strong, V.E.; Russo, P. Complete metastasectomy for renal cell carcinoma: Comparison of five solid organ sites. *J. Surg. Oncol.* **2016**, *114*, 375–379. [CrossRef]
29. Hirota, T.; Tomida, T.; Iwasa, M.; Takahashi, K.; Kaneda, M.; Tamaki, H. Solitary pancreatic metastasis occurring eight years after nephrectomy for renal cell carcinoma: A case report and surgical review. *Int. J. Pancreatol.* **1996**, *19*, 145–153. [CrossRef]
30. Faure, J.P.; Tuech, J.J.; Richer, J.P.; Pessaux, P.; Arnaud, J.P.; Carretier, M. Pancreatic metastasis of renal cell carcinoma: Presentation, treatment and survival. *J. Urol.* **2001**, *165*, 20–22. [CrossRef]
31. Hafez, K.S.; Novick, A.C.; Campbell, S.C. Patterns of tumor recurrence and guidelines for followup after nephron sparing surgery for sporadic renal cell carcinoma. *J. Urol.* **1997**, *157*, 2067–2070. [CrossRef]
32. Zerbi, A.; Ortolano, E.; Balzano, G.; Borri, A.; Beneduce, A.A.; Di Carlo, V. Pancreatic metastasis from renal cell carcinoma: Which patients benefit from surgical resection? *Ann. Surg. Oncol.* **2008**, *15*, 1161–1168. [CrossRef]

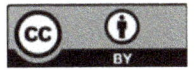

© 2020 by the authors. Licensee MDPI, Basel, Switzerland. This article is an open access article distributed under the terms and conditions of the Creative Commons Attribution (CC BY) license (http://creativecommons.org/licenses/by/4.0/).

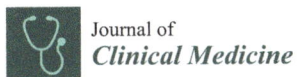 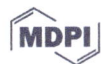

Article

Association of Neutrophil, Platelet, and Lymphocyte Ratios with the Prognosis in Unresectable and Metastatic Pancreatic Cancer

Jessica Allen [1], Colin Cernik [2], Suhaib Bajwa [1], Raed Al-Rajabi [3], Anwaar Saeed [3], Joaquina Baranda [3], Stephen Williamson [3], Weijing Sun [3] and Anup Kasi [3,*]

1. Department of Internal Medicine, School of Medicine, University of Kansas, 3901 Rainbow Blvd, Kansas City, KS 66160, USA; jallen19@kumc.edu (J.A.); sbajwa@kumc.edu (S.B.)
2. Department of Biostatistics and Data Science, University of Kansas, 1450 Jayhawk Blvd, Lawrence, KS 66045, USA; ccernik@kumc.edu
3. University of Kansas Cancer Center, 2650 Shawnee Mission Pkwy, Westwood, KS 66205, USA; ral-rajabi@kumc.edu (R.A.-R.); asaeed@kumc.edu (A.S.); jbaranda@kumc.edu (J.B.); swilliam@kumc.edu (S.W.); wsing2@kumc.edu (W.S.)
* Correspondence: akasi@kumc.edu; Tel.: +1-913-588-1227

Received: 26 August 2020; Accepted: 8 October 2020; Published: 13 October 2020

Abstract: We examined the relationship between the daily rate of change of cancer antigen 19-9 (CA19-9) over the first 90 days of treatment (DRC90) and the pretreatment levels of neutrophils, lymphocytes, and platelets with the overall survival (OS) and progression-free survival (PFS) in patients with stage IV pancreatic ductal adenocarcinoma (PDA) who received chemotherapy. We retrospectively evaluated 102 locally advanced and metastatic PDA patients treated at the University of Kansas Cancer Center (KUCC) between January 2011 and September 2019. We compared the ratio of the pretreatment absolute neutrophil count to the pretreatment absolute lymphocyte count (NLR) and the ratio between the pretreatment platelet count to the pretreatment absolute lymphocyte count (PLR) with the OS and PFS. We compared the DRC90 to the OS and PFS. The ratios were analyzed using the log-rank trend test using the mean of the NLR, PLR, and DRC90 as the threshold for two groups within each variable. Patients with ≥mean NLR (4.6 K/µL) had a significantly lower OS ($p = 0.0444$) and PFS ($p = 0.0483$) compared with patients below the mean. Patients with PLR ≥ mean (3.9 K/µL) did not have a significantly different OS ($p = 0.507$) or PFS ($p = 0.643$) compared with patients below the mean. Patients with DRC90 ≥ mean (−1%) did not have a significantly different OS ($p = 0.342$) or PFS ($p = 0.313$) compared with patients below the mean. Patients with NLR ≥ mean (4.6 K/µL) had a significantly lower OS and PFS compared with patients with NLR below the mean. This implies the possibility of NLR as a prognostic marker in PDA that could guide treatment approaches but still requires validation in a larger cohort.

Keywords: pancreatic cancer; pancreatic ductal adenocarcinoma; pancreatic cancer prognosis

1. Introduction

Pancreatic adenocarcinoma is the third leading cause of death from cancer in the United States with a 5-year survival rate of 9% [1]. There currently no known sufficiently sensitive methods of screening asymptomatic adults for pancreatic adenocarcinoma, and thus, the United States Preventive Services Task Force (USPSTF) currently recommends against screening until symptoms develop [2]. Patients are often diagnosed at later stages, because pancreatic cancer is commonly asymptomatic in the early stages [1]. The effects of this are grim: in patients with stage IV pancreatic adenocarcinoma, the 5-year survival rate drops to 3% [1]. The survival of pancreatic adenocarcinoma has not improved substantially in forty years [3]. Additionally, few risk factors or markers of prognosis have been identified [3].

Individual studies have examined the effect of lymphocytes, neutrophils, and platelets on the overall survival (OS) and progression-free survival (PFS) in patients with pancreatic adenocarcinoma. One study found that a ratio between the pretreatment platelet count to the pretreatment absolute lymphocyte count (PLR) of >240 K/µL, a ratio of the pretreatment absolute neutrophil count to the pretreatment absolute lymphocyte count (NLR) > 5 K/µL, and a daily rate of change of CA19-9 over the first 90 days of treatment (DRC90) > 0.4% were significantly associated with a decreased OS [4]. Another study confirmed that an elevated NLR at or above 3.54 K/µL was significantly associated with a decreased OS [5]. An additional study contradictorily found that NLR > 5 K/µL and CA19-9 at the time of diagnosis ≥ 437 µ/mL were significantly associated with an increased OS and PFS [6]. Further analysis of the effects of the amounts and ratios of immune cells and the rate of tumor marker change in patients at the time of diagnosis on the overall survival is required to ascertain their utility in predicting prognosis and guiding treatment. Thus, in this retrospective study, we analyzed the effect of the NLR, PLR, and DRC90 on the OS and PFS in locally advanced and metastatic pancreatic cancer patients treated at the University of Kansas Cancer Center to add to the existing knowledge regarding the association immune cell ratios have with the prognosis in pancreatic adenocarcinoma.

2. Experimental Section

The study was a retrospective chart review of the characteristics of patients with locally advanced or metastatic pancreatic adenocarcinoma diagnosed between January 2011 and September 2019 from the University of Kansas Cancer Center medical records.

The primary outcomes of interest were the OS and PFS of patients with locally advanced or metastatic pancreatic ductal carcinoma. The NLR and PLR were compared with the OS and PFS. The complete blood cell count closest to the date of the initiation of treatment was used for the neutrophil, lymphocyte, and platelet levels, and patients without a pre-treatment complete blood count (CBC) available were excluded. The DRC90 was calculated and compared with the OS and PFS. The CA19-9 at the time of diagnosis was used as the baseline for measuring the rate of change. The DRC90 was found by calculating the daily percent change of the baseline CA19.9 and the CA19.9 at three months after the treatment initiation. Demographic data, such as the age, gender, race, smoking status, Eastern Cooperative Oncology Group (ECOG) performance status, tumor location, and treatment received, were also collected. All patient data was collected retrospectively via electronic health records and stored on a secure Redcaps database.

The data were deidentified before analysis. Associations between the NLR, PLR, and DRC90 and the OS and PFS were obtained via Kaplan–Meier survival curves and log-rank trend tests using the means of NLR (4.6), PLR (196), and DRC90 (−1%) as the threshold for the two groups within each variable.

3. Results

3.1. Characteristics of Patients

A total of 102 patients diagnosed with locally advanced or metastatic pancreatic cancer with pretreatment complete blood cell counts and pretreatment CA19-9 available, diagnosed between January 2011 and September 2019 from the University of Kansas Cancer Center were included in the study. Patients were split into two groups based on whether they fell at or above the mean NLR, mean PLR, and mean DRC90 or below. The patient characteristics within each group are listed in Table 1.

Table 1. Characteristics of the patients in each group of analysis. The ratio between the pretreatment platelet count to the pretreatment absolute lymphocyte count (PLR), the ratio of the pretreatment absolute neutrophil count to the pretreatment absolute lymphocyte count (NLR), and the daily rate of change of CA19-9 over the first 90 days of treatment (DRC90).

Characteristics	NLR < 4.6 K/μL	NLR ≥ 4.6 K/μL	PLR < 196 K/μL	PLR ≥ 196 K/μL	DRC90 < −1%	DRC90 ≥ −1%
Number	66	35	59	43	66	36
Age (median)	65.5	62	63	64	64	61.5
Gender (%)						
Male	62.0%	60.0%	61.0%	62.8%	60.6%	63.9%
Female	38.0%	40.0%	39.0%	37.20%	39.4%	36.1%
Race						
White	57 (86.4%)	32 (91.4%)	53 (89.8%)	36 (83.7%)	60 (90.9%)	29 (80.6%)
Black or African American	2 (3.0%)	2 (5.7%)	2 (3.4%)	2 (4.7%)	0 (0.0%)	4 (11.1%)
Other	5 (7.6%)	1 (2.9%)	4 (6.8%)	5 (11.6%)	6 (9.1%)	3 (8.3%)
Smoking Status						
Yes	27 (40.9%)	17 (48.6%)	30 (50.8%)	14 (32.6%)	40 (60.6%)	19 (52.8%)
No	37 (56.1%)	17 (48.6%)	27 (45.8%)	28 (65.1%)	25 (37.9)	15 (41.7%)
ECOG Status						
0–1	60 (90.1%)	33 (94.3%)	54 (91.5%)	39 (90.7%)	60 (90.9%)	33 (91.7%)
2 or higher	6 (9.1%)	2 (5.7%)	5 (8.5%)	4 (9.3%)	5 (7.6%)	2 (5.6%)
Tumor Location						
Head	49 (74.2%)	15 (42.3%)	40 (67.8%)	24 (55.8%)	42 (63.6%)	22 (61.1%)
Tail	9 (13.6%)	11 (31.4%)	10 (16.9%)	6 (14.0%)	16 (24.3%)	5 (13.9%)
Body	7 (10.6%)	9 (25.7%)	8 (13.6%)	13 (30.2%)	7 (10.6%)	9 (25.0%)
Neck	1 (1.5%)	0 (0.0%)	1 (1.7%)	0 (0.0%)	1 (1.5%)	0 (0.0%)
Metastatic	46 (69.7%)	33 (94.3%)	46 (78.0%)	34 (79.0%)	54 (81.8%)	33 (91.7%)
Locally Advanced	20 (30.3%)	2 (5.7%)	13 (22.0%)	9 (21.0%)	12 (18.2%)	3 (8.3%)
CA19-9 at the time of diagnosis						
Normal (<38 U/mL)	11 (16.7%)	3 (8.6%)	8 (13.6%)	5 (11.6%)	5 (7.6%)	8 (22.2%)
Abnormal (>38 U/mL)	54 (81.8%)	32 (91.4%)	51 (86.4%)	38 (88.4%)	61 (92.4%)	26 (72.2%)
Treatment Received						
FOLFIRINOX	40 (60.6%)	20 (57.1%)	37 (62.7%)	24 (55.8%)	40 (60.6%)	21 (58.3%)
Gemcitabine/albumin-bound Paclitaxel (Abraxane)	16 (24.2%)	11 (31.4%)	13 (22.0%)	14 (32.6%)	18 (27.3%)	10 (27.8%)
Gemcitabine	4 (6.1%)	0 (0.0%)	4 (6.8%)	0 (0.0%)	2 (3.0%)	2 (5.6%)
Other	6 (9.1%)	4 (11.4%)	5 (8.5%)	5 (11.6%)	6 (9.1%)	3 (8.3%)

3.2. Efficacy

The median progression-free survival for patients with an NLR greater to or equal than the population's mean (4.6 K/μL) was 259 days (95% CI 177–308 days), and the median overall survival was 387 days (95% CI 221–455 days). For patients below the sample's mean NLR (<4.6 K/μL), the median PFS was 339 days (95% CI 207–592 days), and the median OS was 491 days (95% CI 391–527 days). The log-rank test showed that the PFS and OS for patients with an NLR greater than or equal to the mean of 4.6 K/μL and patients with an NLR less than 4.6 K/μL were significantly different ($p = 0.0444$, $p = 0.0483$, respectively), which is shown in Figure 1a,b. An elevated NLR in comparison to the sample population mean was associated with a lower OS and PFS in locally advanced or metastatic pancreatic adenocarcinoma.

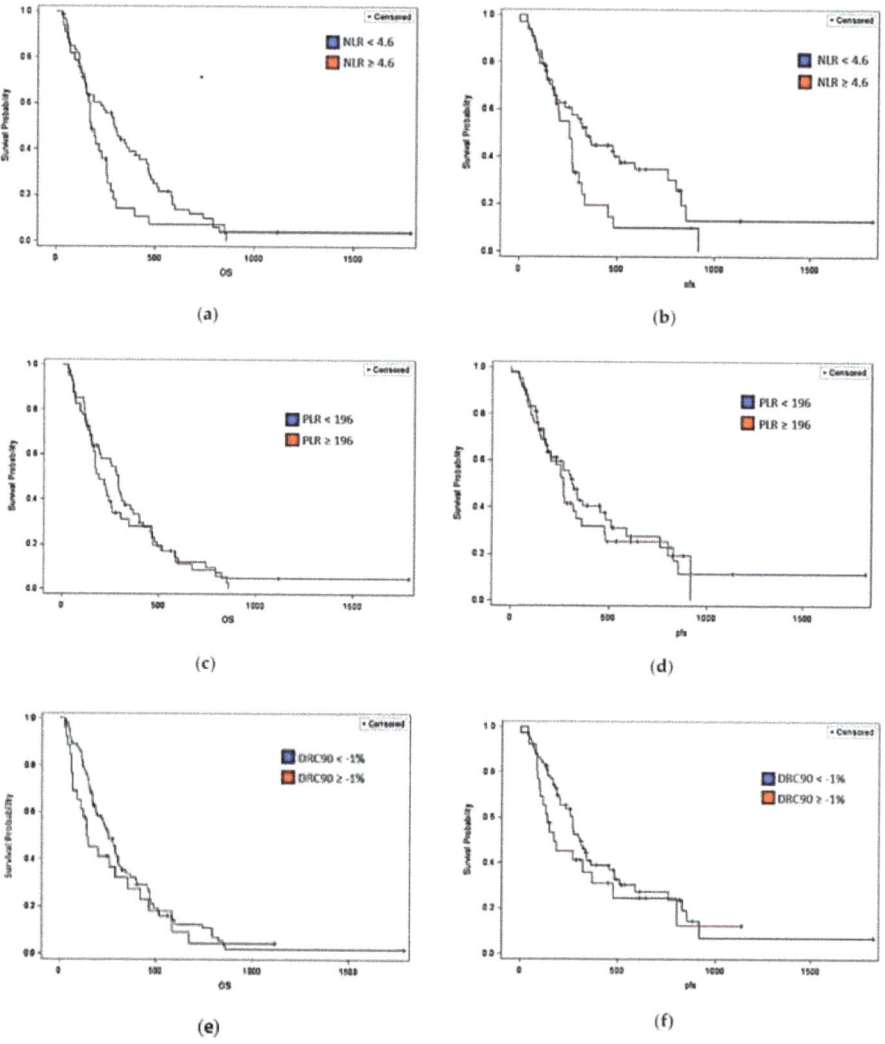

Figure 1. (a) Kaplan–Meier survival curve comparison of the OS of NLR groups; (b) Kaplan–Meier survival curve comparison of the PFS of NLR groups; (c) Kaplan–Meier survival curve comparison of the OS of PLR groups; (d) Kaplan–Meier survival curve comparison of the PFS of PLR groups; (e) Kaplan–Meier survival curve comparison of the OS of DRC90 groups; (f) Kaplan–Meier survival curve comparison of the PFS of DRC90 groups.

The median PFS for patients above the sample's PLR mean of 196 was 267 days (95% CI 177–361 days) and the median OS was 425 days (95% CI 302–494 days). The median PFS for patients below the samples PLR mean was 314 days (95% CI 187–484 days), and the median OS was 477 days (95% CI 381–527 days). The log-rank test did not show significant differences in OS and PFS in patients with a PLR greater than or equal to the sample mean and PLR below the sample mean, as shown in Figure 1c,d.

The median PFS for patients with a DRC90 greater than or equal to the sample mean (−1%) was 176 days (95% CI 101–368 days), and the median OS was 414 days (95% CI 279–547 days). The median PFS for patients with a DRC90 less than the sample mean was 308 days (95% CI 258–455 days), and the median OS was 451 days (95% CI 387–521 days). There was no significant difference in the OS and PFS between the DRC90 groups above the sample mean of −1% and below it, as shown in Figure 1e,f.

4. Discussion

Our findings of a significant association between an elevated NLR and lower OS and PFS agree with the findings of Das et al. and Dede et al., and are contradictory to the findings of Desai et al [4–6]. Thus, three separate studies have now found a significant association between an elevated NLR and lower OS and PFS in patients with locally advanced or metastatic disease, with a combined 283 patients studied. The cutoff NLR value of 4.6 K/μL used to separate groups in this study was lower than the NLR cutoff value of 5 K/μL used by Das et al. and higher than the NLR cutoff value of 3.54 K/μL used by Dede et al. [4,5]. Further investigation into the exact threshold of NLR elevation at which the OS and PFS is negatively affected is warranted in order to guide the treatment of patients with an elevated NLR, as our study further implicates elevated NLR as a negative prognostic factor.

A numerical difference in the PFS and OS was found between the PLR groups, with groups below the mean of 196 showing a PFS of 314 days and an OS of 477 days versus a PFS of 267 and an OS of 425 days in the groups above the sample mean PLR. Although statistical significance was not met, this numerical difference showing a lower PFS and OS in patients with PLR below the sample mean agrees with the statistically significant findings of Das et al., who found an association between an elevated PLR and lower OS and PFS [4].

A numerical difference in the PFS and OS was found between the DRC90 groups, with groups below the mean DRC90 of −1% showing a PFS of 308 days and OS of 451 days versus PFS of 176 and OS of 414 days in the group greater than the mean. Although a statistical difference was not met, this numerical trend agrees with the findings of Das et al. [4].

Our finding of elevated NLR as a poor marker of prognosis agrees with studies done on other forms of cancer [7]. Neutrophils are key components of the innate immune response but have also been implicated in the biogenesis of malignancy via their ability to blunt antitumor T cell responses [8]. Specific subsets of mature neutrophils have shown to play an important role in the escape of tumor cells from antitumor immunity [9]. The current treatment guidelines for metastatic pancreatic adenocarcinoma are largely based on the ECOG status and comorbidity profile [10]. Evidence of the importance of elevated NLR on the outcomes in metastatic pancreatic adenocarcinoma that our study and others provide, as well as larger studies including multiple forms of malignancy, indicate the potential for baseline NLR at the time of diagnosis to factor into treatment guidelines.

The limitations of this study include the retrospective chart review design, the small sample size of analysis ($n = 102$), variability in the treatment regimens received by patients, possible homogeneity due to the sample selection from only one treatment center, and group analysis of both metastatic and locally advanced patients. Our analysis grouped metastatic and locally advanced patients due to sample size limitations, and future studies should analyze these cohorts separately to assess the impact of distant metastasis versus locally advanced disease on outcomes in patients with an elevated NLR.

A large prospective randomized study is needed to confirm our study results, to ascertain the utility of elevated NLR as a prognostic marker in pancreatic cancer, and to further determine what threshold of elevation is universally prognostic. Given the results of our study, which used a threshold NLR of 4.6 K/μL to separate groups, along with the results of Des et al. with their threshold of 5 K/μL and the threshold of 3.54 K/μL used by Dede et al., future studies might start with a threshold below that of Dede et al. to further ascertain at what point an elevated NLR impacts outcomes.

Author Contributions: Conceptualization, A.K. and J.A.; methodology, A.K. and J.A.; software, C.C.; formal analysis, C.C.; investigation; A.K. and J.A.; data curation, J.A. and S.B.; resources, R.A.-R., J.B., A.S., S.W. and W.S.; writing–original draft preparation, J.A.; writing–review and editing, A.K.; supervision, A.K. All authors have read and agreed to the published version of the manuscript.

Funding: This research received no external funding.

Conflicts of Interest: The authors declare no conflict of interest.

References

1. Survival Rates for Pancreatic Cancer. Available online: https://www.cancer.org/cancer/pancreatic-cancer/detection-diagnosis-staging/survival-rates.html#references (accessed on 20 June 2020).
2. Final Recommendation Statement: Pancreatic Cancer: Screening: United States Preventive Services Taskforce. Available online: https://www.uspreventiveservicestaskforce.org/uspstf/document/RecommendationStatementFinal/pancreatic-cancer-screening#:~{}:text=The%20American%20College%20of%20Gastroenterology,degree%20relative)%20and%20suggests%20that (accessed on 20 June 2020).
3. Friess, H.; Demir, I.E. Pancreatic cancer—Lessons from the past decade. *Indian J. Med. Paediatr. Oncol.* **2015**, *36*, 73–76. [CrossRef] [PubMed]
4. Das, A.; McNulty, M.; Higgs, D.; Rogers-Seeley, M.; Fennessy, S.; McGarvey, C.; Dean, A. Correlation of neutrophil -lymphocyte ratio, platelet -lymphocyte ratio and rate of change of CA 19-9 in predicting outcome for metastatic pancreatic cancer. In Proceedings of the World Congress on Gastrointestinal Cancer, Barcelona, Spain, 20–23 June 2019.
5. DeDe, I.; Cetin, M.; Cetin, S. Prognostic value of the neutrophil-lymphocyte ratio and CA 19-9 in predicting survival in patients with metastatic pancreatic cancer. *Ann. Oncol.* **2018**, *29*, viii256. [CrossRef]
6. Desai, J.R.; Colton, B.S.; Wang, H.; Marshall, J.; Kim, S.; Pishvaian, M.J. Neutrophil-to-lymphocyte ratio as a prognostic marker for metastatic pancreatic cancer. *J. Clin. Oncol.* **2018**, *36*, 251. [CrossRef]
7. Mei, Z.; Shi, L.; Wang, B.; Yang, J.; Xiao, Z.; Du, P.; Wang, Q.; Yang, W. Prognostic role of pretreatment blood neutrophil-to-lymphocyte ratio in advanced cancer survivors: A systematic review and meta-analysis of 66 cohort studies. *Cancer Treat. Rev.* **2017**, *58*, 1–13. [CrossRef] [PubMed]
8. Hao, S.; Andersen, M.; Yu, H. Detection of immune suppressive neutrophils in peripheral blood samples of cancer patients. *Am. J. Blood Res.* **2013**, *3*, 239–245. [PubMed]
9. Pillay, J.; Kamp, V.M.; Van Hoffen, E.; Visser, T.; Tak, T.; Lammers, J.-W.; Ulfman, L.H.; Leenen, L.P.; Pickkers, P.; Koenderman, L. A subset of neutrophils in human systemic inflammation inhibits T cell responses through Mac-1. *J. Clin. Investig.* **2012**, *122*, 327–336. [CrossRef] [PubMed]
10. Sohal, D.P.S.; Kennedy, E.B.; Khorana, A.; Copur, M.S.; Crane, C.H.; Garrido-Laguna, I.; Krishnamurthi, S.; Moravek, C.; O'Reilly, E.M.; Philip, P.A.; et al. Metastatic pancreatic cancer: ASCO clinical practice guideline update. *J. Clin. Oncol.* **2018**, *36*, 2545–2556. [CrossRef] [PubMed]

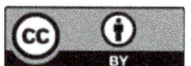

© 2020 by the authors. Licensee MDPI, Basel, Switzerland. This article is an open access article distributed under the terms and conditions of the Creative Commons Attribution (CC BY) license (http://creativecommons.org/licenses/by/4.0/).

Article

Association between Low-Grade Chemotherapy-Induced Peripheral Neuropathy (CINP) and Survival in Patients with Metastatic Adenocarcinoma of the Pancreas

Martina Catalano [1], Giuseppe Aprile [2], Monica Ramello [3], Raffaele Conca [4], Roberto Petrioli [5] and Giandomenico Roviello [6,*]

1. School of Human Health Sciences, University of Florence, Largo Brambilla 3, 50134 Florence, Italy; marti_cat@yahoo.it
2. Department of Oncology, San Bortolo General Hospital, AULSS8 Berica, 36100 Vicenza, Italy; giuseppe.aprile@aulss8.veneto.it
3. Oncology Unit, Department of Medical, Surgical & Health Sciences, University of Trieste, Piazza Ospitale, 34100 Trieste, Italy; monica.ramello@asuits.sanita.fvg.it
4. Division of Medical Oncology, Department of Onco-Hematology, IRCCS-CROB, Referral Cancer Center of Basilicata, via Padre Pio 1, 85028 Rionero, Vulture (PZ), Italy; raffaeleconca@hotmail.it
5. Department of Medicine, Surgery and Neurosciences, Medical Oncology Unit, University of Siena, Viale Bracci-Policlinico "Le Scotte", 53100 Siena, Italy; r.petrioli@ao-siena.toscana.it
6. Department of Health Sciences, University of Florence, Viale Pieraccini 6, 50139 Florence, Italy
* Correspondence: giandomenicoroviello@hotmail.it; Tel.: +39-055-7938313

Abstract: The combination of nab-paclitaxel and gemcitabine demonstrated greater efficacy than gemcitabine alone but resulted in higher rates of chemotherapy-induced peripheral neuropathy (CINP) in patients with metastatic pancreatic cancer (mPC). We aimed to evaluate the correlation between the development of treatment-related peripheral neuropathy and the efficacy of nab-P/Gem combination in these patients. mPC patients treated with nab-paclitaxel 125 mg/m^2 and gemcitabine 1000 mg/m^2 as a first-line therapy were included. Treatment-related adverse events, mainly peripheral neuropathy, were categorized using the National Cancer Institute Common Toxicity Criteria scale, version 4.02. Efficacy outcomes, including overall survival (OS), progression-free survival (PSF), and disease control rate (DCR), were estimated by the Kaplan–Meier model. A total of 153 patients were analyzed; of these, 47 patients (30.7%) developed grade 1–2 neuropathy. PFS was 7 months (95% CI (6–7 months)) for patients with grade 1–2 neuropathy and 6 months (95% CI (5–6 months)) for patients without peripheral neuropathy ($p = 0.42$). Median OS was 13 months (95% CI (10–18 months)) and 10 months (95% CI (8–13 months)) in patients with and without peripheral neuropathy, respectively ($p = 0.04$). DCR was achieved by 83% of patients with grade 1–2 neuropathy and by 58% of patients without neuropathy ($p = 0.03$). In the multivariate analysis, grade 1–2 neuropathy was independently associated with OS (HR 0.65; 95% CI, 0.45–0.98; $p = 0.03$). nab-P/Gem represents an optimal first-line treatment for mPC patients. Among possible treatment-related adverse events, peripheral neuropathy is the most frequent, with different grades and incidence. Our study suggests that patients experiencing CINP may have a more favorable outcome, with a higher disease control rate and prolonged median survival compared to those without neuropathy.

Keywords: pancreas; neuropathy; taxanes; survival

1. Introduction

Metastatic pancreatic cancer (mPC) is associated with poor survival rates, with a worldwide 5-year survival rate lower than 5% [1]. Until recently, patients with advanced pancreatic cancer had limited treatment options. Nab-paclitaxel plus gemcitabine (nab-P/Gem) is a first-line treatment option approved in the US and Europe based on the international phase III MPACT trial results for its proven superiority over gemcitabine [2].

The median overall survival (OS) for nab-P/Gem was 8.5 months compared to 6.7 months for gemcitabine (hazard ratio (HR), 0.72; $p < 0.001$), the median progression-free survival (PFS) was 5.5 months versus 3.7 months (HR, 0.69; $p < 0.001$), and the overall response rate (ORR) was 23% and 7%, respectively ($p < 0.001$). An updated report showed a final OS for nab-P/Gem versus Gem alone of 8.7 months and 6.6 months, respectively (HR, 0.72; $p < 0.001$) [3]. Along with its cost-effectiveness in first-line, a number of retrospective series have confirmed nab-P/Gem as an active, effective, well-tolerated, and cost-effective regimen even in pretreated patients [4–8]. Taxanes are microtubule-stabilizing agents (MTSAs), including polyoxyethylated castor oil-based paclitaxel, docetaxel, and ABI-007 (nab-paclitaxel) used for the treatment of various cancers. ABI-007 is a new polyoxyethylated castor oil-free formulation of paclitaxel developed to overcome the limitations attributed to the solvent Kolliphor EL (previously called Cremophor EL) and improve the therapeutic index and safety profile of solvent-based paclitaxel (sb-P) [9]. Peripheral neuropathy (PN) is the major toxicity related to taxanes [6,10–12]. Although it is not completely clear how taxanes cause PN, in vitro studies have demonstrated that taxanes interrupt axonal transport mediated by microtubules, leading to neuropathy [13]. Other data demonstrate damage to mitochondria that may underlie a metabolic axonal failure in chemotherapy-induced peripheral neuropathy (CIPN) [14,15]. A novel study using the zebrafish model suggested that paclitaxel-induced neuropathy may depend on interactions between skin nerve endings and epidermal basal keratinocytes through the matrix metalloproteinase MMP-13 [16]. Peripheral neuropathy is a troublesome side effect experienced by many cancer patients that should be actively managed during its course and after the end of treatment [17,18]. This specific toxicity can be dose-limiting and may persist indefinitely in some cases [19,20].

In phase II/III trials of various tumor types, nab-paclitaxel regimens demonstrated improved efficacy and tolerability compared with solvent-based taxanes [21,22]. Recent retrospective studies have reported a 30.4% to 56.8% incidence of CIPN during nab-P/Gem combination chemotherapy [2,5,8]. In the MPACT trial, 54% of the patients experienced any-grade CIPN. Subset analysis of the MPACT trial and the report by Cho et al. demonstrated that the development of treatment-related peripheral neuropathy represents an independent, positive predictive factor of OS [8,23]. Although nab-P/Gem combination therapy is now a consolidated treatment in clinical practice, some reports suggest a possible link with long-term prognosis [16,17]. Data regarding its possible association with survival in the real world are still lacking. The aim of our study is to evaluate the correlation between the development of CINP and the efficacy of nab-P/Gem combination therapy in patients with metastatic pancreatic cancer treated in the real world.

2. Materials and Methods

2.1. Eligibility Criteria

Patients investigated in this study derive from the multicenter retrospective study NAPA that evaluated patients with metastatic PC treated with first-line nab-P/Gem according to clinical guidelines. This study involved patients treated at 5 Italian oncological units (after the last amendment that has added another center) with first-line nab-P/Gem between January 2015 and December 2018 [24]. We performed a retrospective study of Italian oncological centers across the North, Central, and South of Italy. This study enrolled adult patients with Eastern Cooperative Oncology Group Performance Status (ECOG-PS) 0–1 and histologically confirmed metastatic adenocarcinoma of the pancreas. Patients were required to have adequate hepatic, hematologic, and renal function (including bilirubin level $\leq$ the upper limit of normal, absolute neutrophil count $\geq 1.5 \times 10^9$/L, platelet count $\geq 100,000$/mm^3, and hemoglobin level ≥ 9 g/dL). Patients who had completed surgery or adjuvant treatments (chemotherapy or radiation therapy) for more than 6 months were evaluated. Patients who had at least one cycle of treatment completed were included. Serious cardiovascular problems (i.e., ejection fraction < 40%, myocardial infarction) or infections represented exclusion criteria. The protocol was approved by the

Institutional Review Board for clinical trials of Tuscany: Section AREA VASTA CENTRO, number:14565_oss; all patients gave their written consent.

2.2. Treatment Schedule and Response Assessments

The initial dose of nab-P/Gem was chosen according to a pivotal study: intravenous infusion of nab-paclitaxel 125 mg/m^2, followed by gemcitabine 1000 mg/m^2 administered intravenously on days 1, 8, and 15 every 4 weeks. A second or additional therapy line was administered according to the single-center experience.

Patients received antiemetic medication at the beginning of each treatment cycle and adequate doses of analgesic drugs to provide optimal pain control. Chemotherapeutic cycles were administered with absolute neutrophil count > 1500/µL, hemoglobin $\geq$ 9 g/dL, and platelets > 100,000/mm^3, granulocyte-olony stimulating factor (G-CSF) was administered according to the local clinical practice. Clinical, radiological, and biochemical pretreatment assessments were performed within 2 weeks from treatment beginning. Blood tests were performed at baseline and before every single drug administration, while measurement of the carbohydrate antigen (CA)19-9 serum level was performed at baseline and every 12 weeks. Tumor response evaluation was performed every 3 months or earlier when clinically required by spiral computed tomography according to the Response Evaluation Criteria in Solid Tumors (RECIST) version 1.1 [25].

2.3. Neuropathy Assessment

Peripheral motor/sensory neuropathy is a disorder characterized by damage or dysfunction of the peripheral motor/sensory nerves. Sensory neuropathy presents as paresthesia, numbness, and pain in the feet and hands [26]. Paresthesia occurs in distal lower extremities with a glove-and-stocking distribution and is most severe on the plantar surface [27]. The severity of most symptoms is mild to moderate, and symptoms generally disappear on cessation of therapy [26,28,29]. Motor neuropathy is usually mild and presents as muscle weakness such as foot drop or difficulty in climbing stairs, decreasing at times fine motor skills [27,30,31]. Neuropathy is graded by subjective complaints of patients and physical examination by clinicians. It was assessed by the National Cancer Institute Common Toxicity Criteria for Adverse Events (NCI-CTCAE) scale, version 4.02 [32]. Grade 1 defines an asymptomatic disorder or loss of deep tendon reflexes or paresthesia where only clinical or diagnostic observations are needed and intervention is not indicated; grade 2 involves moderate symptoms that limit instrumental activities of daily living (ADL); grade 3 involves severe symptoms limiting self-care ADL that need an assistive device; grade 4 involves life-threatening consequences where urgent intervention is indicated. Dose modification, delay, and drug discontinuation related to neuropathy or other adverse events (AE) were performed according to the guidelines.

2.4. Statistical Analysis

This study aimed to evaluate whether the development of neuropathy (grade 1–2) positively correlates with the efficacy and survival of patients with metastatic pancreatic cancer treated with nab-P/Gem as first-line treatment. For this purpose, patients were split into two groups: with or without the development of neuropathy. Patient and tumor characteristics plus treatment data were collected as frequency, percentage of categorical variables, median with 95% confidence interval, and range (for continuous variables). Overall survival was evaluated as the time from nab-P/Gem regimen start to death from any cause or the date of the last follow-up visit. Progression-free survival was evaluated as time from treatment initiation to the date of the disease progression. The Kaplan—Meier method with log-rank test was performed to analyze PFS and OS in relation to the development of grade 1–2 neuropathy. The Cox regression model was used to evaluate the prognostic role of neuropathy and other clinical and/or pathological variables. Statistical analysis was performed using STATA software with a statistical significance threshold agreed upon $p < 0.05$.

3. Results

3.1. Patient Characteristics

From January 2015 to December 2018, 153 patients diagnosed with metastatic PC and treated with first-line nab-P/Gem were retrospectively investigated. Of these, 47 patients (30.7%) developed grade 1–2 neuropathy, and 106 (69.3%) did not develop any neuropathy during treatment. No grade 3 or 4 CIPN was reported. The median age was 67 years (range, 47–84) for the grade 1–2 neuropathy group and 66 years (range, 50–84) for patients without peripheral neuropathy ($p = 0.8$). Eighteen (38.3%) patients with grade 1–2 neuropathy and 37 (34.9%) without neuropathy were 70 or older ($p = 0.7$). Males were more represented in the no peripheral neuropathy group (58.5%) than in patients with PN (55.3 %) without significant differences ($p = 0.7$). Over half of the patients presented with ECOG PS 1 in the two groups (53.2% in patients with CIPN vs. 51.2% in those without CIPN) ($p = 0.8$).

Nineteen (40.4%) patients with neuropathy, and 42 (39.6%) without, presented three or more metastatic sites ($p = 0.5$). Concerning previous treatments, more patients without neuropathy underwent surgery and radiotherapy (11.3% and 25.5%) ($p = 0.2$) than patients with neuropathy (4.3% and 21.3%) ($p = 0.6$) while a biliary stent was previously placed in the 34% and 21.3%, respectively ($p = 0.2$). Basal carbohydrate antigen 19-9 (CA 19-9) levels showed a minimal difference between the two groups ($p = 0.6$). Finally, pain was more present in patients with neuropathy than in the other group (46.8% vs. 34.9%) ($p = 0.2$). Baseline patient characteristics are summarized in Table 1.

Table 1. Patient characteristics.

	All patients ($n = 153$)	Neuropathy G1–2 ($n = 47$)	No Neuropathy ($n = 106$)	p
Age, years				
Mean	67	67.5	66	0.8
Range	50–84	47–84	50–84	
≥70	55 (35.9%)	18 (38.3%)	37 (34.9%)	0.7
ECOG PS				
1	80 (51.2%)	25 (53.2%)	55 (51.2%)	0.8
Sex				
Male	88 (57.5%)	26 (55.3%)	62 (58.5%)	0.7
Number of metastatic sites				
≥3	61 (39.9%)	19 (40.4%)	42 (39.6%)	0.5
Carbohydrate antigen 19-9—U/mL				
Median	547	401	588	
Range	0.8–700,000	1.8–700,000	0.8–129,718	0.6
Previous treatment				
Radiation therapy	14 (9.9%)	2 (4.3%)	12 (11.3%)	0.2
Surgery	37 (24.2%)	10 (21.3%)	27 (25.5%)	0.6
Biliary stent	46 (30.1%)	10 (21.3%)	36 (34%)	0.1
Pain				
Yes	59 (38.6%)	22 (46.8%)	37 (34.9%)	0.2

3.2. Neuropathy and Clinical Outcome

Forty-seven patients (30.7%) developed grade 1–2 neuropathy during treatment. Patients with neuropathy received a mean of six cycles vs. four cycles in patients without neuropathy. Concerning efficacy data, median PFS was 6 months (95% CI (5–6 months)) while median OS was 11 months (95% CI 11 (10–13 months)); no complete responses (CR) were observed, and the disease control rate (DCR) was 66.7% (102 out of 153 patients) among all patients (Table 2).

Table 2. Best response, PFS, and OS according to neutropenia grade.

	All Patients (n= 153)	Neuropathy G1–2 (n = 47)	No Neuropathy (n = 106)	p
PR	58 (37.1%)	16 (34%)	42 (39.6%)	
SD	44 (28.8%)	23 (48.9%)	21 (19.8%)	0.03
DCR (PR + SD)	102 (66.7%)	39 (83%)	63 (58%)	
PD	42 (27.4%)	8 (17%)	34 (32.1%)	
NE	9 (5.9%)	0	9 (8.5%)	
PFS				
M-months	6	7	6	0.42
(95% IC)	(5–6)	(6–7)	(5–6)	
OS				
M-months	11	13	10	0.04
95% IC	(10–13)	(10–18)	(8–13)	
Cycles				
Median	5	6	4	0.03
Range	1–17	2–17	1–17	
Delayed	51 (33.5%)	19 (41.3%)	32 (30.2%)	0.2
Interruption	51 (33.5%)	11 (23.4%)	40 (37.7%)	0.1
Dose reduction	88 (57.5%)	38 (80.8%)	50 (47.2%)	0.01

Patients who developed grade 1–2 neuropathy had a median PFS of 7 months (95% CI (6–7 months)) compared to the PFS of 6 months (95% CI (5–6 months)) for patients without neuropathy (Figure 1, p = 0.42).

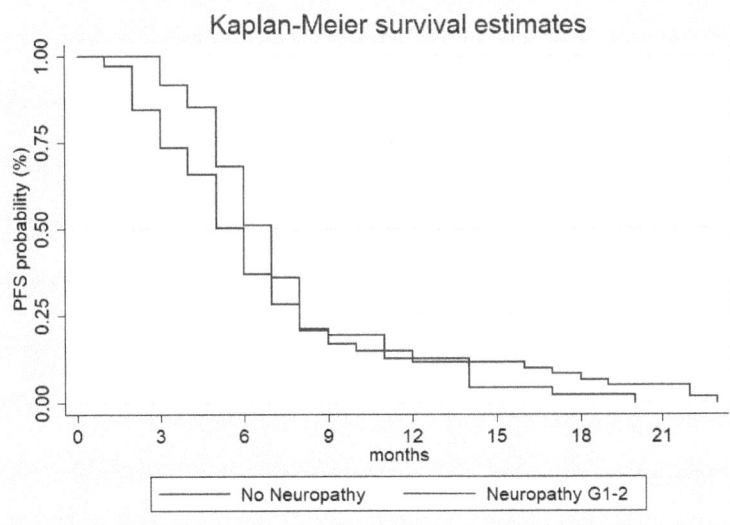

Figure 1. Estimated PFS for nab−Gem according to low-grade CIPN presentation.

Meanwhile, OS was 13 months (95% CI (10–18 months)) and 10 months (95% CI (8–13 months)) in patients with and without neuropathy (Figure 2, p = 0.04).

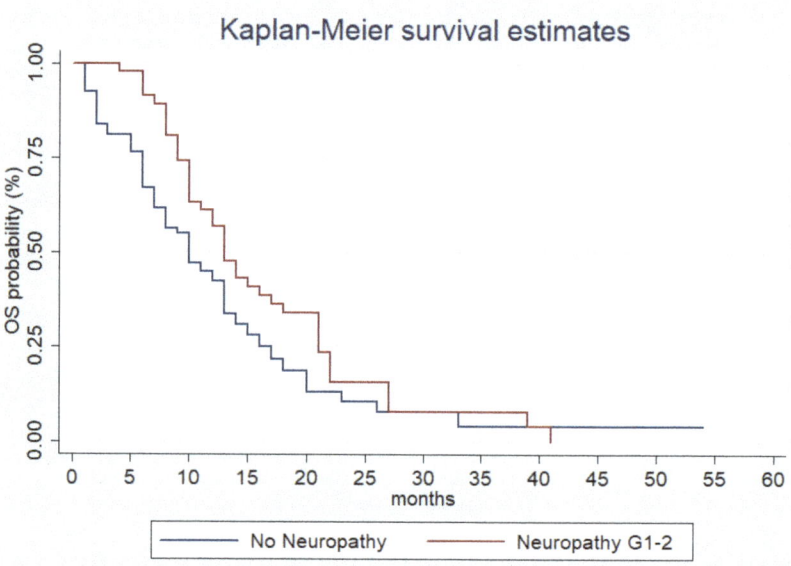

Figure 2. Estimated OS for nab−Gem according to low−grade CIPN presentation.

DCR was achieved in 83% of patients with grade 1–2 neuropathy and in 58% of patients without neuropathy ($p = 0.03$). The results of the univariate analysis for OS show that age ≥ 70, ECOG-PS 1, number of metastatic sites at baseline ≥ 3, and CA 19–9 ≥ 659 U/mL were found to be negative prognostic factors, whereas previous surgery and grade 1–2 neuropathy (HR: 0.62 95% CI 0.46–0.99, $p = 0.05$) were found to be significantly positive prognostic factors (Table 3).

Table 3. Univariate and multivariate analysis for OS.

	HR	IC 95%	p
Univariate			
Age ≥ 70	1.91	1.23–2.90	0.004
ECOG PS (1 vs. 0)	1.45	1.22–3.18	0.05
Sex (male vs. female)	1.20	0.79–1.83	0.48
N. of metastatic sites ≥ 3	4.48	2.54–8.09	<0.001
Carbohydrate antigen 19-9 ≥ 659 U/mL	1.68	1.10–3.22	0.01
Previous radiation therapy	0.47	0.19–1.16	0.1
Previous surgery	0.78	0.49–0.98	0.04
Previous biliary stent	0.84	0.54–1.32	0.4
Pain present	1.50	0.98–2.29	0.06
Neuropathy	0.68	0.46–0.99	0.05
Multivariate			
Age ≥ 70	1.53	1.05–2.21	0.03
ECOG PS (1 vs. 0)	1.24	0.85–1.80	0.26
N. of metastatic sites ≥ 3	3.98	2.22–5.66	<0.001
Carbohydrate antigen 19-9 ≥ 659 U/mL	1.99	1.38–2.88	<0.001
Previous surgery	0.51	0.32–0.82	0.006
Neuropathy	0.65	0.45–0.98	0.03

The multivariate analysis confirms that age ≥ 70, number of metastatic sites, CA 19–9, previous surgery, and grade 1–2 neuropathy were independently associated with OS (Table 3).

4. Discussion

The prognosis of metastatic pancreatic cancer is very poor, with an expected median survival of fewer than 12 months and a long-term survival rate of approximately 5%. Chemotherapy is the only feasible treatment and often correlates with even serious adverse events. In MPACT—the randomized trial that established the efficacy of nab-P/Gem combination therapy in patients with advanced stages of disease—peripheral neuropathy was frequently reported as a distressing chemotherapy-related toxicity. A solvent-free form of nab-paclitaxel was developed to reduce taxane-induced neurotoxicity; nevertheless, this side effect still affects more than 50% of all treated patients [33]. CINP remains a major clinical problem in the treatment of these patients that may require chemotherapy dose reduction or cessation, increasing cancer-related morbidity and mortality [34,35]. Moreover, there is a lack of clinical trials focusing on the treatment of established painful CIPN, and duloxetine remains the only treatment with sufficient evidence recommended in the Clinical Practice Guideline from ASCO [36]. The objective of our study was to investigate the independent prognostic role of treatment-related peripheral neuropathy. We evaluated the association between CINP and treatment outcomes and summarized the current knowledge regarding the significance of this correlation. The incidence and course of CIPN vary across different studies. In recent retrospective studies, the incidence of CIPN ranged from 30% to approximately 60%, but it may be underestimated because of the lack of available methods to properly evaluate, report, and grade neurological toxicities. In the MPACT trial, any-grade peripheral neuropathy was reported in 227 patients randomized to the experimental arm (54%); of these, 70 (17%) experienced grade 3 CIPN, but no grade 4 was reported [23]. Dose reduction or treatment discontinuation were required in 10% and 8% of patients with grade 3 CIPN, respectively [2]. In a Korean cohort study, Cho et al. reported CIPN in more than 50% of patients, and 15 (18.5%) of these patients experienced severe grades of toxicity [8]. In the study by You et al., 13 (14.8%) patients developed grade 2 PN, while 16 (18.2%) developed grade 3 PN; 19.3% and 18.2% of all patients needed dose reduction and discontinuation of treatment due to PN, respectively [37]. In our study, 47 patients (30.7%) experienced grade 1–2 CIPN, and of these, 38 (80.8%) required dose reduction, and 30 (44.7%) discontinued treatment. Unlike other retrospective studies in which the incidence of grade 3 neuropathy ranged from 10% to 30% [4,5,27], no grade 3 CIPN was observed in our cohort.

In MPACT, the development of severe CIPN during treatment with nab-P/Gem was associated with longer survival rates (HR 0.55; 95% CI, 0.39–0.79; $p = 0.0007$), and every increase in grade was associated with a 35% reduction in the risk of death (HR, 0.65; 95% CI, 0.58–0.72; $p < 0.0001$). We also reported a significant association between peripheral neuropathy and overall survival. Indeed, in our analysis, patients receiving nab-P/Gem and developing PN had a significant 3-month longer median OS ($p = 0.04$) compared to those who did report any peripheral neurotoxicity. In our study, baseline differences in patient characteristics likely did not play a role in the observed results, and the association between CIPN with survival was confirmed in the multivariate analysis, adjusted for other prognostic factors. Similarly, the results of other studies were in line with our results. Cho et al. highlighted the presence of neurologic adverse events as independent survival prognostic factors (HR 0.302; 95% CI 0.130–0.702, $p = 0.005$) [8]. You et al. reported a significantly longer survival rate in patients with CIPN compared to those without neuropathy in the naive model (10.13 vs. 15.53 months, $p = 0.007$), although this correlation was not confirmed in the landmark model at 6 months, used to reduce lead time bias (11.4 vs. 15.3 months) ($p = 0.089$) [8,23,37]. Various studies of breast cancer have been conducted to identify clinical or molecular risk factors for the development of chemotherapy-induced neuropathy. Older age, hyperglycemia, and obesity or poor nutritional status, such as single-nucleotide polymorphisms (SNPs) in the FGD4, EPHA5, and FZD3 genes and ABCB1 and GSTP1 polymorphisms, have been associated with the development of taxane-related neuropathy [38–42]. Conversely, in pancreatic cancer, data on risk factors for CIPN are still lacking, and the assessment of risk factors as shown for breast cancer should be considered in future studies. Moreover, the association between the neurologic side effects and OS improvement is not yet clear; a relationship could be due to individual drug sensitivity and increased treatment exposure. Indeed, according to Scheithauer et al., patients who are more chemo-responsive might have a better treatment response and simultaneously more adverse events (AEs) [43]. As stated above, the mechanism by which taxanes cause PN is not fully elucidated, although axonal damage has been identified in some studies. Chemotherapy-related cognitive impairment (CRCI) is another side effect of chemotherapy whose etiology is not well identified but appears to be related to impaired white matter integrity [44]. Moreover, neuroinflammation seems to be another possible explanatory mechanism for cognitive impairment and peripheral neuropathy, as highlighted both in clinical and animal studies [45]. Therefore, CINP and CRCI could be contextually assessed in patients treated with these drugs to evaluate a possible correlation between them and highlight their relationship with efficacy outcomes [45–48].

Although we have demonstrated the favorable impact of CINP on survival, our study has some limitations, mainly owing to its retrospective design, small population sample, and the neuropathy assessment method. Indeed, although the National Cancer Institute's CTCAE is one of the most widely used clinical tools for detecting neuropathy during chemotherapy, it was not specifically developed to assess pain, is not sensitive to change, and has significant inter-rater variability. Methodologies to assess CIPN in clinical trials have therefore been developed to provide improved evaluation tools and patient-reported outcomes. The EORTC QLQ-CINP is a 20-item quality questionnaire that quantifies symptoms and impairments of sensory, motor, and autonomic neuropathy and has been used in large oncology clinical trials [49]. A more recent methodology, the CIPN-R-ODS, was developed with Rasch analysis to build upon disability scales that provide a linear measurement of CIPN-related disability and will likely be utilized in future CIPN clinical trials [50]. Moreover, the Total Neuropathy Score (TNSc) that incorporates quantitative neurological exams and neurophysiology was recently subjected to Rasch analysis in patients with CIPN and could be used to assess outcomes in future clinical trials [51]. Furthermore, other aspects such as mood, pain, depression, and fatigue should be considered contextually through evaluation systems (e.g., Edmonton Symptom Assessment Screen, MD Anderson Symptom Inventory, or EORTC QLQ30) to assess the impact of neuropathy compared to other symptoms in patients' daily living.

Currently, available data on the prognostic value of peripheral neuropathy in patients with mPC who are treated with nab-P/Gem are limited. PN can lead to discontinuation of treatment, affecting the overall response to chemotherapy. Considering the positive correlation between PN and efficacy outcomes, the identification of risk factors for CINP and its management becomes critical; indeed, as demonstrated for other drugs (e.g., Tyrosine Kinase Inhibitor, Anti-Epidermal Growth Factor Receptors), the occurrence of adverse events such as hypertension or skin rash could be used as a surrogate of efficacy [52,53]. Moreover, better knowledge on symptom clusters of CIPN may help to improve symptom management in clinical practice [54]. Therefore, a deeper understanding of the exact mechanism of chemotherapy-induced peripheral neuropathy and assessing its correlation with treatment outcomes in large, prospective trials will help to define the role of PN as a possible surrogate marker for the efficacy of chemotherapy.

5. Conclusions

The combination of nab-P/Gem demonstrated greater efficacy but higher rates of peripheral neuropathy versus gemcitabine in patients with metastatic pancreatic cancer. Although the incidence of PN is lower in solvent-free forms of taxanes such as nab-paclitaxel, it remains the main problem in combination therapy in pancreatic cancer patients. Despite the limitations of this study, our results suggest a positive correlation between nab-P/Gem therapy response and the development of PN. Treatment-related neuropathy might be a predictor of prognosis in patients with metastatic pancreatic cancer treated with nab-paclitaxel, although prospective large-scale trials are needed to confirm these results.

Author Contributions: G.R. had full access to all the data in the study and takes responsibility for the integrity of the data and the accuracy of the data analysis. Study concept and design: G.R., G.A., M.C. Acquisition of data: R.C., Ianza A, M.R., Analysis and interpretation of data: G.R. Drafting of the manuscript: G.R., M.C. Critical revision of the manuscript for important intellectual content: G.A. Statistical analysis: G.R. Administrative, technical, or material support: None. Supervision: R.P. All authors have read and agreed to the published version of the manuscript.

Funding: This research received no external funding.

Institutional Review Board Statement: Institutional Review Board for clinical trials of Tuscany: Section AREA VASTA CENTRO, number:14565_oss. Informed consent was obtained from all individual participants included in the study.

Informed Consent Statement: Informed consent was obtained from all subjects involved in the study.

Data Availability Statement: The data used to support the findings of this study are available from the corresponding author upon reasonable request.

Conflicts of Interest: The authors declare no conflict of interest.

References

1. Howlader, N.; Noone, A.M.; Krapcho, M.; Miller, D.; Bishop, K.; Altekruse, S.F.; Kosary, C.L.; Yu, M.; Ruhl, J.; Tatalovich, Z.; et al. *SEER Cancer Statistics Review*; National Cancer Institute: Bethesda, MD, USA, 2015.
2. Von Hoff, D.D.; Ervin, T.; Arena, F.P.; Chiorean, E.G.; Infante, J.; Moore, M.; Seay, T.; Tjulandin, S.A.; Ma, W.W.; Saleh, M.N.; et al. Increased survival in pancreatic cancer with nab-paclitaxel plus gemcitabine. *N. Engl. J. Med.* **2013**, *369*, 1691–1703. [CrossRef]
3. Goldstein, D.; El-Maraghi, R.H.; Hammel, P.; Heinemann, V.; Kunzmann, V.; Sastre, J.; Scheithauer, W.; Siena, S.; Tabernero, J.; Teixeira, L.; et al. Nab-paclitaxel plus gem-citabine for metastatic pancreatic cancer: Long-term survival from a phase III trial. *J. Natl. Cancer Inst.* **2015**, *107*, dju413. [CrossRef]
4. Kim, G.P.; Parisi, M.F.; Patel, M.B.; Pelletier, C.L.; Belk, K.W. Comparison of treatment patterns, resource utilization, and cost of care in patients with metastatic pancreatic cancer treated with first-line nab-paclitaxel plus gemcitabine or FOLFIRINOX. *Expert Rev. Clin. Pharmacol.* **2017**, *10*, 559–565. [CrossRef]
5. Ottaiano, A.; Capozzi, M.; De Divitiis, C.; Von Arx, C.; Di Girolamo, E.; Nasti, G.; Cavalcanti, E.; Tatangelo, F.; Romano, G.; Avallone, A.; et al. Nab-Paclitaxel and Gemcitabine in Advanced Pancreatic Cancer: The One-year Experience of the National Cancer Institute of Naples. *Anticancer Res.* **2017**, *37*, 1975–1978. [CrossRef] [PubMed]
6. Bertocchi, P.; Abeni, C.; Meriggi, F.; Rota, L.; Rizzi, A.; Di Biasi, B.; Aroldi, F.; Ogliosi, C.; Savelli, G.; Rosso, E.; et al. Gemcitabine Plus Nab-Paclitaxel as Second-Line and Beyond Treatment for Metastatic Pancreatic Cancer: A Single Institution Retrospective Analysis. *Rev. Recent Clin. Trials* **2015**, *10*, 142–145. [CrossRef] [PubMed]
7. Zhang, Y.; Hochster, H.; Stein, S.; Lacy, J. Gemcitabine plus nab-paclitaxel for advanced pancreatic cancer after first-line FOLFIRINOX: Single institution retrospective review of efficacy and toxicity. *Exp. Hematol. Oncol.* **2015**, *4*, 29. [CrossRef]
8. Cho, I.R.; Kang, H.; Jo, J.H.; Lee, H.S.; Chung, M.J.; Park, J.Y.; Park, S.W.; Song, S.Y.; Chung, J.B.; An, C.; et al. Efficacy and treatment-related adverse events of gem-citabine plus nab-paclitaxel for treatment of metastatic pancreatic cancer "in a Korean" population: A single-center cohort study. *Semin Oncol.* **2017**, *44*, 420–427. [CrossRef] [PubMed]
9. Desai, N.; Trieu, V.; Yao, Z.; Louie, L.; Ci, S.; Yang, A.; Tao, C.; De, T.; Beals, B.; Dykes, D.; et al. Increased antitumor activity, intratumor paclitaxel concentrations, and endothelial cell transport of cremophor-free, albumin-bound paclitaxel, ABI-007, compared with cremophor-based paclitaxel. *Clin. Cancer Res.* **2006**, *12*, 1317–1324. [CrossRef]
10. Carrato, A.; García, P.; Lopez, R.; Macarulla, T.; Rivera, F.; Sastre, J.; Gostkorzewicz, J.; Benedit, P.; Pérez-Alcántara, F. Cost-utility analysis of nanoparticle albu-min-bound paclitaxel (nab-paclitaxel) in combination with gemcitabine in metastatic pancreatic cancer in Spain: Results of the PANCOSTABRAX study. *Expert Rev. Pharm. Outcomes Res.* **2015**, *15*, 579–589.
11. Lee, J.J.; Swain, S.M. Peripheral Neuropathy Induced by Microtubule-Stabilizing Agents. *J. Clin. Oncol.* **2006**, *24*, 1633–1642. [CrossRef]
12. Dumontet, C.; Jordan, M.A. Microtubule-binding agents: A dynamic field of cancer therapeutics. *Nat. Rev. Drug Discov.* **2010**, *9*, 790–803. [CrossRef]
13. Komiya, Y.; Tashiro, T. Effects of taxol on slow and fast axonal transport. *Cell Motil. Cytoskelet.* **1988**, *11*, 151–156. [CrossRef] [PubMed]
14. Xiao, W.; Zheng, H.; Bennett, G. Characterization of oxaliplatin-induced chronic painful peripheral neuropathy in the rat and comparison with the neuropathy induced by paclitaxel. *Neuroscience* **2012**, *203*, 194–206. [CrossRef] [PubMed]

15. Zheng, H.; Xiao, W.; Bennett, G. Mitotoxicity and bortezomib-induced chronic painful peripheral neuropathy. *Exp. Neurol.* **2012**, *238*, 225–234. [CrossRef] [PubMed]
16. Lissea, T.S.; Middletona, L.J.; Pellegrinia, A.D.; Martina, P.B.; Spauldinga, E.L.; Lopesa, O.; Brochu, E.A.; Carter, E.V.; Waldron, A.; Rieger, S. Paclitaxel-induced epithelial damage and ectopic MMP-13 expression promotes neurotoxicity in zebrafish. *Proc. Natl. Acad. Sci. USA* **2016**, *113*, E2189–E2198. [CrossRef]
17. Alberti, P.; Cavaletti, G.; Cornblath, D.R. Toxic neuropathies: Chemotherapy Induced Peripheral Neurotoxicity. *Curr. Opin. Neurol.* **2019**, *32*, 676–683. [CrossRef]
18. Loprinzi, C.L.; Lacchetti, C.; Bleeker, J.; Cavaletti, G.; Chauhan, C.; Hertz, D.L.; Kelley, M.R.; Lavino, A.; Lustberg, M.B.; Paice, J.A.; et al. Prevention and Management of Chemotherapy-Induced Peripheral Neuropathy in Survivors of Adult Cancers: ASCO Guideline Update. *J. Clin. Oncol.* **2020**, *38*, 3325–3348. [CrossRef]
19. Rowinsky, E.K.; Chaudhry, V.; Forastiere, A.A.; Sartorius, S.E.; Ettinger, D.S.; Grochow, L.B.; Lubejko, B.G.; Cornblath, D.R.; Donehower, R.C. Phase I and pharmacologic study of paclitaxel and cisplatin with granulocyte colony-stimulating factor: Neuromuscular toxicity is dose-limiting. *J. Clin. Oncol.* **1993**, *11*, 2010–2020. [CrossRef]
20. Park, S.B.; Goldstein, D.; Krishnan, A.V.; Lin, C.S.-Y.; Friedlander, M.L.; Cassidy, J.; Koltzenburg, M.; Kiernan, M.C. Chemotherapy-induced peripheral neurotoxicity: A critical analysis. *CA A Cancer J. Clin.* **2013**, *63*, 419–437. [CrossRef]
21. Gradishar, W.J.; Tjulandin, S.; Davidson, N.; Shaw, H.; Desai, N.; Hawkins, P.B.; O'Shaughnessy, J. Phase III trial of nanoparticle albu-min-bound paclitaxel compared with polyethylated castor oil-based paclitaxel in women with breast cancer. *J. Clin. Oncol.* **2005**, *23*, 7794–7803. [CrossRef]
22. Socinski, M.A.; Bondarenko, I.; Karaseva, N.A.; Makhson, A.M.; Vynnychenko, I.; Okamoto, I.; Hon, J.K.; Hirsh, V.; Bhar, P.; Zhang, H.; et al. Weekly nab-Paclitaxel in Combination With Carboplatin Versus Solvent-Based Paclitaxel Plus Carboplatin as First-Line Therapy in Patients With Advanced Non–Small-Cell Lung Cancer: Final Results of a Phase III Trial. *J. Clin. Oncol.* **2012**, *30*, 2055–2062. [CrossRef]
23. Goldstein, D.; Von Hoff, D.D.; Moore, M.; Greeno, E.; Tortora, G.; Ramanathan, R.K.; Macarulla, T.; Liu, H.; Pilot, R.; Ferrara, S.; et al. Development of peripheral neuropathy and its association with survival during treatment with nab-paclitaxel plus gemcitabine for patients with metastatic adenocarcinoma of the pancreas: A subset analysis from a randomised phase III trial (MPACT). *Eur. J. Cancer* **2016**, *52*, 85–91. [CrossRef] [PubMed]
24. Catalano, M.; Roviello, G.; Conca, R.; D'Angelo, A.; Palmieri, V.E.; Panella, B.; Petrioli, R.; Ianza, A.; Nobili, S.; Mini, E.; et al. Clinical outcomes and safety of pa-tients treated with NAb-Paclitaxel plus Gemcitabine in metastatic pancreatic cancer: The NAPA study. *Curr. Cancer Drug Targets* **2020**, *20*, 887–895. [CrossRef]
25. Eisenhauer, E.; Therasse, P.; Bogaerts, J.; Schwartz, L.; Sargent, D.; Ford, R.; Dancey, J.; Arbuck, S.; Gwyther, S.; Mooney, M.; et al. New response evaluation criteria in solid tumours: Revised RECIST guideline (version 1.1). *Eur. J. Cancer* **2009**, *45*, 228–247. [CrossRef] [PubMed]
26. Valero, V.; Holmes, F.A.; Walters, R.S.; Theriault, R.L.; Esparza, L.; Fraschini, G.; Fonseca, G.A.; Bellet, R.E.; Buzdar, A.U.; Hortobagyi, G.N. Phase II trial of docetaxel: A new, highly effective antineoplastic agent in the management of patients with anthracycline-resistant metastatic breast cancer. *J. Clin. Oncol.* **1995**, *13*, 2886–2894. [CrossRef] [PubMed]
27. Holmes, F.A.; Walters, R.S.; Theriault, R.L.; Buzdar, A.U.; Frye, D.K.; Hortobagyi, G.N.; Forman, A.D.; Newton, L.K.; Raber, M.N. Phase II Trial of Taxol, an Active Drug in the Treatment of Metastatic Breast Cancer. *J. Natl. Cancer Inst.* **1991**, *83*, 1797–1805. [CrossRef] [PubMed]
28. Nabholtz, J.M.; Gelmon, K.; Bontenbal, M.; Spielmann, M.; Catimel, G.; Conte, P.; Klaassen, U.; Namer, M.; Bonneterre, J.; Fumoleau, P.; et al. Multicenter, randomized com-parative study of two doses of paclitaxel in patients with metastatic breast cancer. *J. Clin. Oncol.* **1996**, *14*, 1858–1867. [CrossRef] [PubMed]
29. Hilkens, P.; Verweij, J.; Stoter, G.; Vecht, C.; Van Putten, W.L.; Bent, M.J.V.D. Peripheral neurotoxicity induced by docetaxel. *Neurology* **1996**, *46*, 104–108. [CrossRef]
30. Freilich, R.J.; Balmaceda, C.; Seidman, A.D.; Rubin, M.; DeAngelis, L.M. Motor neuropathy due to docetaxel and paclitaxel. *Neurology* **1996**, *47*, 115–118. [CrossRef]
31. Rowinsky, E.K.; Chaudhry, V.; Cornblath, D.R.; Donehower, R.C. Neurotoxicity of Taxol. *J. Natl. Cancer Inst. Monogr.* **1993**, *15*, 107–115.
32. National Cancer Institute; National Institutes of Health. *Common Terminology Criteria for Adverse Events*; National Institutes of Health. U.S. Department of Health & Human Services: Bethesda, MD, USA, 2020.
33. Peng, L.; Bu, Z.; Ye, X.; Zhou, Y.; Zhao, Q. Incidence and risk of peripheral neuropathy with nab-paclitaxel in patients with cancer: A meta-analysis. *Eur. J. Cancer Care* **2017**, *26*, e12407. [CrossRef]
34. Cavaletti, G.; Marmiroli, P. Chemotherapy-induced peripheral neurotoxicity. *Nat. Rev. Neurol.* **2010**, *6*, 657–666. [CrossRef] [PubMed]
35. De Vos, F.Y.F.L.; Bos, A.M.E.; Schaapveld, M.; De Swart, C.A.M.; De Graaf, H.; Van Der Zee, A.G.J.; Boezen, H.M.; de Vries, E.G.E.; Willemse, P.H.B. A randomized phase II study of paclitaxel with carboplatin ± amifostine as first line treatment in advanced ovarian carcinoma. *Gynecol Oncol.* **2005**, *97*, 60–67. [CrossRef] [PubMed]
36. Chhibber, A.; Mefford, J.; Stahl, E.A.; Pendergrass, S.A.; Baldwin, R.M.; Owzar, K.; Li, M.; Winer, E.P.; Hudis, C.A.; Zembutsu, H.; et al. Polygenic inheritance of paclitaxel-induced sensory peripheral neuropathy driven by axon outgrowth gene sets in CALGB 40101 (Alliance). *Pharm. J.* **2014**, *14*, 336–342. [CrossRef] [PubMed]

37. You, M.S.; Ryu, J.K.; Choi, Y.H.; Choi, J.H.; Huh, G.; Paik, W.H.; Lee, S.H.; Kim, Y.-T. Efficacy of Nab-Paclitaxel Plus Gemcitabine and Prognostic Value of Peripheral Neuropathy in Patients with Metastatic Pancreatic Cancer. *Gut Liver* **2018**, *12*, 728–735. [CrossRef]
38. Schneider, B.P.; Zhao, F.; Wang, M.; Stearns, V.; Martino, S.; Jones, V.; Perez, E.A.; Saphner, T.; Wolff, A.C.; Sledge, G.W., Jr.; et al. Neuropathy Is Not Associated With Clinical Outcomes in Patients Receiving Adjuvant Taxane-Containing Therapy for Operable Breast Cancer. *J. Clin. Oncol.* **2012**, *30*, 3051–3057. [CrossRef]
39. Schneider, B.P.; Li, L.; Radovich, M.; Shen, F.; Miller, K.D.; Flockhart, D.A.; Jiang, G.; Vance, G.; Gardner, L.; Vatta, M.; et al. Genome-Wide Association Studies for Taxane-Induced Peripheral Neuropathy in ECOG-5103 and ECOG-1199. *Clin. Cancer Res.* **2015**, *21*, 5082–5091. [CrossRef]
40. Rivera, E.; Cianfrocca, M. Overview of neuropathy associated with taxanes for the treatment of metastatic breast cancer. *Cancer Chemother. Pharmacol.* **2015**, *75*, 659–670. [CrossRef]
41. Mir, O.; Alexandre, J.; Tran, A.; Durand, J.P.; Pons, G.; Treluyer, J.M.; Goldwasser, F. Relationship between GSTP1 Ile 105Val pol-ymorphism and docetaxel-induced peripheral neuropathy: Clinical evidence of a role of oxidative stress in taxane toxicity. *Ann Oncol.* **2009**, *20*, 736–740. [CrossRef]
42. Robertson, J.; Raizer, J.; Hodges, J.S.; Gradishar, W.; Allen, J.A. Risk factors for the development of paclitaxel-induced neuropathy in breast cancer patients. *J. Peripher. Nerv. Syst.* **2018**, *23*, 129–133. [CrossRef]
43. Scheithauer, W.; Ramanathan, R.K.; Moore, M.; Macarulla, T.; Goldstein, D.; Hammel, P.; Kunzmann, V.; Liu, H.; McGovern, D.; Romano, A.; et al. Dose modification and efficacy of nab-paclitaxel plus gemcitabine vs. gemcitabine for patients with metastatic pancreatic cancer: Phase III MPACT trial. *J. Gastrointest. Oncol.* **2016**, *7*, 469–478. [CrossRef]
44. Lv, L.; Mao, S.; Dong, H.; Hu, P.; Dong, R. Pathogenesis, Assessments, and Management of Chemotherapy-Related Cognitive Impairment (CRCI): An Updated Literature Review. *J. Oncol.* **2020**, 1–11. [CrossRef]
45. Vichaya, E.G.; Chiu, G.S.; Krukowski, K.; Lacourt, T.E.; Kavelaars, A.; Dantzer, R.; Heijnen, C.J.; Walker, A.K. Mechanisms of chemotherapy-induced behavioral toxicities. *Front. Neurosci. Front. Res. Found.* **2015**, *9*, 131. [CrossRef]
46. Šeruga, B.; Zhang, H.; Bernstein, L.J.; Tannock, I.F. Cytokines and their relationship to the symptoms and outcome of cancer. *Nat. Rev. Cancer* **2008**, *8*, 887–899. [CrossRef] [PubMed]
47. Bernstein, L.J.; McCreath, G.A.; Komeylian, Z.; Rich, J.B. Cognitive impairment in breast cancer survivors treated with chemotherapy depends on control group type and cognitive domains assessed: A multilevel meta-analysis. *Neurosci. Biobehav. Rev.* **2017**, *83*, 417–428. [CrossRef]
48. Chovanec, M.; Galikova, D.; Vasilkova, L.; De Angelis, V.; Rejlekova, K.; Obertova, J.; Sycova-Mila, Z.; Palacka, P.; Kalavska, K.; Svetlovska, D.; et al. Chemotherapy-induced peripheral neuropathy (CIPN) as a predictor of decreased quality of life and cognitive impairment in testicular germ cell tumor survivors. *J. Clin. Oncol.* **2020**, *38*, e17063. [CrossRef]
49. Pachman, D.R.; Qin, R.; Seisler, D.K.; Smith, E.M.; Beutler, A.S.; Ta, L.E.; Lafky, J.M.; Wagner-Johnston, N.D.; Ruddy, K.J.; Dakhil, S.R.; et al. Clinical Course of Oxaliplatin-Induced Neuropathy: Results From the Randomized Phase III Trial N08CB (Alliance). *J. Clin. Oncol.* **2015**, *33*, 3416–3422. [CrossRef] [PubMed]
50. Binda, D.; Vanhoutte, E.; Cavaletti, G.; Cornblath, D.; Postma, T.; Frigeni, B.; Alberti, P.; Bruna, J.; Velasco, R.; Argyriou, A.; et al. Rasch-built Overall Disability Scale for patients with chemotherapy-induced peripheral neuropathy (CIPN-R-ODS). *Eur. J. Cancer* **2013**, *49*, 2910–2918. [CrossRef] [PubMed]
51. Binda, D.; Cavaletti, G.; Cornblath, D.R.; Merkies, I.S.J. Sg on behalf of the CI-PeriNomS study group Rasch-Transformed Total Neuropathy Score clinical version (RT-TNSc©) in patients with chemotherapy-induced peripheral neuropathy. *J. Peripher. Nerv. Syst.* **2015**, *20*, 328–332. [CrossRef]
52. Kollmannsberger, C. Sunitinib side effects as surrogate biomarkers of efficacy. *Can. Urol. Assoc. J.* **2016**, *10*, 245–247. [CrossRef] [PubMed]
53. Perez-Soler, R. Rash as a Surrogate Marker for Efficacy of Epidermal Growth Factor Receptor Inhibitors in Lung Cancer. *Clin. Lung Cancer* **2006**, *8*, S7–S14. [CrossRef] [PubMed]
54. Wang, M.; Cheng, H.L.; Lopez, V.; Sundar, R.; Yorke, J.; Molassiotis, A. Redefining chemotherapy-induced peripheral neuropathy through symptom cluster analysis and patient-reported outcome data over time. *BMC Cancer* **2019**, *19*, 1151. [CrossRef] [PubMed]

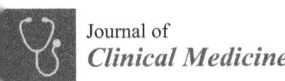

Journal of
Clinical Medicine

Article

The Ratio of C-Reactive Protein to Albumin Is an Independent Predictor of Malignant Intraductal Papillary Mucinous Neoplasms of the Pancreas

Simone Serafini [1], Alberto Friziero [1], Cosimo Sperti [1,*], Lorenzo Vallese [2], Andrea Grego [1], Alfredo Piangerelli [1], Amanda Belluzzi [1] and Lucia Moletta [1]

1 Department of Surgery, Oncology and Gastroenterology, 3rd Surgery Clinic, University of Padua, via Giustiniani 2, 35128 Padua, Italy; simone.serafini@ymail.com (S.S.); alberto.friziero@aopd.veneto.it (A.F.); d.andrea.grego@gmail.com (A.G.); alfredopiange@gmail.com (A.P.); amandabelluzzi@gmail.com (A.B.); lucia.moletta@unipd.it (L.M.)
2 Department of Surgery, SS. Giovanni and Paolo Hospital, Sestiere Castello 6777, 30122 Venice, Italy; l.vallese@gmail.com
* Correspondence: csperti@libero.it; Tel.: +39-049-821-8845

Citation: Serafini, S.; Friziero, A.; Sperti, C.; Vallese, L.; Grego, A.; Piangerelli, A.; Belluzzi, A.; Moletta, L. The Ratio of C-Reactive Protein to Albumin Is an Independent Predictor of Malignant Intraductal Papillary Mucinous Neoplasms of the Pancreas. *J. Clin. Med.* **2021**, *10*, 2058. https://doi.org/10.3390/jcm10102058

Academic Editor: Raffaele Pezzilli

Received: 1 April 2021
Accepted: 7 May 2021
Published: 11 May 2021

Publisher's Note: MDPI stays neutral with regard to jurisdictional claims in published maps and institutional affiliations.

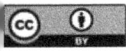

Copyright: © 2021 by the authors. Licensee MDPI, Basel, Switzerland. This article is an open access article distributed under the terms and conditions of the Creative Commons Attribution (CC BY) license (https://creativecommons.org/licenses/by/4.0/).

Abstract: There is growing evidence to indicate that inflammatory reactions are involved in cancer progression. The aim of this study is to assess the significance of systemic inflammatory biomarkers, such as the neutrophil-to-lymphocyte ratio (NLR), the platelet-to-lymphocyte ratio (PLR), the ratio of C-reactive protein to albumin ratio (CAR), the prognostic nutritional index (PNI) and the modified Glasgow prognostic score (mGps) in the diagnosis and prognosis of malignant intraductal papillary mucinous neoplasms (IPMNs) of the pancreas. Data were obtained from a retrospective analysis of patients who underwent pancreatic resection for IPMNs from January 2005 to December 2015. Univariate and multivariate analyses were performed, considering preoperative inflammatory biomarkers, clinicopathological variables, and imaging features. Eighty-three patients with histologically proven IPMNs of the pancreas were included in the study, 37 cases of low-grade or intermediate dysplasia and 46 cases of high-grade dysplasia (HGD) or invasive carcinoma. Univariate analysis showed that obstructive jaundice ($p = 0.02$) and a CAR of >0.083 ($p = 0.001$) were predictors of malignancy. On multivariate analysis, only the CAR was a statistically significant independent predictor of HGD or invasive carcinoma in pancreatic IPMNs, identifying a subgroup of patients with a poor prognosis. Combining the CAR with patients' imaging findings, clinical features and tumor markers can be useful in the clinical management of IPMNs. Their value should be tested in prospective studies.

Keywords: biomarker; C-reactive protein to albumin ratio; inflammation; intraductal papillary mucinous neoplasm; modified Glasgow prognostic score; neutrophyl lymphocite ratio; pancreatic cancer; platelet-to-lymphocyte ratio

1. Introduction

In the pancreas, intraductal papillary mucinous neoplasms (IPMNs) originate from the mucinous epithelium of the pancreatic ductal system. Their incidence is rising, probably due to an increasingly extensive use of cross-sectional imaging, but their management remains controversial. According to the World Health Organization (2010), IPMNs are premalignant lesions showing a broad spectrum of dysplastic changes. According to the different involvement of duct system, IPMNs are divided into main duct type (MD-IPMN), branch duct type (BD-IPMN), and mixed type (MT-IPMN). For the purposes of pathological grading, IPMNs are classified as low-, intermediate- or high-grade dysplasia, or invasive carcinoma. IPMNs with low- and intermediate-grade dysplasia are defined as benign, while the malignant IPMNs include those classified as high-grade dysplasia (HGD) or invasive carcinoma [1]. Benign IPMNs can potentially be managed conservatively, whereas malignant IPMNs require surgical resection in accordance with international guidelines. Malignant IPMNs carry a worse prognosis than benign IPMNs, making it essential to predict the malignant potential of an IPMN accurately at the time of its diagnosis or follow-up. Several clinical and radiological parameters have been considered over time with a view to stratifying the malignant potential of pancreatic IPMNs and thereby facilitate their management. International consensus guidelines (ICG) recommend surgery for cases with one or more "high-risk stigmata" (HRS), while further assessment with endoscopic ultrasonography is suggested for cases with "worrisome features" (WF) [2]. The accuracy of these guidelines in detecting early invasive carcinoma in IPMNs is limited, however [3]. Even conventional tumor markers like CEA and CA 19.9 are not very useful in predicting the risk of malignancy in this setting [4]. There is still a crucial need for markers capable of identifying which IPMNs warrant surgical treatment.

There is growing evidence to indicate that inflammatory reactions and nutritional status are involved in cancer progression. Many host-related inflammatory biomarkers measurable in peripheral blood samples have been investigated as potentially effective prognostic factors in several types of cancer [5–7], including pancreatic adenocarcinoma [8,9]. These serum parameters include, among others, the neutrophil-to-lymphocyte ratio (NLR), the platelet-to-lymphocyte ratio (PLR), the ratio of C-reactive protein to albumin (CAR), the prognostic nutritional index (PNI) and the modified Glasgow prognostic score (mGps). The prognostic impact of these markers in patients with IPMNs has yet to be well established, and the literature reports different results.

The NLR alone was described as an independent predictor of IPMN-associated invasive carcinoma, but its sensitivity was not high enough to distinguish between degrees of dysplasia in IPMNs [10]. On the other hand, a significant prognostic indication of malignancy (both HGD and invasive carcinoma) in IPMNs could only be reached by combining the preoperative NLR and PLR with tumor markers and imaging findings [11,12]. In short, there is still not enough evidence regarding the predictive role of these biomarkers.

Herein we present a retrospective study on a series of patients whose IPMNs were resected in an effort to establish the value of the NLR, PLR, CAR, PNI and mGps in predicting which cases of IPMN are malignant.

2. Materials and Methods

Between January 2005 and December 2015, all consecutive patients with pancreatic IPMNs who underwent surgical resection at our Department were identified using a prospectively maintained database. The data were analyzed retrospectively. The conventional workup included blood tests, tumoral markers, contrast-enhanced magnetic resonance imaging (MRI), bilio-pancreatic endoscopic ultrasound (EUS) and positron emission tomography (PET) with fluorine-18-fluorodeoxyglucose if clinically appropriated. Exclusion criteria were adopted to avoid potential confounding factors, including: a history of other malignancies, autoimmune disease or transplantation requiring immunosuppressant and steroid therapies; cholangitis or other forms of infection; pancreatic endocrine tumors and cystic neoplasms other than IPMNs. Patients diagnosed with metastases were not included. Disease-related symptoms such as visceral abdominal pain, dyspepsia (upper abdominal fullness, nausea, belching) and compression syndrome (experience of feeling full earlier than expected when eating, vomiting) were collected. IPMNs were confirmed on pathological examination of surgical specimens in all cases. The cases were all retrieved from the archives of the Surgical Pathology and Cytopathology Unit at Padova University Hospital (Padova, Italy). Surgical specimens were examined to histologically classify cases as low-, intermediate or HGD or invasive carcinoma, based on the recommendations of the Baltimore consensus [13]. IPMNs were described as main duct (MD), branch duct (BD) or combined type, based on preoperative imaging. Main-duct IPMNs are characterized by involvement of the main pancreatic duct, with or without associated involvement of the branch ducts (in the former case, they are called combined-type IPMNs). They usually present as a dilated (≥1 cm) main pancreatic duct, or as a cystic dilation of the main duct and its branches. Branch-duct IPMNs originate in the side branches of the pancreatic ductal system, appearing as cystic lesions communicating with a main pancreatic duct showing no dilations [14]. All resection procedures were performed by the same surgical team, in accordance with the International Consensus Guidelines of the time [2]. Surgery involved pylorus-preserving pancreaticoduodenectomy (PD) for tumors of the head of the pancreas, or distal pancreatectomy with or without splenectomy, for tumors of the body and tail. Total pancreatectomy was reserved for cases where the resection margins of the pancreas were affected by the tumor. More parenchyma-sparing resections of the pancreas, such as central pancreatectomy and tumor enucleation, were performed in the case of small to medium-sizes lesions localized in the pancreatic body.

Based on the pathological grading of the resected IPMNs, patients were divided into a benign group (IPMNs with low- and intermediate-grade dysplasia) and a malignant group (IPMNs associated with HGD and invasive carcinoma) [1]. Each patient's clinical and pathological records were reviewed, and the following characteristics were included in our analysis: gender; age; abdominal pain; dyspepsia; tumor site; compression syndrome; tumor size; main pancreatic duct (MPD) diameter; cyst diameter; HRS; WF; CEA; CA 19.9; and inflammatory biomarkers, such as the NLR, PLR, CAR, PNI and mGps. Preoperative serum levels of CA 19-9 (RIA, Centocor Inc., Malvern, PA, USA, reference: <37 kU/L) and CEA (EIA Kit, General Biologicals Inc., Taiwan, reference: <5 ng/mL) were recorded. Neutrophil, lymphocyte and platelet counts, and serum albumin levels (g/dL) were obtained from the latest blood sample collected just before surgery. The following indexes were retrospectively calculated: the NLR (the ratio of the absolute neutrophil count to the absolute lymphocyte count in the blood cell count); the PLR (the ratio of the absolute platelet count to the absolute lymphocyte count in the blood cell count); the CAR (the ratio of C-reactive protein [CRP] (mg/dL) to albumin (g/dL); the PNI (calculated as $10 \times$ serum albumin + 0.005 x total lymphocyte counts) and the mGps, which ranged from 0 to 2. Patients with both high CRP levels (>10 mg/L) and hypoalbuminemia (<35 g/L) had a mGps of 2; those with normal CRP and albumin levels scored 0; and those with high CRP levels and normal albumin levels scored 1, in line with recent data [15].

Ethical approval: All procedures performed in studies involving human participants were in accordance with the ethical standards of the institutional and/or national research committee and with the 1964 Helsinki Declaration and its later amendments or comparable ethical standards.

Statistical analyses were run using STATA, version 14.1 (4905 Lakeway Drive College Station, Midtown Dr, TX, 77845, USA). Continuous and categorical variables are reported as medians with the interquartile range (IQR), and as whole numbers (percentages), respectively. The diagnostic accuracy, including sensitivity and specificity, was calculated for each host-derived inflammatory biomarker using the cutoffs obtained from receiver operating characteristic (ROC) curve analysis. The optimal cutoff was identified as the point of intersection nearest the top left-hand corner between the ROC curve and a diagonal line drawn from the top right-hand corner to the bottom left-hand corner of the graph. The sensitivity, specificity, positive predictive value (PPV), negative predictive value (NPV), and accuracy of the inflammatory biomarkers and radiological imaging findings in differentiating between malignant and benign IPMNs were calculated according to the following formulas: sensitivity = true positive (TP)/[TP + false negative (FN)]; specificity = true negative (TN)/[TN + false positive (FP)]; PPV = TP/[TP + FP]; NPV = TN/[TN + FN] and accuracy = [TP + TN]/[TP + TN + FP + FN]. For the univariate analysis, patients were divided into the two groups, with benign and malignant IPMNs. Differences between the characteristics of the patients in these two groups were tested for significance using the Mann-Whitney U test and chi-square test, as appropriate. A multivariate analysis was performed using the logistic regression model, and including significant variables identified in our univariate analysis only. The effect size of the odds ratio (OR) is presented with the 95% confidence interval (CI). Box plot graphs were drawn to represent the distribution of the inflammatory biomarkers of proven prognostic significance.

3. Results

Table 1 shows the clinicopathological features of the whole study cohort, comprising 83 patients with proven IPMNs. The sample was a median 69 years old (range 43–86), and consisted of 45 males and 38 females. No cases of concomitant pancreatic ductal adenocarcinoma were detected. None of the patients received neoadjuvant therapies. Among the 83 patients, 40 patients (48%) had main-duct IPMNs, 10 (12%) had branch-duct IPMNs, and 33 (40%) had combined-type IPMNs. Thirty-seven tumors (44.5%) were benign (30 with low-grade dysplasia, and 7 with intermediate-grade dysplasia), and 46 (55.5%) were malignant (7 with HGD, and 39 with invasive carcinoma). The surgical procedure involved pylorus-preserving PD in 50 patients, distal pancreatectomy with splenectomy in 22, distal pancreatectomy without splenectomy in 7, and total pancreatectomy in one. Tumor enucleation and central pancreatectomy were performed in two and one patient, respectively.

Table 1. Clinicopathological features of the whole cohort. IPMN, intraductal papillary mucinous neoplasm; MD, main duct; BD, branch duct; MPD, main pancreatic duct.

Variables	Whole Cohort (n = 83)
Sex, male n, %	45 (54%)
Female n,%	38 (46%)
Age, median (IQR range), y	69 (62–76)
IPMN type, n (%)	
MD_IPMNs	40 (48%)
BD_IPMNs	10 (12%)
Combined type_IPMNs	33 (40%)
Surgical procedure n (%)	
Pancreaticoduodenectomy	50 (60%)
Distal pancreatectomy + splenectomy	22 (27%)
Spleen-preserving distal pancreatectomy	7 (9%)
Central pancreatectomy	1 (1%)
Total pancreatectomy	1 (1%)
Tumor enucleation	2 (2%)
Histological grade, n (%)	
Low-grade dysplasia	30 (36%)
Intermediate dysplasia	7 (8%)
High-grade dysplasia	7 (8%)
Invasive carcinoma	39 (47%)
High-risk stigmata n (%)	
Obstructive jaundice	18 (22%)
Enhancing solid component	47 (57%)
MPD $\geq$ 10 mm	12 (14%)
Worrisome features n (%)	
Tumor $\geq$ 3 cm	26 (31%)
Pancreatitis	22 (27%)
Enhancing cyst wall	23 (28%)
MPD 5–9 mm	38 (46%)
Abrupt change in caliber of pancreatic duct with distal pancreatic atrophy	39 (47%)

Four inflammatory biomarkers were examined and ROC curve analysis was set to identify the optimal cutoffs for the NLR, PLR and CAR, while the mGps was calculated for each patient. The optimal cutoffs were: 2.38 for the NLR (AUC 0.43, sensitivity of 46% and specificity of 51%); 185.5 for the PLR (AUC 0.51, sensitivity of 37% and specificity of 78%);

0.083 for the CAR (AUC 0.69, sensitivity of 60% and specificity of 70%); and 42.05 for the PNI (AUC 0.46, sensitivity of 52% and specificity of 39%) (Figure 1).

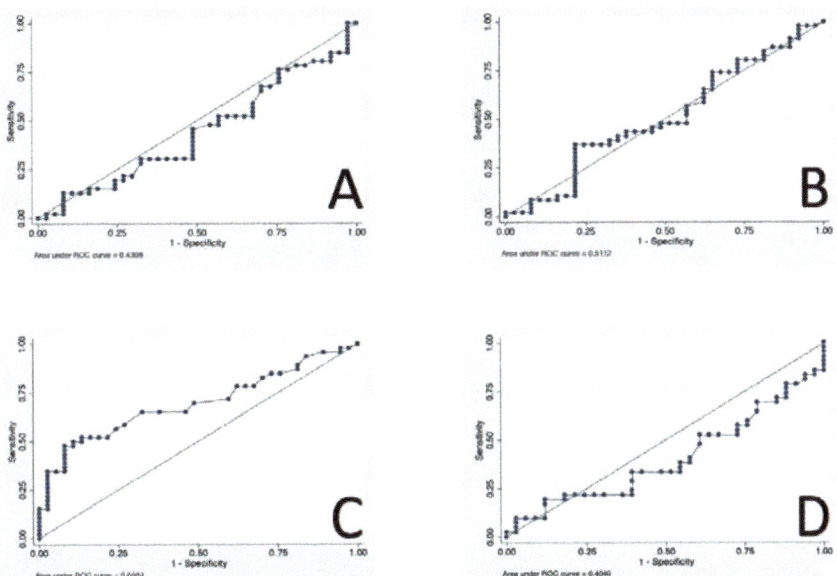

Figure 1. Receiver operator characteristic (ROC) curves of neutrophil-to-lymphocyte ratio (NLR) (**A**), platelet-to-lymphocyte ratio (PLR) (**B**), C-reactive protein to albumin ratio (CAR) (**C**), prognostic nutritional index (PNI) (**D**).

Univariate and multivariate analyses were performed to examine the causal relationship between the presence of IPMNs with a malignant potential and the inflammatory biomarkers (Table 2), inputting patients' preoperative clinicopathological variables and imaging features (Table 3).

Table 2. Clinicopathological features and biomarkers univariate and multivariate analysis for predicting malignant intraductal papillary mucinous neoplasm (IPMNs). Statistically significant values are in bold. OR: odds ratio; CI: confidence interval; NC: not calculated; IQR: interquartile range; MPD: main pancreatic duct; mGps: modified Glasgow prognostic score; NLR: neutrophil-to-lymphocyte ratio; PLR: platelet-to-lymphocyte ratio; CAR: C-reactive protein to albumin ratio; PNI: prognostic nutritional index.

			Univariate	Multivariate	
Variables	Benign IPMNs (n = 37)	Malignant IPMNs (n = 46)	p Value	OR (95% CI)	p Value
Sex, male n (%)	22 (59.46%)	23 (50%)	0.39	NC	
Age, median (IQR)	67.5 (62–73.5)	71 (62–78)	0.18	NC	
Abdominal pain n (%)	21 (56.76%)	18 (39.13%)	0.12	NC	
Dyspepsia n (%)	21 (56.76%)	17 (36.96%)	0.181	NC	
Cephalic location n (%)	27 (72.97%)	27 (58.70%)	0.175	NC	
Compression syndrome n (%)	13 (35.14%)	7 (15.22%)	0.093	NC	
Tumor size cm, median (IQR)	2 (1.8–3)	2.8 (2–3.2)	0.084	NC	
MPD diameter mm, median (IQR)	6 (3–8)	7 (4–8)	0.14	NC	

Table 2. Cont.

Variables	Benign IPMNs (n = 37)	Malignant IPMNs (n = 46)	Univariate p Value	Multivariate OR (95% CI)	p Value
Cyst diameter cm, median (IQR)	3 (2–4)	3 (2–4)	0.69	NC	
High-risk stigmata, n (%)					
Obstructive jaundice	13 (35.14%)	5 (10.87%)	**0.022**	0.37 (0.08–0.158)	0.18
Enhancing mural nodule	25 (67.57%)	22 (47.83%)	0.09	NC	
MPD > 10 mm	7 (18.92%)	5 (10.87%)	0.54	NC	
Worrisome features, n (%)					
Cyst size > 3 cm	12 (32.43%)	14 (30.43%)	0.97	NC	
Pancreatitis	13 (35.14%)	9 (19.57%)	0.27	NC	
Enhancing cyst wall	10 (27.03%)	13 (28.26%)	0.71	NC	
MPD 5–10 mm	17 (45.95%)	21 (45.65%)	0.96	NC	
Abrupt change in caliber of pancreatic duct with distal pancreatic atrophy	17 (45.95%)	22 (47.83%)	0.39	NC	
CA19.9, median (IQR)	4 (2–11)	24 (4–253)	0.42	NC	
CEA, median (IQR)	1 (0–3)	2 (1–5)	0.17	NC	
mGps				NC	
0	31 (83.78%)	37 (80.43%)	0.46		
1	4 (10.81%)	4 (8.70%)	0.52		
2	2 (5.41%)	5 (10.87%)	0.32		
NLR				NC	
<2.38	17 (45.95%)	24 (52.17%)	0.573		
>2.38	20 (54.05%)	22 (47.83%)			
PLR				NC	
<185.5 n %	28 (75.68%)	29 (63.04%)	0.217		
≥185.5 n %	9 (24.32%)	17 (36.96%)			
CAR				7.9 (2.01–31.83)	**0.003**
<0.083 n %	31 (83.78%)	22 (47.83%)	**0.001**		
≥0.083 n %	6 (16.22%)	24 (52.17%)			
PNI				NC	
<42.05 n %	14 (37.84%)	26 (56.52%)	0.15		
>42.05 n %	23 (62.16%)	20 (43.48%)	0.07		

On univariate analysis obstructive jaundice (p value 0.022) and a CAR of >0.083 (p value 0.001) emerged as predictors of malignancy. On multivariate analysis, only the CAR was an independent predictor of malignant IPMN (OR 7.9, IQR 2.01–31.83, p 0.003). No significant differences in gender, age, preoperative abdominal pain, dyspepsia or compression syndrome came to light between patients with benign as opposed to malignant IPMNs. Nor did the two groups differ in terms of tumor size, tumor site, MPD diameter or cyst diameter. The median serum levels of tumor markers CA 19.9 and CEA were not significantly different in the two groups of patients with IPMN. Among the preoperative risk-related parameters considered, the frequency of enhancing mural nodules, MPD ≥ 10 mm, cyst ≥ 3 cm, enhancing cyst walls, pancreatitis, MPD 5–10 mm, and abrupt MPD caliber changes with distal pancreatic atrophy did not differ between the malignant and benign IPMN groups ($p > 0.05$ for all).

The distribution of the CARs in the two groups is represented with a box plot (Figure 2). Most of the patients with benign IPMNs had a CAR lower than the study cutoff, while almost all those with malignant IPMNs had a CAR higher than 0.083.

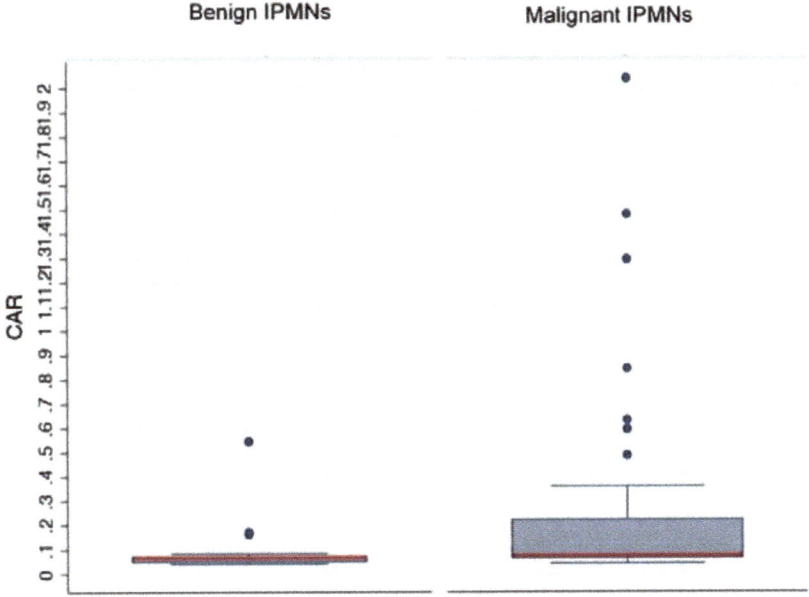

Figure 2. Quantification of CAR values in benign and malignant intraductal papillary mucinous neopla (IPMNs). The red horizontal bar represents the optimal cut off (0.083) obtained with receiver operator characteristic curves analysis and the blue ones represent the 25th and 75th percentiles. CAR: C-reactive protein to albumin ratio.

The sensitivity, specificity, PPV, NPV and accuracy of the CAR in detecting malignancy were 52%, 93%, 91%, 50%, and 66%, respectively, vs. 74%, 50%, 72%, 54%, and 66%, respectively, for the ICG criteria for HRS. Combining the two parameters (patients who demonstrate HRS according to ICG criteria and simultaneously CAR values > 0.083) resulted in a 43% sensitivity, 97% specificity, 94% PPV, 55% NPV, and 63% accuracy for the diagnosis of malignancy.

To judge the prognostic impact of the CAR, we first analyzed that there are no statistically significant differences between the clinicopathological and inflammatory parameters in the patients with high and low CARs, then we examined the association between high CARs and long-term outcomes in the 39 cases of IPMN with invasive carcinoma. Figure 3 shows the survival curves for patients with a high vs. low CAR: those with a higher CAR had a significantly shorter overall survival ($p = 0.004$) than those with a lower CAR.

Table 3. Distribution of clinicopathological features and biomarkers between patients with high and low CAR. CAR: C-reactive protein to albumin ratio; IQR: interquartile range; MPD: main pancreatic duct; CRP: C reactive protein; PNI: prognostic nutritional index; NLR: neutrophil-to-lymphocyte ratio; PLR: platelet-to-lymphocyte ratio.

Variables	CAR ≤ 0.083 (n 53)	CAR ≥ 0.083 (n 30)	p Value
Sex, male n, %	28 (52.83%)	17 (56.67)	0.46
Age, median (IQR)	69.5 (63–76.5)	68 (61–75)	0.42
Abdominal pain n, %	27 (50.94%)	12 (41.38%)	0.28
Dyspepsia n, %	28 (52.83%)	10 (35.71%)	0.11
Cephalic location n, %	36 (67.92%)	18 (60%)	0.31
Compression syndrome n, %	13 (25%)	7 (25.93%)	0.57
Tumour size cm, median (IQR)	3 (2–3.75)	2.5 (1.8–3.3)	0.06
MPD diameter mm, median (IQR)	6 (4–9)	5.5 (3.5–7.5)	0.12
Cyst diameter cm, median (IQR)	3 (2–4)	2.6 (2–3.8)	0.26
High risk stigmata, n (%) Obstructive jaundice	12 (22.64%)	6 (20%)	0.5
Enhancing mural nodule	31 (62%)	16 (53.33%)	0.3
MPD >10 mm	10 (20.41%)	2 (7.14%)	0.11
Worrisome features n (%) Cyst size >3 cm	20 (38.46%)	6 (20.69%)	0.08
Pancreatitis	15 (29.41%)	7 (23.33%)	0.37
Enhancing cyst wall	16 (31.37%)	7 (25%)	0.37
MPD 5–10 mm	22 (44.9%)	16 (57.14%)	0.21
Abrupt change in calibre of pancreatic duct with distal pancreatic atrophy	24 (48.98%)	15 (53.57%)	0.44
CA19.9, median (IQR)	8.5 (2–39)	17.5 (3–107)	0.24
CEA, median (IQR)	1 (0.4–3)	2 (1–4.5)	0.27
Inflammatory biomarkers Neutrophils, median (IQR)	3.7 (2.9–4.7)	3.55 (2.9–5.3)	0.73
Lymphocytes, median (IQR)	1.5 (1.26–2.1)	1.5 (1.2–1.9)	0.62
Platelets, median (IQR)	223 (189–271)	241 (192–296)	0.48
CRP, median (IQR)	3 (2.9–5)	3 (2–4)	0.77
Albumin, median (IQR)	4.2 (4–4.4)	4.2 (4.1–4.4)	0.93
PNI ≥ 42.05, n%	4 (7.55%)	4 (13.33%)	0.31
NLR ≥ 2.38, n%	26 (49.86%)	16 (53.33%)	0.44
PLR ≥ 185.5 n %	13 (24.53%)	13 (43.33%)	0.06

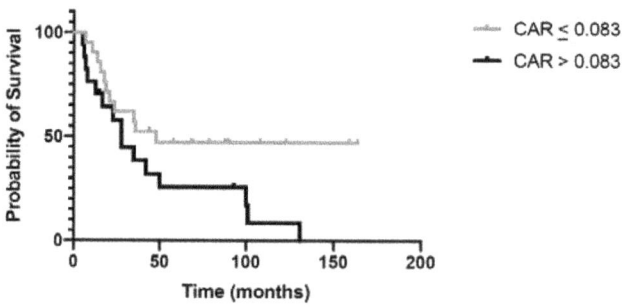

Figure 3. Kaplan–Meier curve for overall survival estimated for patients with C-reactive protein to albumin ratio (CAR) values > 0.083 or ≤ 0.083. CAR > 0.083 was significantly associated with worse survival ($p = 0.004$).

4. Discussion

The present study suggests that the CAR is useful for predicting HGD and invasive carcinoma in patients with IPMNs, and that the value of the CAR in detecting malignancies is independent of the well-established parameters indicated in the international guidelines [2,14,16]. Univariate analysis found obstructive jaundice, and a CAR >0.083 significantly associated with malignant IPMNs, but multivariate analysis showed that only the CAR was an independent predictor of malignant lesions (both HGD and invasive carcinoma). Although the sensitivity of the CAR in detecting malignancies was low, its specificity was higher than that of the ICG criteria for malignant IPMNs. Combining the ICG criteria with the CAR achieved only a slight increase in the specificity and PPV.

The CAR is easily obtained from a simple blood test. It is inexpensive and can be calculated by clinicians both at the initial examination and during the follow-up of patients with IPMNs. Although the CRP preoperative assessment is not a common practice, in our institution, it is included in protocols for research purposes for pancreatic diseases. However, it is becoming more and more common in the standard workup for elective surgery during COVID-19 era. To the best of our knowledge, this is the first study to emphasize the role of the CAR in identifying the malignant potential of IPMNs.

Features previously suggested to predict malignancy (HGD or invasive carcinoma) in IPMNs include: an association with symptoms; cyst wall thickening; mural nodules; MPD dilation; abrupt pancreatic duct caliber changes; lymphadenopathy; and higher than normal CA19-9 or CEA serum levels [17]. The rate of pointless surgical procedures for overestimated pancreatic lesions remains high, however, which is why new, specific biomarkers are needed for a better clinical management of patients with IPMNs. Both the NLR and the PLR have recently been proposed as predictors of an invasive carcinoma in pancreatic cysts [18,19]. High NLRs and PLRs may be due to neutrophilia and a systemic inflammatory response during the development of invasive cancer [20,21], and to a declining lymphocyte counts caused by immune system suppression [22]. The value of the preoperative NLR in predicting the malignant potential of IPMNs has been emphasized by several authors [23–25], but the picture remains unclear. While Hata et al. [26] found the preoperative NLR able to predict cases of IPMN with HGD, it was not helpful in differentiating between high-grade and low-grade lesions in the study by McIntyre et al. [24].

In a series of 318 patients with pancreatic cystic neoplasms (including 86 IPMNs), Goh et al. [27] found that a high preoperative PLR, but not the NLR, was an independent predictor of malignancy. They also found that adding the PLR to the ICG criteria improved the accuracy of the latter in detecting cases of invasive carcinoma.

A systemic inflammatory response has increasingly been recognized as an important factor in the process of carcinogenesis and a cancer's subsequent behavior, with tumor growth appearing to be directly proportional to the degree of inflammation [28,29]. The NLR [23,30,31] or PLR [27], or both [32] have been suggested as useful prognostic markers in patients with pancreatic cancer. A systematic review and meta-analysis conducted by Zhou et al. [33] on 8252 patients with pancreatic cancer showed that a low NLR was significantly associated with better disease-free and overall survival rates than a high NLR. Patients with a low NLR had significantly smaller tumors, better differentiation, earlier-stage disease and low CA 19-9 levels.

The CAR had been previously investigated in pancreatic cancer patients. Haruki et al. [34] found it an independent and significant indicator of poor long-term outcomes after pancreatic resection. Liu et al. [35] also reported finding that a high CAR was an independent factor pointing to a poor prognosis in pancreatic cancer patients. The prognostic implications of inflammatory biomarkers in different types of cancer have also already been reported [36,37].

In our study, the CAR was a predictor of long-term survival in patients with IPMNs associated with invasive carcinoma: patients with a lower CAR had a significantly better survival than those with CAR > 0.083 ($p = 0.004$). This would indicate that the CAR is an important prognostic parameter to consider in the clinical management of patients with IPMNs.

Furthermore, CAR is a new predictive indicator that reflects both inflammatory and nutritional status of cancer patients. This aspects play an important role in carcinogenesis and tumor progression. The real mechanism of the relationship between CAR and survival is unclear. Elevated CRP levels reflect an inflammatory response to tumor necrosis or local tissue damage, which are both factors that condition the stromal microenvironment for the engraftment and growth of metastases [38]. Moreover, PCR has been associated with inhibiting mechanisms of tumor cell apoptosis and an increased production of endothelial growth factors [39]. Likewise, hypoalbuminemia is often observed in patients with malignant diseases and is usually correlated with malnutrition and cachexia, aspects that inevitably affect the poor prognosis of these patients [40,41].

Our study has some limitations that need to be mentioned. First, the design was retrospective, so the possibility of selection bias exists. Second, the sample was small and studies on larger samples will be needed before any definitive conclusions can be drawn. Third, we did not investigate patients whose IPMNs had not been histologically confirmed, or patients who underwent surveillance alone: these patients could be included in future prospective studies. These partial results will have to be validated in further international, randomized multicentric trials in order to increase the number of enrolled patients, reduce selection bias and sample heterogeneity.

5. Conclusions

The preoperative CAR is an independent predictor of HGD or invasive carcinoma in IPMNs and identifies a subgroup of patients with a poor prognosis. Combined with imaging findings, clinical features and tumor markers, the CAR can be useful in the clinical management of IPMNs, and its value should be further investigated in international multicentric randomized clinical studies.

Author Contributions: S.S., conception and design of the study, drafting the article, final approval; A.F., acquisition of data, analysis and interpretation of data, drafting the article, final approval; C.S., conception and design of the study, critical revision, final approval; L.V., acquisition of data, analysis and interpretation of data; A.G., acquisition of data, analysis and interpretation of data; A.P., acquisition of data, analysis and interpretation of data; A.B., acquisition of data, analysis and interpretation of data; L.M., conception and design of the study, critical revision, final approval. All authors have read and agreed to the published version of the manuscript.

Funding: This research received no external funding.

Institutional Review Board Statement: All procedures performed in this study involving human participants were in accordance with the ethical standards of the institutional and/or national research committee and with the 1964 Helsinki Declaration and its later amendments or comparable ethical standards. Ethical review and approval were waived for this study, due to its noninvasive retrospective nature.

Informed Consent Statement: Informed consent was obtained from all subjects involved in the study.

Data Availability Statement: The data presented in this study are available on request from the corresponding author.

Conflicts of Interest: The authors declare no conflict of interest.

References

1. Bosman, F.T.; Carneiro, F.; Hruban, R.H.; Theise, N.D. *WHO Classification of Tumors of the Digestive System*; IARC Press: Lyon, France, 2010.
2. Tanaka, M.; Fernández-del Castillo, C.; Kamisawa, T.; Jang, J.Y.; Levy, P.; Ohtsuka, T.; Salvia, R.; Shimizu, Y.; Tada, M.; Wolfgang, C.L. Revisions of International Consensus Fukuoka Guidelines for the Management of IPMN of the Pancreas. *Pancreatology* **2017**, *17*, 738–753. [CrossRef] [PubMed]
3. Kaimakliotis, P.; Riff, B.; Pourmand, K.; Chandrasekhara, V.; Furth, E.E.; Siegelman, E.S.; Drebin, J.; Vollmer, C.M.; Kochman, M.L.; Ginsberg, G.G.; et al. Sendai and Fukuoka Consensus Guidelines Identify Advanced Neoplasia in Patients with Suspected Mucinous Cystic Neoplasms of the Pancreas. *Clin. Gastroenterol. Hepatol.* **2015**, *13*, 1808–1815. [CrossRef]

4. Kim, J.R.; Jang, J.-Y.; Kang, M.J.; Park, T.; Lee, S.Y.; Jung, W.; Chang, J.; Shin, Y.; Han, Y.; Kim, S.-W. Clinical Implication of Serum Carcinoembryonic Antigen and Carbohydrate Antigen 19-9 for the Prediction of Malignancy in Intraductal Papillary Mucinous Neoplasm of Pancreas. *J. Hepato-Biliary-Pancreat. Sci.* **2015**, *22*, 699–707. [CrossRef] [PubMed]
5. Saito, H.; Kono, Y.; Murakami, Y.; Shishido, Y.; Kuroda, H.; Matsunaga, T.; Fukumoto, Y.; Osaki, T.; Ashida, K.; Fujiwara, Y. Prognostic Significance of the Preoperative Ratio of C-Reactive Protein to Albumin and Neutrophil–Lymphocyte Ratio in Gastric Cancer Patients. *World J. Surg.* **2018**, *42*, 1819–1825. [CrossRef] [PubMed]
6. Gao, J.; Agizamhan, S.; Zhao, X.; Jiang, B.; Qin, H.; Chen, M.; Guo, H. Preoperative C-Reactive Protein/Albumin Ratio Predicts Outcome of Surgical Papillary Renal Cell Carcinoma. *Future Oncol.* **2019**, *15*, 1459–1468. [CrossRef]
7. Xiang, Z.; Hu, T.; Wang, Y.; Wang, H.; Xu, L.; Cui, N. Neutrophil–Lymphocyte Ratio (NLR) Was Associated with Prognosis and Immunomodulatory in Patients with Pancreatic Ductal Adenocarcinoma (PDAC). *Biosci. Rep.* **2020**, *40*, BSR20201190. [CrossRef]
8. Alagappan, M.; Pollom, E.L.; von Eyben, R.; Kozak, M.M.; Aggarwal, S.; Poultsides, G.A.; Koong, A.C.; Chang, D.T. Albumin and Neutrophil-Lymphocyte Ratio (NLR) Predict Survival in Patients with Pancreatic Adenocarcinoma Treated With SBRT. *Am. J. Clin. Oncol.* **2018**, *41*, 242–247. [CrossRef]
9. Shen, Y.; Wang, H.; Li, W.; Chen, J. Prognostic Significance of the CRP/Alb and Neutrophil to Lymphocyte Ratios in Hepatocellular Carcinoma Patients Undergoing TACE and RFA. *J. Clin. Lab. Anal.* **2019**, *33*, e22999. [CrossRef]
10. Gemenetzis, G.; Bagante, F.; Griffin, J.F.; Rezaee, N.; Javed, A.A.; Manos, L.L.; Lennon, A.M.; Wood, L.D.; Hruban, R.H.; Zheng, L.; et al. Neutrophil-to-Lymphocyte Ratio Is a Predictive Marker for Invasive Malignancy in Intraductal Papillary Mucinous Neoplasms of the Pancreas. *Ann. Surg.* **2017**, *266*, 339–345. [CrossRef]
11. Hata, T.; Mizuma, M.; Motoi, F.; Ishida, M.; Morikawa, T.; Nakagawa, K.; Hayashi, H.; Kanno, A.; Masamune, A.; Kamei, T.; et al. An Integrated Analysis of Host- and Tumor-Derived Markers for Predicting High-Grade Dysplasia and Associated Invasive Carcinoma of Intraductal Papillary Mucinous Neoplasms of the Pancreas. *Surg. Today* **2020**, *50*, 1039–1048. [CrossRef]
12. Li, J.A.; Han, X.; Fang, Y.; Zhang, L.; Lou, W.H.; Xu, X.F.; Wu, W.C.; Kuang, T.T.; Wang, D.S.; Rong, Y.F. The value of preoperative CA19-9 combined with platelet-to-lymphocyte ratio in predicting invasive malignancy in intraductal papillary mucinous neoplasms. *Zhonghua Wai Ke Za Zhi* **2019**, *57*, 170–175. [PubMed]
13. Basturk, O.; Hong, S.-M.; Wood, L.D.; Adsay, N.V.; Albores-Saavedra, J.; Biankin, A.V.; Brosens, L.A.A.; Fukushima, N.; Goggins, M.; Hruban, R.H.; et al. A Revised Classification System and Recommendations From the Baltimore Consensus Meeting for Neoplastic Precursor Lesions in the Pancreas. *Am. J. Surg. Pathol.* **2015**, *39*, 1730–1741. [CrossRef]
14. Tanaka, M.; Chari, S.; Adsay, V.; Carlos Castillo, F.-D.; Falconi, M.; Shimizu, M.; Yamaguchi, K.; Yamao, K.; Matsuno, S. International Consensus Guidelines for Management of Intraductal Papillary Mucinous Neoplasms and Mucinous Cystic Neoplasms of the Pancreas. *Pancreatology* **2006**, *6*, 17–32. [CrossRef] [PubMed]
15. Laird, B.J.; Kaasa, S.; McMillan, D.C.; Fallon, M.T.; Hjermstad, M.J.; Fayers, P.; Klepstad, P. Prognostic Factors in Patients with Advanced Cancer: A Comparison of Clinicopathological Factors and the Development of an Inflammation-Based Prognostic System. *Clin. Cancer Res.* **2013**, *19*, 5456–5464. [CrossRef]
16. Tanaka, M.; Fernández-del Castillo, C.; Adsay, V.; Chari, S.; Falconi, M.; Jang, J.-Y.; Kimura, W.; Levy, P.; Pitman, M.B.; Schmidt, C.M.; et al. International Consensus Guidelines 2012 for the Management of IPMN and MCN of the Pancreas. *Pancreatology* **2012**, *12*, 183–197. [CrossRef] [PubMed]
17. Kwon, W.; Han, Y.; Byun, Y.; Kang, J.S.; Choi, Y.J.; Kim, H.; Jang, J.-Y. Predictive Features of Malignancy in Branch Duct Type Intraductal Papillary Mucinous Neoplasm of the Pancreas: A Meta-Analysis. *Cancers* **2020**, *12*, 2618. [CrossRef]
18. Goh, B.K.P.; Tan, D.M.Y.; Chan, C.-Y.; Lee, S.-Y.; Lee, V.T.W.; Thng, C.-H.; Low, A.S.C.; Tai, D.W.M.; Cheow, P.-C.; Chow, P.K.H.; et al. Are Preoperative Blood Neutrophil-to-Lymphocyte and Platelet-to-Lymphocyte Ratios Useful in Predicting Malignancy in Surgically-Treated Mucin-Producing Pancreatic Cystic Neoplasms?: NLR and PLR in Pancreatic Cysts. *J. Surg. Oncol.* **2015**, *112*, 366–371. [CrossRef] [PubMed]
19. Arima, K.; Okabe, H.; Hashimoto, D.; Chikamoto, A.; Kuroki, H.; Taki, K.; Kaida, T.; Higashi, T.; Nitta, H.; Komohara, Y.; et al. The Neutrophil-to-Lymphocyte Ratio Predicts Malignant Potential in Intraductal Papillary Mucinous Neoplasms. *J. Gastrointest. Surg.* **2015**, *19*, 2171–2177. [CrossRef] [PubMed]
20. Hamada, S.; Masamune, A.; Shimosegawa, T. Inflammation and Pancreatic Cancer: Disease Promoter and New Therapeutic Target. *J. Gastroenterol.* **2014**, *49*, 605–617. [CrossRef] [PubMed]
21. Sadot, E.; Basturk, O.; Klimstra, D.S.; Gönen, M.; Lokshin, A.; Do, R.K.G.; D'Angelica, M.I.; DeMatteo, R.P.; Kingham, T.P.; Jarnagin, W.R.; et al. Tumor-Associated Neutrophils and Malignant Progression in Intraductal Papillary Mucinous Neoplasms: An Opportunity for Identification of High-Risk Disease. *Ann. Surg.* **2015**, *262*, 1102–1107. [CrossRef]
22. Inman, K.S. Complex Role for the Immune System in Initiation and Progression of Pancreatic Cancer. *World J. Gastroenterol.* **2014**, *20*, 11160. [CrossRef]
23. Arima, K.; Okabe, H.; Hashimoto, D.; Chikamoto, A.; Tsuji, A.; Yamamura, K.; Kitano, Y.; Inoue, R.; Kaida, T.; Higashi, T.; et al. The Diagnostic Role of the Neutrophil-to-Lymphocyte Ratio in Predicting Pancreatic Ductal Adenocarcinoma in Patients with Pancreatic Diseases. *Int. J. Clin. Oncol.* **2016**, *21*, 940–945. [CrossRef] [PubMed]
24. McIntyre, C.A.; Pulvirenti, A.; Lawrence, S.A.; Seier, K.; Gonen, M.; Balachandran, V.P.; Kingham, T.P.; D'Angelica, M.I.; Drebin, J.A.; Jarnagin, W.R.; et al. Neutrophil-to-Lymphocyte Ratio as a Predictor of Invasive Carcinoma in Patients with Intraductal Papillary Mucinous Neoplasms of the Pancreas. *Pancreas* **2019**, *48*, 832–836. [CrossRef] [PubMed]

25. Ohno, R.; Kawamoto, R.; Kanamoto, M.; Watanabe, J.; Fujii, M.; Ohtani, H.; Harada, M.; Kumagi, T.; Kawasaki, H. Neutrophil to Lymphocyte Ratio Is a Predictive Factor of Malignant Potential for Intraductal Papillary Mucinous Neoplasms of the Pancreas. *Biomark. Insights* **2019**, *14*, 117727191985150. [CrossRef]
26. Hata, T.; Mizuma, M.; Motoi, F.; Ishida, M.; Morikawa, T.; Takadate, T.; Nakagawa, K.; Hayashi, H.; Kanno, A.; Masamune, A.; et al. Diagnostic and Prognostic Impact of Neutrophil-to-Lymphocyte Ratio for Intraductal Papillary Mucinous Neoplasms of the Pancreas With High-Grade Dysplasia and Associated Invasive Carcinoma. *Pancreas* **2019**, *48*, 99–106. [CrossRef] [PubMed]
27. Goh, B.K.P.; Teo, J.-Y.; Allen, J.C.; Tan, D.M.Y.; Chan, C.-Y.; Lee, S.-Y.; Tai, D.W.M.; Thng, C.-H.; Cheow, P.-C.; Chow, P.K.H.; et al. Preoperative Platelet-to-Lymphocyte Ratio Improves the Performance of the International Consensus Guidelines in Predicting Malignant Pancreatic Cystic Neoplasms. *Pancreatology* **2016**, *16*, 888–892. [CrossRef] [PubMed]
28. Bhatti, I.; Peacock, O.; Lloyd, G.; Larvin, M.; Hall, R.I. Preoperative Hematologic Markers as Independent Predictors of Prognosis in Resected Pancreatic Ductal Adenocarcinoma: Neutrophil-Lymphocyte versus Platelet-Lymphocyte Ratio. *Am. J. Surg.* **2010**, *200*, 197–203. [CrossRef] [PubMed]
29. Ahmad, J.; Grimes, N.; Farid, S.; Morris-Stiff, G. Inflammatory Response Related Scoring Systems in Assessing the Prognosis of Patients with Pancreatic Ductal Adenocarcinoma: A Systematic Review. *Hepatobiliary Pancreat. Dis. Int.* **2014**, *13*, 474–481. [CrossRef]
30. Stotz, M.; Gerger, A.; Eisner, F.; Szkandera, J.; Loibner, H.; Ress, A.L.; Kornprat, P.; A Zoughbi, W.; Seggewies, F.S.; Lackner, C.; et al. Increased Neutrophil-Lymphocyte Ratio Is a Poor Prognostic Factor in Patients with Primary Operable and Inoperable Pancreatic Cancer. *Br. J. Cancer* **2013**, *109*, 416–421. [CrossRef]
31. Shusterman, M.; Jou, E.; Kaubisch, A.; Chuy, J.W.; Rajdev, L.; Aparo, S.; Tang, J.; Ohri, N.; Negassa, A.; Goel, S. The Neutrophil-to-Lymphocyte Ratio Is a Prognostic Biomarker in An Ethnically Diverse Patient Population with Advanced Pancreatic Cancer. *J. Gastrointest. Cancer* **2020**, *51*, 868–876. [CrossRef]
32. Asari, S.; Matsumoto, I.; Toyama, H.; Shinzeki, M.; Goto, T.; Ishida, J.; Ajiki, T.; Fukumoto, T.; Ku, Y. Preoperative Independent Prognostic Factors in Patients with Borderline Resectable Pancreatic Ductal Adenocarcinoma Following Curative Resection: The Neutrophil-Lymphocyte and Platelet-Lymphocyte Ratios. *Surg. Today* **2016**, *46*, 583–592. [CrossRef] [PubMed]
33. Zhou, Y.; Wei, Q.; Fan, J.; Cheng, S.; Ding, W.; Hua, Z. Prognostic Role of the Neutrophil-to-Lymphocyte Ratio in Pancreatic Cancer: A Meta-Analysis Containing 8252 Patients. *Clin. Chim. Acta* **2018**, *479*, 181–189. [CrossRef]
34. Haruki, K.; Shiba, H.; Shirai, Y.; Horiuchi, T.; Iwase, R.; Fujiwara, Y.; Furukawa, K.; Misawa, T.; Yanaga, K. The C-Reactive Protein to Albumin Ratio Predicts Long-Term Outcomes in Patients with Pancreatic Cancer After Pancreatic Resection. *World J. Surg.* **2016**, *40*, 2254–2260. [CrossRef]
35. Liu, Z.; Jin, K.; Guo, M.; Long, J.; Liu, L.; Liu, C.; Xu, J.; Ni, Q.; Luo, G.; Yu, X. Prognostic Value of the CRP/Alb Ratio, a Novel Inflammation-Based Score in Pancreatic Cancer. *Ann. Surg. Oncol.* **2017**, *24*, 561–568. [CrossRef] [PubMed]
36. Kinoshita, A.; Onoda, H.; Imai, N.; Iwaku, A.; Oishi, M.; Tanaka, K.; Fushiya, N.; Koike, K.; Nishino, H.; Matsushima, M. The C-Reactive Protein/Albumin Ratio, a Novel Inflammation-Based Prognostic Score, Predicts Outcomes in Patients with Hepatocellular Carcinoma. *Ann. Surg. Oncol.* **2015**, *22*, 803–810. [CrossRef] [PubMed]
37. Proctor, M.J.; Morrison, D.S.; Talwar, D.; Balmer, S.M.; O'Reilly, D.S.J.; Foulis, A.K.; Horgan, P.G.; McMillan, D.C. An Inflammation-Based Prognostic Score (MGPS) Predicts Cancer Survival Independent of Tumour Site: A Glasgow Inflammation Outcome Study. *Br. J. Cancer* **2011**, *104*, 726–734. [CrossRef] [PubMed]
38. Wong, V.K.H.; Malik, H.Z.; Hamady, Z.Z.R.; Al-Mukhtar, A.; Gomez, D.; Prasad, K.R.; Toogood, G.J.; Lodge, J.P.A. C-Reactive Protein as a Predictor of Prognosis Following Curative Resection for Colorectal Liver Metastases. *Br. J. Cancer* **2007**, *96*, 222–225. [CrossRef]
39. Yang, J.; Wezeman, M.; Zhang, X.; Lin, P.; Wang, M.; Qian, J.; Wan, B.; Kwak, L.W.; Yu, L.; Yi, Q. Human C-Reactive Protein Binds Activating Fcgamma Receptors and Protects Myeloma Tumor Cells from Apoptosis. *Cancer Cell* **2007**, *12*, 252–265. [CrossRef] [PubMed]
40. Kanda, M.; Fujii, T.; Kodera, Y.; Nagai, S.; Takeda, S.; Nakao, A. Nutritional Predictors of Postoperative Outcome in Pancreatic Cancer. *Br. J. Surg.* **2011**, *98*, 268–274. [CrossRef] [PubMed]
41. Okumura, S.; Kaido, T.; Hamaguchi, Y.; Fujimoto, Y.; Masui, T.; Mizumoto, M.; Hammad, A.; Mori, A.; Takaori, K.; Uemoto, S. Impact of Preoperative Quality as Well as Quantity of Skeletal Muscle on Survival after Resection of Pancreatic Cancer. *Surgery* **2015**, *157*, 1088–1098. [CrossRef]

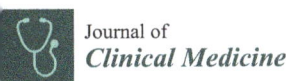 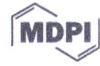

Article

Rate of Post-Operative Pancreatic Fistula after Robotic-Assisted Pancreaticoduodenectomy with Pancreato-Jejunostomy versus Pancreato-Gastrostomy: A Retrospective Case Matched Comparative Study

Marco V. Marino [1,2,*], Adrian Kah Heng Chiow [3], Antonello Mirabella [1], Gianpaolo Vaccarella [1] and Andrzej L. Komorowski [4]

1. Department of General and Emergency Surgery, Azienda Ospedaliera Ospedali Riuniti Villa Sofia-Cervello, 90127 Palermo, Italy; antonellomirabella@gmail.com (A.M.); janpaol@yahoo.it (G.V.)
2. Department of General and Oncologic Surgery, Università degli Studi di Palermo, 90127 Palermo, Italy
3. Hepatopancreatobiliary Unit, Department of Surgery, Changi General Hospital, Singapore 529889, Singapore; adrian.chiow.k.h@singhealth.com.sg
4. Department of General Surgery, College of Medicine, University of Rzeszow, 35-959 Rzeszow, Poland; z5komoro@cyf-kr.edu.pl
* Correspondence: marco.vito.marino@gmail.com

Abstract: Background: Different techniques of pancreatic anastomosis have been described, with inconclusive results in terms of pancreatic fistula reduction. Studies comparing robotic pancreaticogastrostomy (PG) and pancreaticojejunostomy (PJ) are scarcely reported. Methods: The present study analyzes the outcomes of two case-matched groups of patients who underwent PG ($n = 20$) or PJ ($n = 40$) after pancreaticoduodenectomy. The primary aim was to compare the rate of post-operative pancreatic fistula. Results: Operative time (375 vs. 315 min, $p = 0.34$), estimated blood loss (270 vs. 295 mL, $p = 0.44$), and rate of clinically relevant post-operative pancreatic fistula (12.5% vs. 10%, $p = 0.82$) were similar between the two groups. PJ was associated with a higher rate of intra-abdominal collections (7.5% vs. 0%, $p = 0.002$), but lower post-pancreatectomy hemorrhage (2.5% vs. 10%, $p = 0.003$). PG was associated with a lower rate of post-operative pancreatic fistula (POPF) (33.3% vs. 50%, $p = 0.003$) in the high-risk group of patients. Conclusions: The outcomes of post-operative pancreatic fistula are comparable between the two reconstruction techniques. PG may have a lower incidence of POPF in patients with high-risk of pancreatic fistula.

Keywords: robotic pancreatic surgery; pancreato-gastrostomy; pancreatic fistula

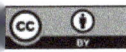

1. Introduction

Pancreaticoduodenectomy (PD) is a complex operation associated with significant post-operative mortality (1–6%) [1] and morbidity rate (10–45%) [2], even at high-volume pancreatic centers [3].

The management of the pancreatic remnant is still controversial, and multiple reconstructive techniques have been reported [4,5]. The main goal of each technique is to minimize the occurrence of post-operative pancreatic fistula (POPF), and its consequence on patient outcomes [6]. Pancreaticojejunostomy (PJ), including pancreatic invagination or duct-to-mucosa anastomosis [7,8], and pancreaticogastrostomy (PG) are the most commonly used reconstructive techniques [9]. Technical details are mainly based on surgeon's preference, in the attempt to define the ideal technique to reduce POPF [5].

Current evidence does not show any conclusive advantage of one technique over another. To date, there are no specific recommendations on how to manage the pancreatic stump after pancreaticoduodenectomy [10]. Minimal invasive pancreatic surgery is gaining an increased interest worldwide both for distal pancreatectomy [11] and pancreaticoduodenectomy [12,13]. Robotic pancreaticoduodenectomy (RPD) may mitigate some risk factors of POPF, such as blood loss [14]. However, to date, few comparative studies have been performed comparing RPD with PG and PJ [15]. The present study aims to compare the post-operative outcomes of PG and PJ after RPD.

2. Materials and Methods

A retrospective analysis of a prospectively maintained database including all RPD carried out between August 2014 and October 2019 at the Department of General Surgery, of our Tertiary Care Center was performed.

Patients with a preoperative diagnosis of benign tumor or localized and resectable malignant tumor at the periampullary region who did not meet any of the exclusion criteria (Table 1) were selected for RPD and they were included in the study. All pancreatic anastomoses in RPD until 2018 were PJ. Subsequently, the PG anastomosis technique was adopted as the only method for pancreatic reconstruction during RPD. The same surgeon performed all the anastomoses during the time period of the study.

Table 1. Exclusion criteria from the study.

Unsuitability for pneumoperitoneum
ASA score > III
Body mass index (BMI) < 35 kg/m^2
Borderline or Locally advanced tumours
Intraperitoneal or extraperitoneal metastases
Tumor size > 5 cm
Patients who underwent total pancreatectomy
Patients requiring concomitant organ or vascular resection
Conversion to open

Abbreviation: ASA, American Society of Anaesthesiologists.

The study was approved by the Institutional Review Board of the hospital. Informed written consent was obtained from all participants and the study has been carried out following the declaration of Helsinki guidelines.

2.1. Study Endpoints

The primary outcome of the present study was to compare the effectiveness of the robotic PG reconstruction versus PJ in patients undergoing RPD in terms of POPF rate.

Secondary outcomes were the length of hospital stay, duration of surgical intervention, time needed to complete the pancreatic anastomosis, rate of surgical re-intervention and of overall post-operative complications. The study compared the results of patients who underwent PG (n = 20) and PJ (n = 40). The two groups were further case-matched using four variables, in accordance with the POPF scoring system of Callery et al. (soft pancreatic texture, disease pathology, pancreatic duct diameter <3 mm, intraoperative blood loss) [16–18]. Based on gland texture, pathology, pancreatic duct diameter, and intraoperative blood loss, the patients were scored according to the fistula risk score (FRS) from a total of 0–10 points. They were then subclassified into negligible risk (0 points), low risk (1–2 points), intermediate risk (3–6 points) and high risk (7–10 points) [16]. The patient population was also classified and case-matched according to the recent ISGPS classification for parenchyma risk factors proposed by Schuh et al. [19].

A risk analysis was performed to confirm all potential risk factors for POPF.

2.2. Definitions

POPF was defined and graded using the revised consensus guidelines by the International Study Group for Pancreatic Fistula (ISGPF) [20].

The pancreatic texture was assessed on the resected pancreatic specimens and classified as hard or soft. Pancreatic duct diameter was measured by intraoperative ultrasound and confirmed on the cutting surface of the remnant pancreas using a ruler.

Post-operative complications were graded according to the Clavien-Dindo classification system, and Grade III or higher were regarded as significant complications [21]. The highest grade of complication was considered in patients with more than one complication.

Biliary fistula, delayed gastric emptying, and post-pancreatectomy hemorrhage were classified using international definitions [22–24]. Intra-abdominal abscess or fluid collection were diagnosed based on post-operative ultrasound or computed tomography (CT) scans [25].

Operative time was defined as the time from skin incision to wound dressing. Intraoperative blood loss was quantified by measuring the amount of fluid obtained from the suction device.

Mortality was defined as a death that occurred within 90 days after surgery.

2.3. Surgical Technique

Our surgical technique for a fully robotic-assisted pylorus-preserving RPD was previously described elsewhere [26].

The PJ was fashioned with an end-to-side duct-to-mucosa two-layer anastomosis with interrupted sutures (Cattell Warren technique). A continuous 3/0 V-loc™ (Covidien; Mansfield, MA, USA) suture was placed between the seromuscular layer of the jejunum and the posterior capsule of the pancreatic remnant. Then, the jejunum was opened, and the pancreatic duct was secured to the jejunal mucosa using 5/0 polypropylene interrupted sutures (PROLENE®). A 3/0 V-loc™ self-fixating running suture finally approximated the anterior jejunal seromuscular layer and the anterior aspect of the pancreatic remnant (Supplementary Video S1 Part A).

For the trans-gastric PG anastomosis, a 2.5-cm longitudinal gastrostomy was performed on the anterior wall of the stomach, and the pancreas was invaginated into the gastric lumen through a small opening on the posterior gastric wall, enlarged to approximately half of the pancreatic diameter. The pancreatic remnant was pulled holding the stay sutures previously placed as described by Giulianotti et al. during robotic PD [27]. Then, the pancreatic parenchyma was sutured to the gastric mucosa using interrupted 4/0 polydioxanone (PDS II®) sutures. The anterior gastrotomy was closed with a 3/0 PDS running suture (Supplementary Video S1 Part B).

In all cases, an internal not secured 5-French (duct size < 4 mm) or 7-French (4–8 mm duct size) silastic pediatric feeding tube was inserted into the pancreatic duct to assure its patency.

Finally, an abdominal (12 French) closed-suction drain was placed behind the pancreatic anastomosis reaching also the anterior aspect of the hepaticojejunostomy.

2.4. Statistical Analysis

Continuous variables were expressed as mean values ± standard deviation (SD) or as median and interquartile range (IQRs) where appropriate. Categorical data were presented as frequency and percentages. Fisher's exact test and Pearson Chi square test and the Mann-Whitney U test were used to define associations between categorical and continuous variables, respectively. Univariate analysis was carried out to identify all significant factors which have been reported to influence POPF: age, gender (male), body mass index >25 Kg/m^2, diabetes mellitus, and cardiovascular disease [28,29].

SPSS 19.0 (SPSS Inc, Chicago, IL, USA) was used for the statistical analysis. A p value < 0.05 was considered statistically significant. Variables with $p < 0.10$ were included in the multivariate analysis.

3. Results

A total of 60 patients underwent RPD during the study period. Twenty patients underwent PG, while 40 patients underwent PJ. Table 2 shows the preoperative features and final pathology data. Pancreatic ductal adenocarcinoma was the most common indication for surgery (48.3%). In the same period, a total of 282 patients who underwent open PD did not meet the criteria for RPD.

Table 2. Demographic, pre-operative characteristics and risk factors variables for post-operative pancreatic fistula (POPF) of patient undergoing robotic pancreatojejunostomy (PJ) and pancreatogastrostomy (PG).

Variables	PJ ($n = 40$)	PG ($n = 20$)	Overall ($n = 60$)	p Value
Age, years, median (IQR)	63.2 (55.6–71.4)	61.9 (53.8–68.5)	62.9 (54.1–71.1)	0.688
Sex, n (%)				
• Male	27 (67.5%)	13 (65%)	40 (66.7%)	0.627
• Female	13 (32.5%)	7 (35%)	20 (33.3%)	0.799
BMI, Kg/m^2, mean (±SD)	25.1 ± 3.4	24.8 ± 2.8	25 ± 3.2	0.824
ASA score, mean (±SD)	2.5 ± 0.06	2.2 ± 0.04	2.4 ± 0.7	0.856
Pathology				
• Malignant	30 (75%)	15 (75%)	45 (75%)	1
• PDAC	21	8	29	
• IPMN Cancer	3	2	5	
• Ampullary Carcinoma	2	2	4	
• Cholangiocarcinoma	2	2	4	
• Duodenal Carcinoma	1	1	2	
• NEC	1	/	1	
• Benign	10 (25%)	5 (25%)	15 (25%)	1
• IPMN	4	2	6	
• Serous cystic Neoplasm	3	1	4	
• MCN	2	1	3	
• Chronic Pancreatitis	1	1	2	
Tumor size, cm, mean (±SD)	2.86 ± 1.7	2.55 ± 1.4	2.8 ± 1.6	0.822
Neoadjuvant CHT, n (%)	6 (15%)	2 (10%)	8 (13.3%)	0.479
Pancreatic texture, n (%)				
• Soft	16 (40%)	8 (40%)	24 (40%)	1
• Hard	24 (60%)	12 (60%)	36 (60%)	
Wirsung duct diameter, median ± SD	3.4 ± 2.4	2.9 ± 2.5	3.2 ± 2.4	0.627
• ≥3 mm, n (%)	31 (77.5%)	14 (70%)	45 (75%)	0.669
• <3 mm, n (%)	9 (22.5%)	6 (30%)	15 (25%)	0.611
ISGPS classification				
• A	19 (47.5%)	9 (45%)	28 (46.7%)	0.821
• B	5 (12.5%)	3 (15%)	8 (13.3%)	0.793
• C	12 (30%)	5 (25%)	17 (28.3%)	0.645
• D	4 (10%)	3 (15%)	7 (11.7%)	0.612
Mean CRS-POPF ± SD	4.6 ± 2.2	5.1 ± 1.8	4.7 ± 2.1	0.433
Histopathology, n (%)				
• Ampullary/Duodenal/Cystic	8 (20%)	5 (25%)	13 (21.7%)	0.523
• PDAC/IPMN/others	32 (80%)	15 (75%)	47 (78.3%)	
Estimated blood loss				
• ≥500 mL	8 (20%)	4 (20%)	12 (20%)	1
• <500 mL	32 (80%)	16 (80%)	48 (80%)	
Categories of POPF risk, n (%)				
• Negligible	6 (15%)	2 (10%)	8 (13.3%)	0.788
• Low	16 (40%)	6 (30%)	22 (%)	
• Intermediate	14 (35%)	9 (45%)	23 (35%)	
• High	4 (10%)	3 (15%)	7 (11.7%)	

BMI: Body Mass Index, ASA: American Society of Anesthesiologists, PDAC: Pancreatic Ductal Adenocarcinoma, IPMN: Intraductal Papillary Mucinous Neoplasm, NET: Neuroendocrine Cancer, MCN: Mucinous Cystic Neoplasm, CHT: Chemotherapy, CRS: Clinical risk score, POPF: Post-operative pancreatic fistula.

Patients in the PJ and PG groups had similar risk factors for POPF development. The fistula risk score (FRS) was distributed as follows: eight patients (13.3%) had a negligible risk, 24 (40%) low risk, 21 (35%) moderate risk, and seven (11.7%) patients had high risk, without any difference between PJ and PG groups.

The overall operative time (median ± SD) was 355 min ± 103. Patients who underwent PG had similar operative time compared to PJ (315 vs. 375 min, $p = 0.345$).

The fashioning of PJ required a longer time in comparison to PG (32 ± 11 vs. 25 ± 14 min, $p = 0.002$). The median (IQR) estimated blood loss was 275 mL (180–600). No statistically significant difference was observed between the two groups (270 vs. 295 mL, $p = 0.442$).

A total of seven patients experienced a clinically significant POPF (11.7%), with a similar rate after PG and PJ (12.5% vs. 10%, $p = 0.820$).

A 18.3% rate of severe complications was reported, with the two group of patients showing a similar morbidity rate (20% vs. 15%, $p = 0.542$). Two patients in the PJ group underwent a reoperation due to the onset of clinically relevant POPF and ascites which required the disassembly of the pancreatic anastomosis and the fashioning of a new PJ. In the PG group, a patient with post-operative bleeding required a surgical revision after the failure of endoscopic approach.

The post-operative hospital stay was comparable between the two groups (14 ± 4 vs. 11 ± 6 days, $p = 0.223$). The overall mortality rate was 5% (Table 3).

Table 3. Postoperative outcomes of patients who underwent PJ vs. PG reconstruction.

Variables	PJ (n = 40)	PG (n = 20)	Overall (n = 60)	p Value
Operative time, min, median ± SD	375 ± 102	315 ± 110	355 ± 103	0.345
Time of the anastomoses, min, median ± SD	32 ± 11	25 ± 14	30.2 ± 12	0.002
Estimated blood loss, ml, median (IQR)	270 (180–600)	295 (200–700)	275 (180–600)	0.442
Intraoperative blood transfusion, n (%)	3 (7.5%)	1 (5%)	4 (6.7%)	0.766
Post-operative complications, n (%)	19 (47.5%)	9 (45%)	28 (46.6%)	0.635
• Grade < III	−11 (27.5%)	−6 (30%)	−17 (28.3%)	0.826
• Grade ≥ III	−8 (20%)	−3 (15%)	−11 (18.3%)	0.542
• Biochemical leak	5 (12.5%)	3 (15%)	8 (13.3%)	0.524
CR-POPF	5 (12.5%)	2 (10%)	7 (11.7%)	0.827
• Grade B	−3 (7.5%)	−1 (5%)	−4 (6.7%)	0.789
• Grade C	−2 (5%)	−1 (5%)	−3 (5%)	0.977
Delayed gastric emptying, n (%)	2 (5%)	1 (5%)	3 (5%)	0.928
Grade C Postoperative hemorrhage, n (%)	1 (2.5%)	2 (10%)	3 (5%)	0.338
Pancreatitis, n (%)	1 (2.5%)	/	1 (1.4%)	0.782
Bile leakage, n (%)	1 (2.5%)	1 (5%)	2 (3.3%)	0.654
Ascites, n (%)	1 (2.5%)	/	1 (1.4%)	0.782
Intra-abdominal collection, n (%)	3 (7.5%)	/	3 (4.3%)	0.002
Length of hospital stays, days, median ± SD	14 ± 4	11 ± 6	15.8 ± 5	0.223
Readmission, n (%)	4 (10%)	1 (5%)	5 (8.3%)	0.524
Reoperation, n (%)	2 (5%)	1 (5%)	3 (5%)	0.928
Mortality 90-days, n (%)	2 (5%)	1 (5%)	3 (5%)	0.928

CR-POPF: Clinically Relevant Postoperative pancreatic fistula.

The case-matched analysis according to the four variables of the clinical risk score for POPF (soft pancreatic texture, pancreatic duct diameter < 3 mm and intraoperative blood loss > 500 mL and histopathology), showed that PJ was associated with longer anastomotic time (46 vs. 25 min, *p* = 0.002), but not with an increased risk of POPF. PJ was associated with a higher rate of intrabdominal collection (*p* = 0.002), but a lower rate of post-pancreatectomy hemorrhage (*p* = 0.003) (Table 4).

Table 4. Comparison of postoperative results of PJ and PG cohorts matched for the four variables (histopathology, pancreatic texture, pancreatic duct diameter, intraoperative blood loss) of the clinical risk score for post-operative pancreatic fistula (POPF).

Variables	PJ (*n* = 20)	PG (*n* = 20)	*p* Value
Histopathology, *n* (%)			
- PDAC/IPMN	14 (70%)	15 (75%)	0.855
- Ampullary, Duodenal, Cystic	6 (30%)	5 (25%)	0.793
Pancreatic texture, *n* (%)			
- Soft	13 (65%)	13 (65%)	1
- Hard	7 (35%)	7 (35%)	1
Pancreatic duct diameter, mm, *n* (%)			
- ≥3	13 (65%)	14 (70%)	0.643
- <3	7 (35%)	6 (30%)	0.635
ISGPS Classification			
- A	9 (45%)	9 (45%)	1
- B	3 (15%)	3 (15%)	1
- C	5 (25%)	5 (25%)	1
- D	3 (15%)	3 (15%)	1
Intraoperative blood loss, mL, *n* (%)			
- ≥500	5 (25%)	4 (20%)	0.617
- <500	15 (75%)	16 (80%)	0.539
Median Operative time, min (IQR)	330 (270.2–395.8)	315 (265–382)	0.75
Anastomotic time, min (IQR)	46 (28–52)	25 (18–40)	0.002
Morbidity rate, *n* (%)	11 (55%)	9 (45%)	0.721
- Minor	5 (25%)	6 (30%)	0.586
- Major	6 (30%)	3 (15%)	0.324
Biochemical Leak, *n* (%)	4 (20%)	3 (15%)	0.721
CR–POPF, *n* (%)	3 (15%)	2 (10%)	0.478
Delayed gastric emptying, *n* (%)	1 (5%)	1 (5%)	1
Post-pancreatectomy hemorrhage, *n* (%)	/	2 (10%)	0.003
Intra-abdominal collection, *n* (%)	3 (15%)	/	0.002
Reoperation, *n* (%)	2 (10%)	1 (5%)	0.474
Median length of hospital stays, days (IQR)	14.2 (12.4–22)	11.5 (9.5–19)	0.165

In the univariate analysis, risk factors for POPF were BMI, pancreatic duct diameter, the texture of the pancreas, and estimated blood loss. PJ was not associated with an increased risk of POPF (Table 5). Three out of seven patients experienced a CR-POPF in the high-risk group (Figure 1).

In the stratified analysis according to the clinical risk score, there was no significant difference for cases included in the low-risk group (PG 0% vs. PJ 6.3%, *p* = 0.445) and intermediate-risk (PJ 14.3% vs. PG 14.3%, *p* = 1.000) in terms of POPF. In contrast, PG was associated with a lower rate of POPF in the high-risk group (PG 33.3% vs. PJ 50%, *p* = < 0.05).

Table 5. Risks factors for POPF.

Variables	CR-POPF (n = 7)	No-POPF (n = 53)	Univariate p Value	Odds Ratio	95% CI
Age					
• ≥65 years	4	27	0.76		
• <65 years	3	26			
Sex					
• Male	4	36	0.57		
• Female	3	17			
BMI					
• ≥25 Kg/m²	5	14	<0.05	6.96	(1.2–40.1)
• <25 Kg/m²	2	39			
Diabetes					
• YES	1	10	0.77		
• NO	6	43			
ASA score					
• ≥3	3	29	0.55		
• <3	4	24			
Pancreatic duct diameter					
• ≥3 mm	2	43			
• <3 mm	5	10	<0.05	10.7	(1.8–63.6)
Underlying pathology					
PDAC/IPMN/etc.	4	43	0.16		
Ampullary/Cystic/Duodenal	3	10			
Tumor size					
• ≥2.5 cm	2	21	0.59		
• <2.5 cm	5	33			
Texture of the pancreas					
• Soft	6	18	<0.05	11.66	(1.3–104.4)
• Hard	1	35		-	
Operative time					
• ≥355 min	4	34	0.71		
• <355 min	3	19			
Blood loss					
• ≥500 mL	5	7	<0.05	10.95	(2.1–56.3)
• <500 mL	2	46		-	
Reconstruction type					
• PJ	5	35	0.77		
• PG	2	18			

BMI: Body Mass Index, ASA: American Society of Anesthesiologist, PDAC: Pancreatic ductal adenocarcinoma, IPMN: Intraductal Papillary Mucinous Neoplasm, PJ: Pancreatojejunostomy, PG: Pancreatogastrostomy.

At six months follow-up, three patients in the PG group were readmitted for vague abdominal pain, dyspepsia, abdominal distension associated with changes in bowel habit. No sign of anastomotic stricture was observed during the diagnostic tests.

In the PJ group we observed two hospital readmissions in patients experiencing fever and associated fatigue. In both cases, an abdominal collection was detected at diagnostic CT-scan.

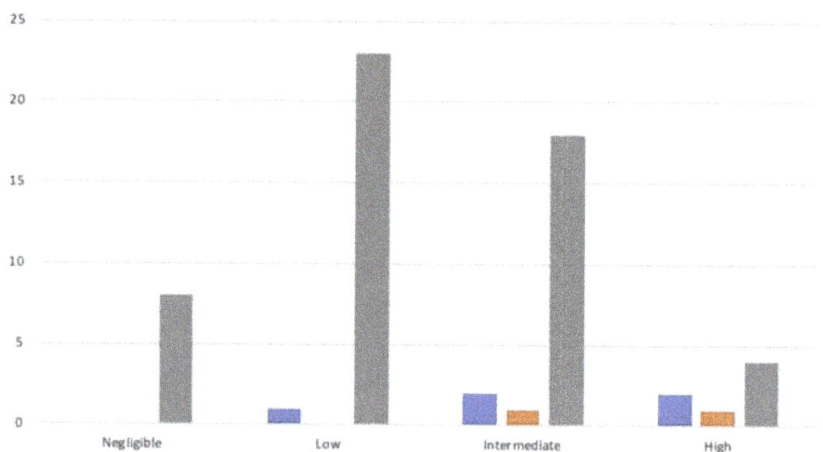

Figure 1. Rate of the clinically relevant postoperative pancreatic fistula (CR-POPF) in a subgroup analysis.

4. Discussion

Despite significant advancements in the operative techniques and improvements in perioperative surgical care, more than 20% of patients still develop a POPF after PD [30].

To date, there is no gold standard technique for pancreatic anastomosis and experience-related methods are connected to the surgeon expertise, so that "the best anastomosis is probably the one with which the surgeon is most familiar".

A recent systematic review comparing open PG versus PJ concluded that the two techniques are equivalent in terms of overall post-operative outcomes, nevertheless PJ seemed associated with a slight reduction of post-operative bleeding (9.3% vs. 13.8%), but it showed a higher risk of developing intra-abdominal abscess (14.7% vs. 8.0%) compared to PG [10]. This was also a consistent finding in our study.

Open PD still represents the gold standard in case of resectable pancreatic head tumors, whereas minimally invasive PD is currently performed in selected high-volume centers [31].

In our experience, the decision for the shift in the reconstruction strategy from the conventional PJ technique to the PG has to be found in the emerging evidence from multicenter randomized controlled trials showing that the incidence of POPF is lower in patients undergoing PG than in those undergoing PJ [32,33]. However, our results showed that both techniques are equally feasible and safe, with similar morbidity rate and length of in-hospital stay.

Significant efforts have been directed at identifying risk factors of POPF after PD. Callery et al. validated a model for predicting clinically significant POPF after PD by using four parameters: pancreatic texture, pathology, pancreatic duct diameter, and intra-operative blood loss which are incorporated into a convenient scoring system of risk categories [16].

Some risk factors, such as soft pancreatic texture, small pancreatic duct diameter and higher BMI are no modifiable because they are inherent to the patient. Conversely, the anastomotic technique is the only factor that can hypothetically modify the risk of POPF after PD. In the present study, the rate of POPF after PG and PJ was not statistically different overall, although subgroup analysis showed lesser POPF in PG in patients with high FRS.

A broad Cochrane systematic review published in 2017 concluded that PG may have little or no difference compared to PJ in the overall risk of any surgical complications and particularly in POPF formation, mortality and length of post-operative hospital stay, concluding that there was no reliable evidence to support the use of PG over PJ [10].

A recent meta-analysis including 11 RCTs that enrolled a total of 1765 patients concluded that POPF was related to a significantly lower morbidity rate in the PG group than in the PJ group (OR = 0.67, p = 0.002). In contrast, clinically significant POPF rates were not significantly different between the two groups (OR = 0.61, p = 0.09). PJ was also associated with a statistically significant lower incidence of post-operative bleeding compared with PG (OR = 1.47, p = 0.03), whereas the rate of delayed gastric emptying was not significantly different (OR = 1.09, p = 0.54) [34].

The RPD is gaining momentum among the pancreatic surgeon community, and recently the correlation between robotic approach and POPF was investigated [35]. Although the benefits shown in terms of lower estimated blood loss and shorter length of hospital stay, RPD failed to demonstrate a significant reduction in the POPF compared to open PD [12,36].

A multi-institutional study using data from the American College of Surgeons National Surgical Quality Improvement Program concluded that patients undergoing minimally invasive PD had higher rates of clinically relevant POPF compared to open PD (15.3% vs. 13.0%, p = 0.03), but the surgical technique was not an independent factor associated with POPF on the adjusted multivariate analysis (OR 1.05, 95% CI 0.87–1–26) [37]. Conversely, in tha high volume center, the RPD was associated to lower CR-POPF when compared to OPD (6.7% vs. 15.8%, p < 0.001) [38].

The present study found similar results between the two anastomosis techniques in terms of operative time and estimated blood loss, although PJ required longer operative time for its fashioning. From a technical point view, the PJ was more challenging for the higher number of sutures required and for the difficulties in exposing the posterior row of the anastomosis. On the other hand, the PG required a major traction on the pancreatic stump that may cause bleeding from pancreatic surface. This may account for the higher rate of post-operative collection, but lower post-operative hemorrhage noted for PJ compared to PG in our study.

Since 2013, the fistula risk score was developed to assess the risk of clinically relevant POPF. While widely used, recent studies have found that not all factors were statistically significant especially with respect to blood loss suggesting that newer predictive models maybe necessary [18]. This includes alternative FRS comprising of pancreatic texture, pancreatic duct diameter and body mass index (BMI) [39]. Recently, Polanco et al. found that high BMI, high estimated blood loss, smaller tumor size and small duct diameter are the main predictors for POPF in RPD [40].

In the present study, the univariate analysis revealed that the pancreatic duct diameter, as well as soft consistency of the pancreas, higher BMI and higher blood loss, were associated with increased risk of POPF. The diameter of the pancreatic duct and the soft texture of the pancreas influenced the rate of POPF heavily, as demonstrated by the fact that 66.6% of patients who developed a POPF had a pancreatic duct diameter <3 mm and 55.6% of patients had a soft pancreatic texture. The soft pancreas is more susceptible to ischemia and injury. Moreover, soft texture is generally associated with a small pancreatic duct, and a preserved exocrine function, resulting in increased activation and secretion of pancreatic juice [41]. A narrowed pancreatic duct is not only more challenging to reconstruct, but anastomoses in such cases are also more likely to either occlude or dehisce [40]. In our study, the rate of POPF after PG is significantly lower in patients with high risk of POPF as the PG obviates the need to anastomose the pancreatic duct compared to the PJ duct to mucosa technique. Further studies are needed to determine better predictive models for POPF. A large adequately powered well designed RCT comparing PG versus PJ in robotic PD from experienced centers may be the next step to consider the validity of our findings and further shed light to the optimal method for reconstruction in this complex surgery.

Our retrospective cohort study has several limitations. It has been carried out at a single-institution and included a small cohort of patients. The case matched study design reduced the number of involved procedures in the analysis. Furthermore, the study compares only one type of PJ compared to PG and its findings may not be applicable to PJ reconstruction via other techniques. However, the bias related to variations in the surgical technique and the post-operative management is minimal as the same pancreatic team performed all the RPD in this series. A major experience and a growing number of cases performed by the team in the near future will add more validity to the conclusions drawn. A comparison among the outcomes of other experienced centers could lead to a standardization of this complex and emerging surgical technique.

5. Conclusions

The present study showed that the rate of POPF after robotic PG and PJ were equivalent with a lower rate of POPF after PG for patients at high risk of POPF.

Supplementary Materials: The following are available online at https://www.mdpi.com/article/10.3390/jcm10102181/s1, Video S1: Robotic-assisted PJ vs PG: a video technique; (Part A) pancreato-jejunostomy (PJ) and (Part B) pancreato-gastrostomy (PG).

Author Contributions: Conception and design: M.V.M., A.K.H.C.; Administrative support: A.K.H.C., A.L.K.; Provision of study materials or patients: M.V.M., A.M., G.V.; Collection and assembly of data: M.V.M., A.M., A.L.K., G.V.; Data analysis and interpretation: All authors; Manuscript writing: All authors; All authors have read and agreed to the published version of the manuscript.

Funding: This research received no external funding.

Institutional Review Board Statement: The study was conducted in accordance with the ethical standards of the 1964 Helsinki Declaration and its later amendments or comparable ethical standards. The study was conducted after the approval of the Institutional Review Board of Hospital (protocol code N°45GJU00; approved on 27 March 2017).

Informed Consent Statement: Informed consent was obtained from all subjects involved in the study.

Data Availability Statement: Data are available on request.

Conflicts of Interest: Marco V. Marino has been involved as a Consultant in Company CAVA Robotic International LCC. All other authors declare no conflict of interest.

References

1. Testini, M.; Piccinni, G.; Lissidini, G.; Gurrado, A.; Tedeschi, M.; Franco, I.; Di Meo, G.; Pasculli, A.; De Luca, G.; Ribezzi, M.; et al. Surgical management of the pancreatic stump following pancreato-duodenectomy. *J. Visc. Surg.* **2016**, *153*, 193–202. [CrossRef]
2. McMillan, M.T.; Malleo, G.; Bassi, C.; Allegrini, V.; Casetti, L.; Drebin, J.A.; Esposito, A.; Landoni, L.; Lee, M.K.; Pulvirenti, A.; et al. Multicenter, Prospective Trial of Selective Drain Management for Pancreatoduodenectomy Using Risk Stratification. *Ann. Surg.* **2017**, *265*, 1209–1218. [CrossRef] [PubMed]
3. Tran, T.B.; Dua, M.M.; Worhunsky, D.J.; Poultsides, G.A.; Norton, J.A.; Visser, B.C. The First Decade of Laparoscopic Pancreaticoduodenectomy in the United States: Costs and Outcomes Using the Nationwide Inpatient Sample. *Surg. Endosc.* **2016**, *30*, 1778–1783. [CrossRef]
4. Traverso, L.W.; Longmire, W.P., Jr. Preservation of the pylorus in pancreaticoduodenectomy. *Surg. Gynecol. Obstet.* **1978**, *146*, 959–962. [CrossRef] [PubMed]
5. Crippa, S.; Cirocchi, R.; Randolph, J.; Partelli, S.; Belfiori, G.; Piccioli, A.; Parisi, A.; Falconi, M. Pancreaticojejunostomy is comparable to pancreaticogastrostomy after pancreaticoduodenectomy: An updated meta-analysis of randomized controlled trials. *Langenbeck's Arch. Surg.* **2016**, *401*, 427–437. [CrossRef] [PubMed]
6. Menahem, B.; Guittet, L.; Mulliri, A.; Alves, A.; Lubrano, J. Pancreaticogastrostomy is superior to pancreaticojejunostomy for prevention of pancreatic fistula after pancreaticoduodenectomy: An updated meta-analysis of randomized controlled trials. *Ann. Surg.* **2015**, *261*, 882–887. [CrossRef]
7. Bai, X.; Zhang, Q.; Gao, S.; Lou, J.; Li, G.; Zhang, Y.; Ma, T.; Zhang, Y.; Xu, Y.; Liang, T. Duct-to-Mucosa vs Invagination for Pancreaticojejunostomy after Pancreaticoduodenectomy: A Prospective, Randomized Controlled Trial from a Single Surgeon. *J. Am. Coll. Surg.* **2016**, *222*, 10–18. [CrossRef]

8. Xu, J.; Zhang, B.; Shi, S.; Qin, Y.; Ji, S.; Xu, W.; Liu, J.; Liu, L.; Liu, C.; Long, J.; et al. Papillary-like main pancreatic duct invaginated pancreaticojejunostomy versus duct-to-mucosa pancreaticojejunostomy after pancreaticoduodenectomy: A prospective randomized trial. *Surgery* **2015**, *158*, 1211–1218. [CrossRef]
9. Zhu, F.; Wang, M.; Wang, X.; Tian, R.; Shi, C.; Xu, M.; Shen, M.; Han, J.; Luo, N.; Qin, R. Modified Technique of Pancreaticogastrostomy for Soft Pancreas with Two Continuous Hemstitch Sutures: A Single-Center Prospective Study. *J. Gastroint. Surg.* **2013**, *17*, 1306–1311. [CrossRef]
10. Cheng, Y.; Lai, M.; Wang, X.; Tu, B.; Cheng, N.; Gong, J. Pancreaticogastrostomy versus pancreaticojejunostomy reconstruction for the prevention of pancreatic fistula following pancreaticoduodenectomy. *Cochrane Database Syst. Rev.* **2016**, *12*, CD012257. [CrossRef]
11. Marino, M.V.; Mirabella, A.; Ruiz, M.G.; Komorowski, A.L. Robotic-Assisted versus Laparoscopic Distal Pancreatectomy: The Results of a Case-Matched Analysis from a Tertiary Care Center. *Dig. Surg.* **2020**, *37*, 229–239. [CrossRef] [PubMed]
12. Podda, M.; Gerardi, C.; Di Saverio, S.; Marino, M.V.; Davies, R.J.; Pellino, G.; Pisanu, A. Robotic-assisted versus open pancreaticoduodenectomy for patients with benign and malignant periampullary disease: A systematic review and meta-analysis of short-term outcomes. *Surg. Endosc.* **2020**, *34*, 2390–2409. [CrossRef] [PubMed]
13. Beane, J.D.; Zenati, M.; Hamad, A.; Hogg, M.E.; Zeh, H.J., III; Zureikat, A.H. Robotic pancreatoduodenectomy with vascular resection: Outcomes and learning curve. *Surgery* **2019**, *166*, 8–14. [CrossRef] [PubMed]
14. Bao, P.Q.; Mazirka, P.O.; Watkins, K.T. Retrospective Comparison of Robot-Assisted Minimally Invasive Versus Open Pancreaticoduodenectomy for Periampullary Neoplasms. *J. Gastroint. Surg.* **2014**, *18*, 682–689. [CrossRef]
15. Topal, B.; Fieuws, S.; Aerts, R.; Weerts, J.; Feryn, T.; Roeyen, G.; Bertrand, C.; Hubert, C.; Janssens, M.; Closset, J. Belgian Section of Hepatobiliary and Pancreatic Surgery. Pancreaticojejunostomy versus pancreaticogastrostomy reconstruction after pancreaticoduodenectomy for pancreatic or periampullary tumours: A multicenter randomised trial. *Lancet Oncol.* **2013**, *14*, 655–662. [CrossRef]
16. Callery, M.P.; Pratt, W.B.; Kent, T.S.; Chaikof, E.L.; Vollmer, C.M. A Prospectively Validated Clinical Risk Score Accurately Predicts Pancreatic Fistula after Pancreatoduodenectomy. *J. Am. Coll. Surg.* **2013**, *216*, 1–14. [CrossRef] [PubMed]
17. McMillan, M.T.; Ecker, B.L.; Behrman, S.W.; Callery, M.P.; Christein, J.D.; Drebin, J.A.; Fraker, D.L.; Kent, T.S.; Lee, M.K.; Roses, R.E.; et al. Externalized Stents for Pancreatoduodenectomy Provide Value Only in High-Risk Scenarios. *J. Gastrointest. Surg.* **2016**, *20*, 2052–2062. [CrossRef]
18. Shubert, C.R.; Wagie, A.E.; Farnell, M.B.; Nagorney, D.M.; Que, F.G.; Lombardo, K.R.; Truty, M.J.; Smoot, R.L.; Kendrick, M.L. Clinical Risk Score to Predict Pancreatic Fistula after Pancreatoduodenectomy: Independent External Validation for Open and Laparoscopic Approaches. *J. Am. Coll. Surg.* **2015**, *221*, 689–698. [CrossRef]
19. Schuh, F.; Mihaljevic, A.L.; Probst, P.; Trudeau, M.T.; Müller, P.C.; Marchegiani, G.; Besselink, M.G.; Uzunoglu, F.; Izbicki, J.R.; Falconi, M.; et al. A Simple Classification of Pancreatic Duct Size and Texture Predicts Postoperative Pancreatic Fistula. *Ann. Surg.* **2021**. Epub ahead of print. [CrossRef]
20. Bassi, C.; Marchegiani, G.; Dervenis, C.; Sarr, M.; Abu Hilal, M.; Adham, M.; Allen, P.; Andersson, R.; Asbun, H.J.; Besselink, M.G.; et al. The 2016 update of the International Study Group (ISGPS) definition and grading of postoperative pancreatic fistula: 11 Years After. *Surgery* **2017**, *161*, 584–591. [CrossRef]
21. Clavien, P.A.; Barkun, J.; De Oliveira, M.L.; Vauthey, J.N.; Dindo, D.; Schulick, R.D.; De Santibañes, E.; Pekolj, J.; Slankamenac, K.; Bassi, C.; et al. The Clavien-Dindo classification of surgical complications: Five-year experience. *Ann. Surg.* **2009**, *250*, 187–196. [CrossRef] [PubMed]
22. Peng, S.Y.; Wang, J.W.; Lau, W.Y.; Cai, X.J.; Mou, Y.P.; Liu, Y.B.; Li, J.T. Conventional versus binding pancreaticojejunostomy after pancreaticoduodenectomy: A prospective randomized trial. *Ann. Surg.* **2007**, *245*, 692–698. [CrossRef] [PubMed]
23. Wente, M.N.; Bassi, C.; Dervenis, C.; Fingerhut, A.; Gouma, D.J.; Izbicki, J.R.; Neoptolemos, J.P.; Padbury, R.T.; Sarr, M.G.; Traverso, L.W.; et al. Delayed gastric emptying (DGE) after pancreatic surgery: A suggested definition by the International Study Group of Pancreatic Surgery (ISGPS). *Surgery* **2007**, *142*, 761–768. [CrossRef] [PubMed]
24. Wente, M.N.; Veit, J.A.; Bassi, C.; Dervenis, C.; Fingerhut, A.; Gouma, D.J.; Izbicki, J.R.; Neoptolemos, J.P.; Padbury, R.T.; Sarr, M.G.; et al. Postpancreatectomy hemorrhage (PPH)–An International Study Group of Pancreatic Surgery (ISGPS) definition. *Surgery* **2007**, *142*, 20–25. [CrossRef]
25. Kawai, M.; Tani, M.; Terasawa, H.; Ina, S.; Hirono, S.; Nishioka, R.; Miyazawa, M.; Uchiyama, K.; Yamaue, H. Early removal of prophylactic drains reduces the risk of intra-abdominal infections in patients with pancreatic head resection: Prospective study for 104 consecutive patients. *Ann. Surg.* **2006**, *244*, 1–7. [CrossRef]
26. Marino, M.V.; Podda, M.; Ruiz, M.G.; Fernandez, C.C.; Guarrasi, D.; Fleitas, M.G. Robotic-assisted versus open pancreaticoduodenectomy: The results of a case-matched comparison. *J. Robot. Surg.* **2019**, *14*, 493–502. [CrossRef] [PubMed]
27. Giulianotti, P.C.; Gonzalez-Heredia, R.; Esposito, S.; Masrur, M.; Gangemi, A.; Bianco, F.M. Trans-gastric pancreaticogastrostomy reconstruction after pylorus-preserving robotic Whipple: A proposal for a standardized technique. *Surg. Endosc.* **2018**, *32*, 2169–2174. [CrossRef]
28. Hu, B.-Y.; Wan, T.; Zhang, W.-Z.; Dong, J.-H. Risk factors for postoperative pancreatic fistula: Analysis of 539 successive cases of pancreaticoduodenectomy. *World J. Gastroenterol.* **2016**, *22*, 7797–7805. [CrossRef]

29. Pedrazzoli, S. Pancreatoduodenectomy (PD) and postoperative pancreatic fistula (POPF): A systematic review and analysis of the POPF-related mortality rate in 60,739 patients retrieved from the English literature published between 1990 and 2015. *Medicine* **2017**, *96*, e6858. [CrossRef]
30. Vollmer, C.M., Jr.; Sanchez, N.; Gondek, S.; McAuliffe, J.; Kent, T.S.; Christein, J.D.; Callery, M.P.; Pancreatic Surgery Mortality Study Group. Pancreatic Surgery Mortality Study Group. A root-cause analysis of mortality following major pancreatectomy. *J. Gastrointest. Surg.* **2012**, *16*, 89–102. [CrossRef]
31. Boggi, U.; Napoli, N.; Costa, F.; Kauffmann, E.F.; Menonna, F.; Iacopi, S.; Vistoli, F.; Amorese, G. Robotic-assisted pancreatic resections. *World J. Surg.* **2016**, *40*, 2497–2506. [CrossRef]
32. Figueras, J.; Sabater, L.; Planellas, P.; Muñoz-Forner, E.; Lopez-Ben, S.; Falgueras, L.; Sala-Palau, C.; Albiol, M.; Ortega-Serrano, J.; Castro-Gutierrez, E. Randomized clinical trial of pancreaticogastrostomy versus pancreaticojejunostomy on the rate and severity of pancreatic fistula after pancreaticoduodenectomy. *BJS* **2013**, *100*, 1597–1605. [CrossRef]
33. Keck, T.; Wellner, U.F.; Bahra, M.; Klein, F.; Sick, O.; Niedergethmann, M.; Wilhelm, T.J.; Farkas, S.A.; Börner, T.; Bruns, C.; et al. Pancreatogastrostomy Versus Pancreatojejunostomy for RECOnstruction After PANCreatoduodenectomy (RECOPANC, DRKS 00000767). *Ann. Surg.* **2016**, *263*, 440–449. [CrossRef]
34. Jin, Y.; Feng, Y.-Y.; Qi, X.-G.; Hao, G.; Yu, Y.-Q.; Li, J.-T.; Peng, S.-Y. Pancreatogastrostomy vs pancreatojejunostomy after pancreaticoduodenectomy: An updated meta-analysis of RCTs and our experience. *World J. Gastrointest. Surg.* **2019**, *11*, 322–332. [CrossRef] [PubMed]
35. Marino, M.V.; Podda, M.; Pisanu, A.; di Saverio, S.; Fleitas, M.G. Robotic-assisted Pancreaticoduodenectomy: Technique Description and Performance Evaluation after 60 Cases. *Surg. Laparosc. Endosc. Percutaneous Tech.* **2020**, *30*, 156–163. [CrossRef] [PubMed]
36. McMillan, M.T.; Zureikat, A.H.; Hogg, M.E.; Kowalsky, S.J.; Zeh, H.J.; Sprys, M.H.; Vollmer, C.M. A Propensity Score–Matched Analysis of Robotic vs Open Pancreatoduodenectomy on Incidence of Pancreatic Fistula. *JAMA Surg.* **2017**, *152*, 327–335. [CrossRef] [PubMed]
37. Kantor, O.; Talamonti, M.S.; Pitt, H.A.; Vollmer, C.M.; Riall, T.S.; Hall, B.L.; Wang, C.-H.; Baker, M.S. Using the NSQIP Pancreatic Demonstration Project to Derive a Modified Fistula Risk Score for Preoperative Risk Stratification in Patients Undergoing Pancreaticoduodenectomy. *J. Am. Coll. Surg.* **2017**, *224*, 816–825. [CrossRef] [PubMed]
38. Cai, J.; Ramanathan, R.; Zenati, M.S.; Al Abbas, A.; Hogg, M.E.; Zeh, H.J.; Zureikat, A.H. Robotic Pancreaticoduodenectomy Is Associated with Decreased Clinically Relevant Pancreatic Fistulas: A Propensity-Matched Analysis. *J. Gastrointest. Surg.* **2019**, *24*, 1111–1118. [CrossRef]
39. Mungroop, T.H.; Van Rijssen, L.B.; Van Klaveren, D.; Smits, F.J.; Van Woerden, V.; Linnemann, R.J.; De Pastena, M.; Klompmaker, S.; Marchegiani, G.; Ecker, B.L.; et al. Alternative fistula risk score for pancreatoduodenectomy (a-FRS): Design and international external validation. *Ann. Surg.* **2019**, *269*, 937–943. [CrossRef]
40. Polanco, P.M.; Zenati, M.S.; Hogg, M.E.; Shakir, M.; Boone, B.A.; Bartlett, D.L.; Zeh, H.J.; Zureikat, A.H. An analysis of risk factors for pancreatic fistula after robotic pancreaticoduodenectomy: Outcomes from a consecutive series of standardized pancreatic reconstructions. *Surg. Endosc.* **2016**, *30*, 1523–1529. [CrossRef]
41. Lee, S.E.; Jang, J.Y.; Lim, C.S.; Kang, M.J.; Kim, S.H.; Kim, M.A.; Kim, S.W. Measurement of pancreatic fat by magnetic resonance imaging: Predicting the occurrence of pancreatic fistula after pancreatoduodenectomy. *Ann. Surg.* **2010**, *251*, 932–936. [CrossRef] [PubMed]

MDPI
St. Alban-Anlage 66
4052 Basel
Switzerland
Tel. +41 61 683 77 34
Fax +41 61 302 89 18
www.mdpi.com

Journal of Clinical Medicine Editorial Office
E-mail: jcm@mdpi.com
www.mdpi.com/journal/jcm

www.ingramcontent.com/pod-product-compliance
Lightning Source LLC
LaVergne TN
LVHW070643100526
838202LV00013B/872